T0257637

Encyclopedia of Diabetes: Complications in Type 1 Diabetes

Volume 10

Encyclopedia of Diabetes: Complications in Type 1 Diabetes
Volume 10

Edited by **Rex Slavin, Windy Wise and Roy Marcus Cohn**

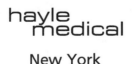

New York

Published by Hayle Medical,
30 West, 37th Street, Suite 612,
New York, NY 10018, USA
www.haylemedical.com

Encyclopedia of Diabetes: Complications in Type 1 Diabetes
Volume 10
Edited by Rex Slavin, Windy Wise and Roy Marcus Cohn

International Standard Book Number: 978-1-63241-152-5 (Hardback)

Contents

Preface

This book was inspired by the evolution of our times; to answer the curiosity of inquisitive minds. Many developments have occurred across the globe in the recent past which has transformed the progress in the field.

The book contains reviews regarding the pathogenesis of Type-1 Diabetes, which is a classic autoimmune disease. Genetic factors are responsible but they cannot describe the rapid, even overwhelming extent of this disease. It is important to comprehend etiology and pathogenesis of this disease. The complexities related to Type-1 Diabetes include a number of clinical problems. Several veterans in this field have analyzed a number of topics for consideration that are appropriate for clinicians as well as researchers alike. The book has been organized under two sections: Diabetes Onset and Cardiovascular Complications.

This book was developed from a mere concept to drafts to chapters and finally compiled together as a complete text to benefit the readers across all nations. To ensure the quality of the content we instilled two significant steps in our procedure. The first was to appoint an editorial team that would verify the data and statistics provided in the book and also select the most appropriate and valuable contributions from the plentiful contributions we received from authors worldwide. The next step was to appoint an expert of the topic as the Editor-in-Chief, who would head the project and finally make the necessary amendments and modifications to make the text reader-friendly. I was then commissioned to examine all the material to present the topics in the most comprehensible and productive format.

I would like to take this opportunity to thank all the contributing authors who were supportive enough to contribute their time and knowledge to this project. I also wish to convey my regards to my family who have been extremely supportive during the entire project.

Editor

Part 1

Diabetes Onset

Early and Late Onset Type 1 Diabetes: One and the Same or Two Distinct Genetic Entities?

Laura Espino-Paisan, Elena Urcelay,
Emilio Gómez de la Concha and Jose Luis Santiago
Clinical Immunology Department, Hospital Clínico San Carlos,
Instituto de Investigación Sanitaria San Carlos (IdISSC),
Spain

1. Introduction

Type 1 diabetes is a complex autoimmune disease in which genetic and environmental factors add up to induce an autoimmune destruction of the insulin-producing pancreatic β cells. Although type 1 diabetes is popularly associated to an onset in infancy or adolescence, it can begin at any age. The reasons behind this temporal difference in the onset of the disease are probably a mixture of genetic and environmental factors, just as the induction of the disease itself. Despite the great progress that the study of the genetics of type 1 diabetes has experienced in the last years, the genetic factors that could modify the age at diagnosis of type 1 diabetes have not been analyzed so deeply. This knowledge would be interesting to discover new routes to delay the disease onset and preserve the β cell mass as long as possible. In this chapter, we will review the characteristics of adult-onset type 1 diabetes patients and afterwards we will focus on the studies in type 1 diabetes genetics and the reported associations of genetics and age at onset of the disease. Finally, we will present an analysis of ten genetic associations in a group of Spanish patients with early and late onset of type 1 diabetes.

2. Diagnostic criteria for diabetes and further classification of the disease

Type 1 diabetes is the most prevalent chronic disease in childhood and it is also the most frequent form of diabetes in subjects diagnosed before age 19 (Duncan, 2006). Adults can also suffer from type 1 diabetes, given that the prevalence rate does not vary greatly with age, but the diagnosis of the disease in adult age is complicated by the higher prevalence of type 2 diabetes, which is the most frequent form of diabetes in adulthood (American Diabetes Association [ADA], 2010). Classical diabetes classifications used to categorize patients by their age at diagnosis or insulin requirement. Thus, type 1 diabetes was termed juvenile diabetes or insulin-dependent diabetes mellitus (IDDM) and type 2 diabetes could be diabetes of the adult or non-insulin dependent diabetes mellitus (NIDDM). However, type 2 diabetes can begin as an insulin-dependent condition or at an early age, type 1 diabetes can begin at any age, and a certain form of adult onset autoimmune diabetes termed latent autoimmune diabetes of the adult (LADA) is non-insulin-dependent by definition at the time of diagnosis, nevertheless it is an autoimmune form of diabetes. Therefore, cataloging the different forms of diabetes is not so simple and classifications based in age at diagnosis or insulin requirement are no longer employed. Hence, we will review the diagnostic criteria for diabetes and define what can be considered adult-onset type 1 diabetes.

According to the most recent classification of the American Diabetes Association (ADA, 2010), the diagnostic criteria for diabetes are 1) levels of glycosilated haemoglobin over 6.5%, 2) fasting plasma glucose levels over 126 mg/dl, defining fasting state as no caloric intake for at least eight hours, 3) plasma glucose over 200 mg/dl at two hours during an oral glucose tolerance test (OGTT) or 4) random plasma glucose over 200 mg/dl in a patient with classic symptoms of hyperglycemia (poliuria, polidypsia or glucosuria). Patients with type 1, type 2 diabetes or LADA must feet these criteria. Then, further classification of the patient should be considered.

2.1 Type 1 diabetes

Type 1 diabetes accounts for 5-10% of the total cases of diabetes and it is the 90% of the cases of diabetes diagnosed in children (ADA, 2010). The disease is an autoimmune condition characterized by the destruction of the pancreatic β cells by autoreactive T lymphocytes. Hyperglicemia manifests when 60-90% of the β cell mass has been lost. As a result of the autoimmune insult, antibodies against pancreatic islets are synthesized and can be detectable in serum (see table 1). These antibodies precede in several years the clinical symptoms. They are not pathogenic (Wong et al, 2010), but its detection helps in the classification of the patient as type 1 diabetes, especially when the disease is diagnosed in adulthood. Antibodies against pancreatic antigens are positive at diagnosis in 90% of type 1 diabetes patients. Obesity is quite uncommon in these patients, but not incompatible with the disease. Patients are frequently insulin-dependent since diagnosis and insulin-replacement therapy is ultimately necessary for survival. Also, C-peptide levels (a measure of β cell activity) are usually low or undetectable. When untreated, type 1 diabetes leads to diabetic ketoacidosis, a life-threatening condition derived from the use of fat deposits (ADA, 2010).

Adult-onset type 1 diabetes patients tend to have a softer disease onset, with a lower frequency of diabetic ketoacidosis and a slower loss of insulin secretion capacity (Hosszufalusi et al, 2003; Leslie et al, 2006). These characteristics lead to think that a slower autoimmune reaction is taking place in the patient with adult onset.

	Autoantibody	Antigen expression
IAA	Anti-insulin antibodies	Pancreas
GADA	Anti-glutamate decarboxilase antibodies	Pancreas/nervous system
IA2-A	Anti-insulinoma associated 2 antibodies	Pancreas
ICA	Anti-islet cell antibodies (several antigens)	Pancreas
SCL38A	Antibodies against the zinc channel ZnT8	Pancreas

Table 1. Autoantibodies against pancreatic antigens in type 1 diabetes.

2.2 Type 2 diabetes

Type 2 diabetes includes 90-95% of the total cases of diabetes and accounts for 80-85% of the cases diagnosed in adulthood (ADA, 2010). The disease is a result of a combination of peripheral insulin resistance and relative insulin deficiency that develops into hyperglycemia. The hyperglycemia in type 2 diabetes appears gradually, usually with absence of the classic symptoms (polyuria, polydipsia) and can go undetected for long time before diagnosis. The etiologic factors of type 2 diabetes are unknown and probably this trait, more than type 1 diabetes, is composed of several different diseases with the common clinical manifestation of hyperglycemia. However, there is no proof of an implication of an autoimmune response, and thus autoantibodies against pancreatic antigens are always negative (ADA, 2010). Patients are usually obese and non-insulin dependent, although insulin can become a necessary therapy for a good control of hyperglycemia in some cases. However, insulin treatment in type 2 diabetes is not required for survival. C-peptide levels can be lower than in healthy controls, reflecting the relative insulin deficiency, but they are higher than in type 1 diabetes patients and decrease more gradually with time (Hosszufalusi et al, 2003). Diabetic ketoacidosis is quite rare and tends to develop due to underlying conditions, such as an infection (ADA, 2010).

2.3 Latent autoimmune diabetes of the adult (LADA)

Early after the discovery of antibodies against pancreatic antigens in the serum of type 1 diabetic subjects, it was noticed by clinicians that 10% of patients first diagnosed with type 2 diabetes tested positive for type 1 diabetes antibodies (mainly GADA and ICA) (Palmer et al, 2005). Those patients slowly but relentlessly progressed to insulin-dependency and showed signs of pancreatic islet dysfunction such as a progressive decrease of C-peptide levels. These characteristics defined a new category in the diabetes spectra called the latent autoimmune diabetes of the adult, and abbreviated LADA. Diagnostic criteria for these patients are age at diagnosis over 30 years, presence of antibodies against pancreatic islets, with a higher frequency of single positivity and GADA or ICA antibodies than type 1 diabetes patients, and no requirement of insulin for at least six months since diagnosis (Palmer et al, 2005; Leslie et al, 2006). There seems to exist a similar but milder genetic background to that of type 1 diabetic patients (Hosszufalusi et al, 2003; Palmer et al, 2005), and some researchers think of LADA as a slower and less aggressive form of type 1 diabetes, to the point that this condition is usually termed type 1.5 diabetes. Debate exists over LADA being an entity of its own or just a less aggressive form of type 1 diabetes at an older age (Hosszufalusi et al, 2003; Palmer et al, 2005; Leslie et al, 2006; Steck & Eisenbarth, 2008). Anyway, this group of patients poses a very interesting subset for testing β cell preserving therapies in an autoimmune form of diabetes due to its slow progression to insulin-dependency.

2.4 The diagnosis of an adult-onset diabetic patient

When recruiting patients for genetic studies, a careful evaluation of adult-onset patients must be carried out to avoid misclassification. In most cases, the three more common forms of diabetes in adults can be distinguished with a test for antibodies against pancreatic antigens at diagnosis and the requirement for insulin therapy (see table 2).

	Adult-onset type 1 diabetes	Type 2 diabetes	LADA
Insulin requirement	Ultimately needed for survival	Useful for improved glycemic control in some cases	Not for the first 6 months after diagnosis. Patients eventually evolve to insulin-dependency
Corporal phenotype	Usually lean	Usually obese	Variable
Antibodies	2 or more positive	Negative	At least 1 positive High frequency of GADA+ and/or ICA+
C-peptide levels	Low or absent	Normal or slightly decreased	Low
Diabetic ketoacidosis	Present	Rare	Rare
T-cell response against pancreatic islet antigens	Positive	Negative	Positive
Type 1 diabetes HLA susceptibility	Present	Absent	Present
% of total adult diabetes	5-10%	80-85%	5-10%

Table 2. Summary of the characteristics of the three more common forms of diabetes in adulthood: adult-onset type 1 diabetes, type 2 diabetes and LADA (Leslie et al, 2006; ADA, 2010).

The subgroup of adult-onset type 1 diabetic patients is relatively easy to separate from the other two clinical manifestations of diabetes in adulthood: patients should be insulin-dependent since diagnosis, positive for at least two type 1 diabetes autoantibodies and usually of lean body type. However, many genetic studies in the last years have excluded the adult subset of type 1 diabetic patients as a precaution to avoid contamination with type 2 diabetic patients. This conservative measure has excluded a group of patients that could give us important information about the genetics of the disease: the existence of genes that modify the progression of the disease, together with unknown environmental factors, which would be the causatives of the fast immune β cell destruction in a child and the slower destruction in an adult patient.

From now on, we will focus on the genetics of type 1 diabetes and the study of the influence of genetics in age at disease onset.

3. Genetic studies in type 1 diabetes

The existence of a genetic basis that influences the development of type 1 diabetes is known since the first studies associated alleles and haplotypes in the Human Leukocyte Antigen (HLA) complex with type 1 diabetes risk in the late 70s (Nerup et al, 1974). Familial studies have been able to quantify the genetic basis of the disease in a range between 30-70% of the total contributing factors, being the remainder due to environmental factors (Redondo et al, 2001a; Pociot et al, 2010). Half of this genetic contribution is due to alleles and haplotypic combinations in the HLA region (Erlich et al, 2008), which is the strongest genetic modifier of type 1 diabetes risk. The rest of the genetic load is composed of genes with smaller effects, some of which have been unveiled in the last thirty years through different approaches developed as the technology for DNA study evolved. These studies ranged from the association studies of candidate genes to the complex hypothesis-free genome-wide association studies. In this section, we will briefly review the methodology employed in these studies and its importance in the unraveling of the type 1 diabetes genetic component.

3.1 Association studies of candidate genes

The association studies are suited for the detection of variants with moderate or low effects on the disease, as long as the studied variants are relatively frequent in the population of study (minor allele frequency over 5%) (Pociot et al, 2010; Steck & Rewers, 2011). Association can be measured in a case-control design (study of the differences between a set of unrelated patients and healthy controls) or a family design (analysis of deviations in the theoretical 50% transmission of the variant from healthy parents to patients). Previous to the massive knowledge that the Human Genome Project provided to genetic studies in humans, association studies had to focus on the selection of candidate genes, which limited these studies to genes with known function and biased the selection by what was known (or believed) about the pathogenesis of the disease at the moment. Nevertheless, this approach discovered the five classical regions associated with type 1 diabetes and detailed in table 3.

First reported	Gene	Function
1970-1980 (Nerup et al, 1974)	HLA class II	Antigen presentation in antigen-presenting cells.
1984 (Bell et al, 1984)	INS	Expression levels in the thymus regulate the presence of insulin-reactive T cells.
1996 (Nistico et al, 1996)	CTLA4	Modulator of inactivation of the immune response. Constitutively expressed in regulatory T cells, a lymphocyte subset specialized in the suppression of autoimmunity.
2004 (Bottini et al, 2004)	PTPN22	Suppressor of signals through the TCR. Susceptibility variant is believed to favor the survival of auto-reactive T cells in the thymus.
2005 (Vella et al, 2005)	IL2RA	Alpha subunit of the high affinity IL2 receptor. Constitutively expressed in regulatory T cells, it is essential for the maintenance of this cell subset.

Table 3. Classical type 1 diabetes associated genes discovered through association studies of candidate genes. TCR: T cell receptor.

3.2 The genome wide association studies

The first genome-wide association study was published in 2007 (The Wellcome Trust Case-Control Consortium [WTCCC], 2007). Samples from seven diseases (among them type 1 and type 2 diabetes) were collected, recruiting 2000 cases of each disease and a common subset of 3000 healthy controls. This single study described four new regions strongly associated with type 1 diabetes, almost the same number of regions that the previous association studies had taken three decades to discover.

Genome-wide association studies were possible thanks to the great development in the knowledge of human genetics and in the techniques to study DNA, derived from initiatives such as the Human Genome Project. The design of a genome-wide study is based on the analysis of over 500.000 single nucleotide polymorphisms (SNPs) throughout the genome in each subject recruited. The study design is usually a case-control approach, but both case-control and family studies are commonly used to replicate the stronger associations in the recent genome-wide studies (Hakonarson et al, 2007; Barrett et al, 2009). Since their object of analysis is the whole genome, these kind of studies are hypothesis-free and are able to detect associations in regions and genes that a candidate gene study would have never considered, such as regions with genes of unknown function and genes in routes not classically considered to take part in the pathogenesis of the disease. Thus, from the four regions associated with type 1 diabetes and described in the WTCCC study (WTCCC, 2007), one (16p13) covered a gene of unknown function, and two (12q13 and 12q24) pointed to regions with several candidate genes.

Despite the advantage that poses the hypothesis-free design, the genome-wide association studies have a great disadvantage in return: the high number of polymorphisms studied implies an elevated number of statistical comparisons and an increased probability of obtaining false-positive associations. Therefore, these studies are subject to a strong statistical correction (WTCCC, 2007), and, depending on the number of markers analyzed, p values should be as low as 10^{-7} to be considered statistically significant (Todd et al, 2007). Moreover, the results obtained (especially those that are borderline significant) should be replicated in independent populations to assure that the result is not a false positive and it is not influenced by population variability (McCarthy et al, 2008). At this stage is where follow-up studies take place. Follow-up studies select associations from genome-wide studies for replication purposes, being the more interesting those that are borderline significant.

Genome-wide association studies and their follow-up have been successful in uncovering associations of high to moderate effect (odds ratio over 1.15) in variants with a minor allele frequency over 5%. Now, the remainder of the genetic component in type 1 diabetes is proposed to reside in rare variants with high effect and common variants with low effect on the disease (Pociot et al, 2010). Due to the stringent statistical correction required, genome-wide studies are not suitable for detecting these associations and new approaches will be necessary. Despite their limitations, in just five years genome-wide studies have revealed ten times more genetic regions than the older approaches did in thirty years, providing fifty genetic regions associated with type 1 diabetes. A brief summary of these regions can be consulted in table 4.

3.3 The problem with age at diagnosis

Although type 1 diabetes has a similar prevalence in all ages, the restriction to pediatric patients has been a popular criterion for recruitment of patients in studies on the genetics of the disease, as it is shown in table 5. Its purpose is to avoid the inclusion of misdiagnosed

Chromosome	Candidate gene	OR	Reference study	Published age-at-onset analysis
1p13.2	PTPN22	2.05	(Smyth et al. 2008)	Yes
1q31.2	RGS1	0.89	(Smyth et al. 2008)	
1q32.1	IL20-IL10-IL19	0.84	(Barrett et al. 2009)	
2q11.2	Several	--	(Barrett et al. 2009)	
2q24.2	IFIH1	0.86	(Smyth et al. 2008)	
2q32.2	STAT4	1.10	(Fung et al. 2009)	Yes
2q33.2	CTLA4	0.82	(Smyth et al. 2008)	
3p21.31	CCR5	0.85	(Smyth et al. 2008)	
4p15.2	AC111003.1	1.09	(Barrett et al. 2009)	
4q27	IL2-IL21	1.13	(Barrett et al. 2009)	
6p21	HLA	0.02-49.2	(Ounissi-Benkalha and Polychronakos 2008)	Yes
6q15	BACH2	1.13	(Cooper et al. 2008)	
6q22.32	CENPW	1.17	(Barrett et al. 2009)	
6q23.3	TNFAIP3	0.90	(Fung et al. 2009)	
6q25.3	TAGAP	0.92	(Smyth et al. 2008)	
7p15.2	Several	0.88	(Barrett et al. 2009)	
7p12.1	COBL	0.77	(Barrett et al. 2009)	
9p24.2	GLIS3	0.88	(Barrett et al. 2009)	
10p15.1	IL2RA	0.62	(Smyth et al. 2008)	Yes
10p15.1	PRKCQ	0.69	(Lowe et al. 2007)	
10q22.3	ZMIZ1	--	(Barrett et al. 2009)	
10q23.31	RNLS	0.75	(Barrett et al. 2009)	
11p15.5	INS	0.42	(Smyth et al. 2008)	Yes
12p13.31	CLEC2D-CD69	1.09	(Barrett et al. 2009)	
12q13.3	CYP27B1	1.22	(Bailey et al. 2007)	
12q13.2	ERBB3	1.31	(Barrett et al. 2009)	Yes
12q24.12	SH2B3	1.28	(Smyth et al. 2008)	Yes
13.32.3	GRP183	1.15	(Heinig et al. 2010)	
14q24.1	Several	0.86	(Barrett et al. 2009)	
14q32.2	Several	1.09	(Barrett et al. 2009)	
14q32.2	Several	0.90	(Wallace et al. 2009)	
15q14	RASGRP1	1.21	(Qu et al. 2009)	
15q25.1	CTSH	0.86	(Smyth et al. 2008)	
16p13.13	CLEC16A	0.81	(Smyth et al. 2008)	Yes
16p11.2	IL27	0.86	(Barrett et al. 2009)	
16q23.1	Several	1.28	(Barrett et al. 2009)	
17q12	Several	0.87	(Barrett et al. 2009)	
17q21.2	SMARCE1	0.95	(Barrett et al. 2009)	

Table 4. Summary of the 50 chromosomal regions currently associated with type 1 diabetes (continues in next page). The odds ratio in the table has been extracted from the reference study. Data come from the on-line database www.t1dbase.org, belonging to the Type 1 Diabetes Genetics Consortium (T1DGC). The reference study does not correspond with the published age-at-onset study. Genes CLEC16A and SH2B3 were analyzed in Todd et al (2007) and where not associated with age at onset. The rest of the age-at-onset associations are reviewed in section 4.

Chromosome	Candidate gene	OR	Reference study	Published age-at-onset analysis
18p11.21	PTPN2	1.28	(Smyth et al. 2008)	Yes
18q22.2	CD226	1.16	(Smyth et al. 2008)	
19p13.2	TYK2	0.86	(Wallace et al. 2009)	
19q13.32	Several	0.86	(Barrett et al. 2009)	
19q13.4	FUT2	--	(Barrett et al. 2009)	
20p13	Several	0.90	(Barrett et al. 2009)	
21q22.3	UBASH3A	1.13	(Smyth et al. 2008)	
22q12.2	Several	1.10	(Barrett et al. 2009)	
22q12.3	IL2RB	--	(Barrett et al. 2009)	
22q13.1	C1QTNF6	1.11	(Cooper et al. 2008)	
Xp22.2	TLR8	0.84	(Barrett et al. 2009)	
Xq28	Several	1.16	(Barrett et al. 2009)	

Table 4 (continuation). Summary of the 50 chromosome regions currently associated with type 1 diabetes.

patients (type 2 diabetics or LADA patients) within adult-onset diabetic patients. However, enough criteria exist to discriminate type 1 diabetic patients from the remainder of diabetic adults, and the exclusion of adult type 1 diabetes patients limits the knowledge of the genetics of the disease only to its early onset. Adult-onset patients show signs of a slower immune reaction to β cells. The factors that cause a rapid destruction of β cells in a child but a slower degeneration in an adult-onset patient are unknown, nevertheless they are probably a mixture of genetic and environmental factors. Some hypotheses may explain the different speed in clinical manifestations: the genetic load of adult-onset diabetes could be composed of a lower number of associated genes than in the early-onset patients, or could be the same genes but with less effect in the adult disease, or maybe the adult-onset population has genes associated that are exclusive of adult-onset. Besides, the simple replication in adult-onset patients of associations found in pediatric type 1 diabetes is interesting to prove that, from a genetic perspective, adult-onset patients are as much type 1 diabetes as the pediatric-onset ones.

Four genome-wide studies and a series of follow-up have been published in type 1 diabetes in the last five years (table 5). Two included systematically some adult-onset patients in their populations; however most of these studies lacked an analysis of the influence of genetics in the age of diagnosis. The characteristics of the four genome-wide and some selected follow-up and major genetic studies, and the populations included in them, can be consulted in table 5.

The two populations that recruit late-onset patients deserve a more detailed commentary. The GoKinD (Genetics of kidneys in diabetes) population, included in Cooper et al in 2008, belongs to a United States project that aims at studying the genetics of kidney diseases in type 1 diabetes. Selection criteria for type 1 diabetes were age at diagnosis before 31 years, insulin therapy needed within the first year of diagnosis and not interrupted for any reason ever since. Patients had a minimum disease duration of 10 years. Analysis of the influence of genetics in age at diagnosis was not carried out in this genome-wide study.

Study	Year of publication	Population	Age limit for selection of participants	Study of genetics and age at diagnosis
(1) WTCCC	2007	2000 cases, British	Diagnosis before 17 years	No
(2) Todd et al	2007 Follow-up from WTCCC	4000 cases and 2997 British families	Diagnosis before 17 years	Yes
(3) Hakonarson et al	2007	563 cases and 1422 families from Britain, the US and Australia	Most diagnosed before 18 years	No
(4) Cooper et al	2008	GoKinD population 1785 US cases	Diagnosis before 31 years	No
(5) Smyth et al	2008 Major genetic study	8064 cases and 3064 families from US, Finland, Ireland, Norway and Romania	Diagnosis before 17 years	No
(6) Barrett et al	2009	T1DGC population 3983 cases and 2319 families from Britain, the US and Australia	Diagnosis before 35 years	No

Table 5. Genome-wide and major genetic studies performed in type 1 diabetes. Studies 2, 4 and 6 performed metanalysis with the WTCCC data. Also, the last genome-wide carried out by Barrett et al (study 6) performed a meta-analysis of the three larger genome-wide studies (1, 4 and 6) performed in type 1 diabetes.

The T1DGC (Type 1 Diabetes Genetics Consortium) is an initiative constituted in 2002 with the aim of providing resources to the research in type 1 diabetes. Since 2007, the consortium has published several studies on type 1 diabetes genetics (Erlich et al, 2008; Hakonarson et al, 2008; Howson et al, 2009; Qu et al, 2009) and, although the genome-wide study in which the T1DGC population was genotyped did not include an age-at-onset analysis, this group is lately including age-at-onset analyses in their publications and some of their studies have provided the first evidences of influence of genetics in age at onset of the post-genome wide era (Hakonarson et al, 2008). The selection criteria for adult patients are year at diagnosis under 35 years and uninterrupted insulin treatment for at least 6 months (Hakonarson et al, 2007). However, despite the wider limit in age at onset in this population, the majority of the patients included are pediatric, as reflected in the mean age at onset (around ten years) found in the published studies (Hakonarson et al, 2008; Howson et al, 2009).

4. Reported genetic associations of genes and age-at-diagnosis

The influence of genetics in age at onset of type 1 diabetes has been analyzed in some studies. However, initiatives to replicate these first studies or to establish a protocol to analyze the genetics or early and late onset are lacking, and therefore there is disparity in the definition and selection of late-onset type 1 diabetes patients, and in the statistical methods employed to analyze the associations. In this section, we will review some selected studies on the influence of genetics in age at diagnosis of type 1 diabetes.

- Familial studies: analysis in monozygotic twins with one member affected with type 1 diabetes have shown that the probability of developing the disease in the non-affected twin is considerably higher (38%) when the affected twin developed type 1 diabetes at an early age (under 24 years) than when the affected twin developed the disease after 25 years of age (6% risk for the non-affected twin) (Redondo et al, 2001b). This observation might suggest that early-onset type 1 diabetes has a stronger genetic component (responsible of the higher concordance rate) than the same disease with a late onset.

- HLA associations to age at onset: several studies (Redondo et al, 2001a; Leslie et al, 2006; Klinker et al, 2010) have pointed out to the higher risk and earlier onset of type 1 diabetes in patients that are heterozygote for the HLA class II risk haplotypes *DRB1*03* and *DRB1*04-DQB1*03:02*. On the other hand, the influence of HLA class I alleles in age at diagnosis has been thoroughly studied, and alleles *B*39* and *A*24* have been consistently associated to an earlier onset of the disease (Valdes et al, 2005; Nejentsev et al, 2007). The *B*39* allele, for example, precipitates the age of diagnosis in four years (Valdes et al, 2005).

- *IL12B*: the gene *IL12B* codes for the p40 subunit of the interleukin 12, also shared with interleukin 23. A 2004 study (Windsor et al, 2004) carried out in an Australian cohort including early and late onset patients found association of a polymorphism in position +1188 of the gene with late-onset of the disease (over 25 years). Neither associations on the *IL12B* gene with type 1 diabetes nor the described age-at-onset association have been replicated in recent studies.

- *CAPSL-IL7R*: this region was first associated with type 1 diabetes in a study of non-synonymous polymorphisms, finding a marker in the *CAPSL* gene that was highly associated with the disease (Smyth et al, 2006). Another polymorphism in the *IL7R* gene has been associated to type 1 diabetes and multiple sclerosis (Hafler et al, 2007; Todd et al, 2007). Our group undertook a replication study on both polymorphisms briefly after the discovery of the first signal (Santiago et al, 2008). We found association with type 1 diabetes in both polymorphisms and also described that both markers were associated with an earlier onset, an effect more noticeable in the *IL7R* polymorphism.

- Region 12q13 (*ERBB3* gene): in a replication study of borderline significant signals from a previous genome-wide (Hakonarson et al, 2007), the T1DGC found evidence of the association of three 12q13 polymorphisms with age at diagnosis (Hakonarson et al, 2008). The influence of this region on age at onset of type 1 diabetes has been subsequently analyzed in two independent studies (Awata et al, 2009; Wang et al, 2010) that, with different statistical methodology, did not replicate the effect seen in the first study. Finally, we have studied several signals in this region and found an age-at-diagnosis effect stronger than the previously described, with homozygotes for the susceptibility allele having an age at onset five years earlier than carriers of protective alleles (Espino-Paisan et al, 2011b).

- Region 2q32 (*STAT4* gene): a study in 2008 described an association of polymorphisms in the *STAT4* gene with type 1 diabetes patients with an onset earlier than 8 years (Lee et al, 2008). Among the polymorphisms studied was rs7574865, which we will include in our study on age at onset in section 5. This study was carried out in a pediatric Korean population, therefore population differences have to be taken in consideration, given that the genetics of Asian and Caucasian type 1 diabetes patients present some important differences (Ikegami et al, 2007).

- Insulin gene: the T1DGC group analyzed several classical type 1 diabetes genes (Howson et al, 2009) and found association of the susceptibility variant in the insulin gene to an onset of type 1 diabetes two years earlier than the protective allele. However, this effect was not replicated in one of the cohorts included in the study. We will analyze the same polymorphism in our study in section 5.

- IL2RA: a Finnish study analyzed several classical type 1 diabetes genes in a group with late-onset of the disease (Klinker et al, 2010). They found associations of the insulin, PTPN22, IFIH1 and CTLA4 genes with late-onset patients, and replicated the age-at-onset effect of the DRB1*03-DRB1*04-DQB1*03:02 heterozygote. They also found that IL2RA was associated with an earlier disease onset. However, the T1DGC studied the IL2RA gene and did not find any effect in age at onset, although they did not include the stronger association in the gene that the Finnish study did analyze (Howson et al, 2009). Our group conducted a replication study in polymorphisms in the IL2RA gene and we found them associated to both early and late disease onset (Espino-Paisan et al, 2011c).

- PTPN22: a German group studied the C1858T polymorphism in the PTPN22 gene and found that the susceptibility polymorphism was associated to an earlier onset of the disease in a group of pediatric-onset patients (Kordonouri et al, 2010). Patients with the susceptibility polymorphism had an onset of the disease two years earlier than homozygotes for the protective allele. However, this observation was not replicated in the T1DGC study (Howson et al, 2009). We will study this polymorphism in our group of pediatric and adult patients in section 5.

- PTPN2: our group studied the influence in age at disease onset of two polymorphisms in the PTPN2 gene that had been previously associated with type 1 diabetes (Todd et al, 2007; WTCCC, 2007). We found that one of the studied polymorphisms was associated with an earlier disease onset, with carriers of the susceptibility allele having a disease onset almost three years earlier than homozygotes for the protective allele (Espino-Paisan et al, 2011a).

5. A practical study: Genetic analysis of a population with early and late-onset type 1 diabetes patients

We have selected ten chromosome regions (five classical genes and five genome-wide discoveries) previously studied in type 1 diabetes to test their association with pediatric and late-onset patients. We will briefly review their role in the pathogenesis of the disease and compare our results with the previous reported associations.

5.1 Population of study and methods

A total of 444 type 1 diabetes patients (47% female) were included in this study. All patients were recruited from the Madrid area (Spain), all where Caucasoid and diagnosed according to the criteria of the American Diabetes Association (ADA, 2010). Age at diagnosis was available for 415 patients and ranged from 1 to 65 years. Mean age at onset of the population was 18.6±11.1 years and median age at onset was 16 years. All patients were insulin-dependent since diagnosis and had been on uninterrupted insulin treatment for at least 6 months. Adult patients diagnosed over 35 years were included on the basis of positivity to autoantibodies, lean body type and insulin-dependency status. Also, a maximum of 888 ethnically matched controls (53.7% female) with no history of type 1 diabetes in first degree relatives were recruited.

Genes in the HLA complex were genotyped by two SSOP (Sequence Specific Oligonucleotide Probe) procedures: dot-blot hybridization and Luminex technology. The remaining genes were studied through genotyping of single nucleotide polymorphisms by TaqMan Assays in a 7900HT fast real-time PCR system (Applied Biosystems Foster City, CA, USA). The call rate for each SNP was 95%. A summary of these studied polymorphisms can be consulted in table 6.

Chromosome	Candidate gene	SNP	Assay reference	Control MAF
1p13	PTPN22	rs2476601	By design	T (0.06)
2q24	IFIH1	rs1990760	C___2780299_30	G (0.46)
2q32.3	STAT4	rs7574865	C__29882391_10	T (0.21)
2q33.2	CTLA-4	rs231775	C___2415786_20	T (0.29)
		rs3087243	C___3296043_10	G (0.48)
6q23.3	TNFAIP3	rs10499194	C___1575581_10	T (0.32)
9q33.2	TRAF1	rs2269059	C__15875924_10	A (0.07)
11p15.5	INS	rs689	C___1223317_10	A (0.28)
12p13.31	CLEC2D	rs11052552	C__32169467_10	G (0.49)
16p13.13	CLEC16A	rs2903692	C__15941578_10	A (0.42)

Table 6. Summary of the genotyped SNPs in each gene. MAF: minor allele frequency.

No statistically significant deviations from Hardy-Weinberg equilibrium were found in the control subset for each polymorphism. A case-control analysis was performed to asses association of the selected variants with type 1 diabetes. Differences were calculated through Chi-square and Fisher's exact tests when necessary. Analysis of age at onset was performed through a stratified and a continuous approach. For the stratified analysis, cases were classified in early-onset (age at diagnosis under 17 years) or late-onset (age at diagnosis over 16 years) and compared with Chi-square test or Fisher's exact test. Associations were estimated by the odds ratio (OR) with 95% confidence interval. All Chi-square and Fisher's exact test comparisons were calculated with Epi Info v.5 (CDC, Atlanta, USA). For the continuous analysis approach, ages at onset associated to each allele were compared with the non-parametric U Mann-Whitney test implemented in SPSS v.15.0 (Chicago, Illinois, USA).

5.2 Selected genes and results
5.2.1 Classical type 1 diabetes associations
Class II HLA alleles (chromosome 6p21): class II HLA binds extra-cellular antigens processed by antigen presenting cells and presents them to CD4+ helper T cells. The proposed mechanism in the pathogenesis of type 1 diabetes takes place at the negative selection process during lymphocyte thymic maturation (Redondo et al, 2001a; Ounissi-Benkalha and Polychronakos, 2008). Negative selection occurs when a T cell with an autoreactive T cell receptor (TCR) binds a HLA molecule loaded with an autoantigen. This union sends a strong activation signal through the TCR that is deleterious to the autoreactive T cell. Theoretically, susceptibility HLA alleles bind pancreatic antigens less efficiently, lowering the activation signal to non-deleterious levels and allowing the autoreactive T cell to escape from thymic selection.

The HLA associations detected in our group in the case-control analysis and the study on age at onset can be consulted in table 7. Due to the high number of alleles and haplotypic combinations in this region, and the low frequency of some of them, a stratified analysis would imply a marked loss of statistical power, so we choose to perform only the continuous analysis. We did not find evidence of an influence in age at diagnosis in any of the haplotypic combinations included, which means that our adult-onset patients have the same HLA contribution to type 1 diabetes than our pediatric patients. Of notice, there are two haplotypes with a marked difference in the mean age at diagnosis: the DRB1*04-DQB1*03:02 homozygote (carriers have an onset three years earlier) and carriers of the protective haplotype DRB1*15:01-DQB1*06:02 (carriers have an onset ten years later than non carriers). None of these comparisons are statistically significant, but it could be a problem of low statistical power since both genotypes are quite infrequent. A larger sample would be needed to elucidate the possible associations.

Many studies describe the DRB1*03-DRB1*04 heterozygote as associated with earlier age at diagnosis of type 1 diabetes, and also as the haplotypic combination that confers a higher risk to the disease. In our population we do not see an age effect (p=0.9). Moreover, the DRB1*03-DRB1*04 heterozygote does not confer the higher risk, but the DRB1*04 homozygote, the DRB1*03 or DRB1*04 carrier, and the DRB1*03 homozygote.

Insulin gene (chromosome 11p15): the insulin gene is also proposed to participate in the generation of autoreactive T cells in the thymus. The polymorphism associated with type 1 diabetes is a VNTR (variable number of tandem repeats) that locates upstream of the INS gene and modifies its expression in the thymus (Pugliese et al, 1997; Vafiadis et al, 1997). Alleles in this VNTR range from 26 to 210 repetitions of a consensus sequence and are usually classified in three groups: short class I alleles (26 to 64 repetitions), intermediate class II alleles (64 to 139 repetitions, infrequent in Caucasian and Asian populations) and large class III alleles (140 to 210 repetitions). Large alleles are associated with protection from type 1 diabetes and are related to a higher expression of insulin in the thymus (Vafiadis et al, 1997). This is thought to favor the negative selection of insulin-reactive T cells, a theory that would be consistent with the lower levels of insulin antibodies detected in patients that carry the large class III alleles (Hermann et al, 2005). We have selected a polymorphism (rs689) in linkage disequilibrium with the two main classes of alleles that is usually employed in genetic studies (Hermann et al, 2005; Todd et al, 2007; Smyth et al, 2008) as a proxy to the VNTR genotyping.

Genotype	Case-control analysis			
	Genotype frequency		p	OR
	T1D	Controls		
DR4-DQ8 homozygote	0.052	0.002	6.0×10^{-8}	33.59 (5.40-1386)
DR3-DQ2 carrier or DR4-DQ8 carrier	0.894	0.384	2.1×10^{-61}	13.24 (9.27-18.96)
DR3-DQ2 carrier	0.143	0.015	3.1×10^{-16}	11.19 (5.31-24.41)
DR3-DQ2 DR4-DQ8	0.249	0.031	1.6×10^{-26}	10.36 (6.11-17.75)
DR4-DQ8 – X (not DR3)	0.256	0.123	3.7×10^{-8}	2.43 (1.74-3.39)
DR3-DQ2 – X (not DR4)	0.369	0.221	2.0×10^{-7}	2.03 (1.53-2.69)
DR2-DQ6 – X	0.011	0.186	4.5×10^{-19}	0.05 (0.02-0.12)

Table 7. Case-control analysis of selected HLA haplotypes. Comparisons were calculated with Chi-square and Fisher's exact test when necessary. HLA haplotypes have been abbreviated: DR4-DQ8 (*DRB1*04-DQA1*03:01-DQB1*03:02*), DR3-DQ2 (*DRB1*03-DQA1*05:01-DQB1*02:01*), DR2-DQ6 (*DRB1*15:01-DQA1*01:02-DQB1*06:02*). T1D: type 1 diabetes.

Genotype	Continuous analysis		
	Mean age at onset		P
	Carrier	Non carrier	
DR4-DQ8 homozygote	15.9 (11.5)	18.6 (11.1)	0.2
DR3-DQ2 carrier Or DR4-DQ8 carrier	18.3 (11.1)	19.4 (10.2)	0.4
DR3-DQ2 carrier	17.5 (11.2)	18.6 (11.0)	0.2
DR3-DQ2 DR4-DQ8	18.0 (10.7)	18.6 (11.2)	0.9
DR4-DQ8 – X (not DR3)	18.0 (10.5)	18.9 (11.5)	0.7
DR3-DQ2 – X (not DR4)	18.8 (11.9)	18.4 (11.5)	0.9
DR2-DQ6 – X	28.0 (13.7)	18.5 (11.0)	0.2

Table 7 (continuation). Analysis of age at onset in selected HLA haplotypes. Comparisons were calculated with the U Mann-Whitney test. HLA haplotypes: DR4-DQ8 (*DRB1*04-DQA1*03:01-DQB1*03:02*), DR3-DQ2 (*DRB1*03-DQA1*05:01-DQB1*02:01*), DR2-DQ6 (*DRB1*15:01-DQA1*01:02-DQB1*06:02*). T1D: type 1 diabetes.

In our study, we replicate the association previously described in the *INS* gene and we do not find effects on age at onset in the stratified and continuous analysis. Results are provided in table 8.

Gene	CASE-CONTROL AND AGE-STRATIFIED ANALYSES			CONTINUOUS ANALYSIS Mean age at onset		
	MAF	p	OR	Major allele	Minor allele	P
INS						
T1D-control	0.175	0.282	8.3x10⁻⁹	0.54 (0.43-0.67)	19.3 (11.8)	18.0 (10.7)	0.4
Pediatric-adult T1D	0.162	0.177	0.6			
CTLA4 rs231775						
T1D-control	0.328	0.299	0.1	1.14 (0.96-1.37)	18.4 (10.9)	18.9 (11.4)	0.6
Pediatric-adult T1D	0.323	0.339	0.6			
CTLA4 rs3087243						
T1D-control	0.477	0.518	0.05	0.85 (0.72-1.00)	18.9 (11.0)	17.8 (10.8)	0.2
Pediatric-adult T1D	0.493	0.451	0.2			
PTPN22						
T1D-control	0.115	0.064	7x10⁻⁶	1.91 (1.42-2.56)	18.4 (11.2)	19.0 (10.6)	0.4
Pediatric-adult T1D	0.113	0.127	0.5			
IFIH1						
T1D-control	0.373	0.409	0.1	0.86 (0.70-1.06)	17.2 (10.3)	17.2 (10.6)	0.9
Pediatric-adult T1D	0.373	0.394	0.6			

Table 8. Analysis of classical gene associations in type 1 diabetes. Minor allele frequency (MAF) is provided in case-control and age-stratified analyses, and comparisons were calculated with Chi-square and Fisher's exact test when necessary. In the continuous analysis, mean ages at onset associated to each allele and the p value from the U Mann-Whitney test are presented. *INS*: insulin gene. T1D: type 1 diabetes.

CTLA4 (chromosome 2q33): this gene encodes a negative regulator of lymphocytic activation. Its expression is induced in activated lymphocytes, but it is also constitutively expressed in regulatory T cells, a lymphocyte subpopulation specialized in the suppression of autoimmunity. Also, a soluble form of CTLA4 is secreted in the serum, and it is believed that this form contributes to the downregulation of activation in the immune system (Ueda et al, 2003). Several polymorphisms have been identified and associated with type 1 diabetes (Ueda et al, 2003; Qu et al, 2009). We have selected two functional polymorphisms: one aminoacidic change related to lower membrane expression of the protein (rs231775) and a polymorphism in the 3′ end that is related to higher expression of soluble CTLA4 (rs3087243), which also is one of the strongest associations with type 1 diabetes in the gene (Ueda et al, 2003; Qu et al, 2009).

We replicate the association described in *CTLA4* rs3087243. Differences in *CTLA4* rs231775 do not reach statistical signification, but this could be due to low statistical power to detect the previously described association (Ueda et al, 2003). We do not find effects of any of the polymorphisms on age at onset. Results can be consulted in table 8.

PTPN22 (chromosome 1p13): this gene encodes a lymphoid-specific phosphatase called LYP, which is an important downregulator of T cell activation through the TCR. We selected the classical non-synonymous polymorphism C1858T that causes a substitution from arginine to tryptophan in the aminoacid 620 of the encoded protein (Bottini et al, 2004). The mutant form shows a higher phosphatase activity, and therefore it suppresses T cell activation more efficiently. Its role in type 1 diabetes is believed to be at the thymic selection process, where the mutant PTPN22 would lower the activation signal sent to the autoreactive T cell through its TCR, thus contributing to its survival (Bottini et al, 2006). It also has been proposed that the increased suppression of activation associated to the mutant form could affect negatively the activation of regulatory T cells (Bottini et al, 2006).

We replicate the association previously described in the *PTPN22* gene and we do not find effects on age at onset in the stratified and continuous analysis. Results can be consulted in table 8.

IFIH1/MDA5 (chromosome 2q24): certain viral infections such as that caused by Enterovirus are more prevalent in type 1 diabetes patients than in the healthy population, and it has been proposed that they could participate in the development or acceleration of the immune response against the β cell (Hober & Sauter 2010). The helicase IFIH1 recognizes viral double stranded RNA (dsRNA) and it is expressed in the cytoplasm of several cells, including β cells. In the presence of a viral infection, IFIH1 binds the dsRNA and induces the synthesis of pro-inflammatory cytokines. Functional experiments show that protection from type 1 diabetes is achieved through a lower performance of the sentinel role of IFIH1 that would end up in lower activation of the immune system in response to the viral infection (Colli et al, 2010).

We detect a lower frequency of the minor allele of *IFIH1* in type 1 diabetes patients respect to controls; however this difference is not statistically significant, probably due to low statistical power of our study. We do not find effects on age at diagnosis of type 1 diabetes in the stratified and continuous analysis. Results are provided in table 8.

5.2.2 Genome-wide associations

Region 2q32 (STAT4): the gene *STAT4* is an interesting candidate for type 1 diabetes. Member of a family of transcription factors, STAT4 activates the transcription of several genes including IFN-γ in response to interleukin-12 signaling. The pathway IL12-STAT4-IFNγ polarizes the immune response to a Th1 type, the kind of response that is thought to be responsible of the type 1 diabetes autoimmune reaction (Raz et al, 2005). We have selected a polymorphism that was first discovered associated with rheumatoid arthritis (Remmers et al, 2007). Our group studied this polymorphism in several autoimmune diseases and described its association with type 1 diabetes (Martinez et al, 2008), as it can be seen in table 9. Influence of this polymorphism in age at onset has been previously studied in a pediatric-onset Korean population, as we described in section 4. We performed a stratified and continuous analysis of age at onset and we did not find evidences of the influence of this polymorphism in age at onset of the disease. Results can be consulted in table 9.

Gene	CASE-CONTROL AND AGE-STRATIFIED ANALYSES				CONTINUOUS ANALYSIS		
	MAF		p	OR	Mean age at onset		P
					Major allele	Minor allele	
2q32 (STAT4)							
T1D-control	0.240	0.192	0.01	1.33 (1.05-1.68)	17.6 (10.6)	16.7 (9.4)	0.6
Pediatric-adult T1D	0.237	0.250	0.7	--			
6q23 (TNFAIP3)							
T1D-control	0.282	0.321	0.05	0.83 (0.69-1.01)	18.7 (11.1)	17.8 (10.6)	0.3
Pediatric-adult T1D	0.297	0.271	0.4	--			
9q33 (TRAF1)							
T1D-control	0.085	0.071	0.2	--	18.4 (11.1)	21.2 (10.5)	0.02
Pediatric-adult T1D	0.063	0.104	0.04	--			
12p13 (CLEC2D)							
T1D-control	0.462	0.504	0.06	0.85 (0.71-1.01)	17.6 (10.7)	18.5 (11.0)	0.4
Pediatric-adult T1D	0.471	0.460	0.8	--			
16p13 (CLEC16A)							
T1D-control	0.368	0.416	0.05	0.82 (0.66-1.01)	16.9 (9.7)	18.0 (11.5)	0.5
Pediatric-adult T1D	0.359	0.394	0.4	--			

Table 9. Analysis of selected gene associations from genome-wide studies in type 1 diabetes. Minor allele frequency (MAF) is provided in case-control and pediatric vs adult onset analyses, and comparisons are calculated with Chi-square and Fisher's exact test when necessary. In the continuous analysis, mean ages at onset associated to each allele and the p value from the U Mann-Whitney test are presented. T1D: type 1 diabetes.

Region 6q23 (TNFAIP3): two polymorphisms located in an intergenic space adjacent to the *TNFAIP3* gene have been associated to several autoimmune diseases, among them type 1 diabetes (Fung et al, 2009). We have selected the polymorphism that shows a stronger association with the disease. The gene *TNFAIP3* is expressed in β cells and serves as an anti-inflammatory mechanism by its downregulation of the NF-κB activation (Liuwantara et al, 2006); therefore, it poses an interesting candidate gene in the pathogenesis of type 1 diabetes. To our knowledge, this is the first time that this region is studied in relation to its influence in age at onset.

In our study, we replicate the association previously seen in type 1 diabetes and we do not find differences in age at onset either in the stratified or continuous analyses. Results are provided in table 9.

Region 9q33 (TRAF1): this region was first associated to rheumatoid arthritis (Kurreeman et al, 2007). Our group took part in a collaborative study that analyzed this region in several autoimmune diseases and found association with type 1 diabetes, among others

(Kurreeman et al, 2010). As an extension of the cited study, we selected and studied new polymorphisms in the *TRAF1* gene and analyzed their influence in age at onset of the disease. We present in table 9 the results obtained in one polymorphism that has not been previously studied in type 1 diabetes. Like *TNFAIP3*, the gene *TRAF1* is expressed in β cells and protects them against cytokine-mediated apoptosis in an inflammatory environment (Sarkar et al, 2009).

The polymorphism in *TRAF1* shows interesting data (table 9). We do not see statistical differences in the case-control analysis, but the age-stratified analysis shows an elevation of the minor allele frequency only in the adult-onset patients, that is statistically significant when compared to pediatric patients (p=0.04) and to controls (OR=1.52 [1.00-2.31]; p=0.04). On the other hand, the pediatric patients are similar to controls (p=0.6). The continuous analysis confirms the difference observed in the stratified analysis, showing an age at onset associated to the minor allele (mean 21.2) that is almost three years higher than the age at onset associated to the major allele (mean 18.4). Therefore, there seems to exist an association in this gene that is exclusive of our adult-onset type 1 diabetes patients.

Region 12p13 (CLEC2D): first associated with type 1 diabetes in the WTCCC study (WTCCC, 2007), it includes several genes. Polymorphisms associated with the disease (WTCCC, 2007; Barrett et al, 2009) have been identified in the surroundings of two genes with immunological function: *CLEC2D* and *CD69*. We will focus on the polymorphism near *CLEC2D* (coding the NK receptor LLT1), which was the strongest signal reported by the WTCCC (WTCCC, 2007) in this region. To date, the influence of region 12p13 on age at onset has not been studied.

In our study, we detect a trend towards association with type 1 diabetes of the studied polymorphism. We do not find differences in age at onset in the stratified and continuous analyses. Results are provided in table 9.

Region 16p13 (CLEC16A): this region was one of the most strongly associated with type 1 diabetes in the WTCCC (WTCCC, 2007) and was also discovered independently in a parallel study (Hakonarson et al, 2007). It covers a gene of unknown function termed *CLEC16A*, which is expressed in antigen presenting cells and NK cells, but little else is known about this gene or its possible role in the pathogenesis of the disease. Our group replicated the association detected in the WTCCC study (Martinez et al, 2010). Here we will analyze its influence in age at onset.

We replicate the association previously seen in type 1 diabetes. We do not find differences in age at onset in the stratified and continuous analyses. Results are provided in table 9.

5.3 Discussion

In this study we analyzed ten genetic regions, five of them classical type 1 diabetes genes and another five extracted from recent genome-wide studies. The analysis of age at onset (either age-stratified or considering age as a continuum) did not provide statistical differences in nine of the ten regions studied, therefore we propose that our adult-onset patients have the same genetic background in the studied genes that our pediatric-onset patients. Hence there is no reason to exclude these late-onset patients from genetic studies on type 1 diabetes. The results we observe in the classical type 1 diabetes susceptibility genes (table 8) are concordant with a recent Finnish study (Klinker et al, 2010) that analyzes these genes in late-onset patients and finds the same associations previously described in pediatric-onset type 1 diabetes. Also, a recent study from the T1DGC (Howson et al, 2009) that replicated 19 genes, including *PTPN22*, *IFIH1* and *CTLA4*, studied age at onset in each one and did not find statistical differences, supporting the idea that the classical genetic associations to type 1 diabetes are shared between the early and late onset patients.

Interestingly, in our population we do not find differences in the HLA associations with early and late onset. It has been described before that the *DRB1*03-DRB1*04* heterozygote is the combination that confers a higher risk and it is associated with an earlier age at onset of type 1 diabetes (Redondo et al, 2001a; Leslie et al, 2006; Klinker et al, 2010). However, in our population the heterozygote is the fourth combination in risk conferred to the disease after the *DRB1*04-DQB1*03:02* homozygote, the *DRB1*03* or *DRB1*04-DQB1*03:02* carrier and the *DRB1*03* homozygote, and we do not see an effect on age at diagnosis of the heterozygote. This could be due to populational differences, quite important in the HLA complex. It is well known that not all the *DRB1*03* haplotypes confer the same susceptibility to the disease. An extended conserved haplotype marked by *B*18-DRB1*03-DQB1*02:01* is described to confer higher susceptibility among the *DRB1*03*-carrying haplotypes (Johansson et al, 2003; Urcelay et al, 2005). This haplotype is more frequent in the Mediterranean area and its frequency descends in Northern Europe. Therefore, it could be possible that the higher frequency of this high risk haplotype enhances the risk conferred by being a *DRB1*03* homozygote in a Mediterranean population such as the Spanish.

A recent study with the T1DGC family cohort (Howson et al, 2009) found a mild effect of the insulin gene in age at diagnosis of the disease, with the susceptibility allele conferring an onset two years earlier than the protective allele. We do not see an effect on age at diagnosis (continuous analysis, p=0.4). Moreover, in the aforementioned Finnish report, the authors also studied the *INS* gene and found association in late onset patients (Klinker et al, 2010). It is possible that our study lacks statistical power to detect a difference of two years in the age at diagnosis. However, the authors of the T1DGC study tried to replicate their findings in a case series of 900 patients and did not find the effect they saw in the family cohort, opening the door to the possibility that the described effect is a false positive.

Finally, we find that *TRAF1* is only associated to late-onset type 1 diabetes. Although our study is limited by low statistical power and would require replication in an independent late onset type 1 diabetes cohort, this is an interesting finding that would justify the study of the late-onset patients as a distinct set among the type 1 diabetes patients.

From the study of these ten genetic regions in our group composed of early and late onset patients, we propose that there are no major genetic differences between patients with an early and a late onset of type 1 diabetes.

6. Conclusions

Although the knowledge on the genetics of type 1 diabetes has experienced a great development in the last years, it has not provided many hints on the basis of the genetic components that could modify the age at onset of the disease. Several studies have approached the subject, but few of the reported associations have been properly replicated in independent populations. Also, the heterogeneity in the methodology of the published studies should be discussed: some studies select only paediatric patients. If the influence of a genetic region reaches a peak in the paediatric age and then decreases with time, a study with paediatric and adult patients would better estimate the difference than a study with only paediatric patients in which the difference may be seen, but also may be smaller than it really is. The majority of the published studies analyze the age at diagnosis of type 1 diabetes as a continuous variable, but some studies adopt a stratified analysis that implies the fragmentation of the patients in two or more groups and the individual analysis of each subgroup. This strategy defines artificial groups with limits that do not have a biological justification, and makes it more likely to produce false results in underpowered studies. We recommend the age-stratified analysis as a screening method or as a confirmation analysis, but we consider the analysis of age as a continuous variable a more accurate method to detect differences, given that it only takes into consideration the genotype studied and the ages at onset of all the patients carrying this genotype. Therefore, we propose that age at diagnosis of type 1 diabetes should be studied in groups that include paediatric and adult onset patients, and that the statistical analysis should include at least one method that considers age at diagnosis as a continuum.

Despite the improvements that can be incorporated to age-at-onset analysis, what is known to date about the influence of the genetics on the early and late onset of type 1 diabetes allows us to formulate a tentative answer to the question that gives title to this chapter: are early and late onset type 1 diabetes the same or two distinct genetic entities? Our data, presented in section 5, and the previous studies reviewed in section 4 suggest that there are no major differences in the genetic component of paediatric and adult patients. Both share the risk conferred by the main type 1 diabetes risk modifiers such as the HLA, the insulin gene or *PTPN22*. However, two points have to be taken into consideration: first, minor differences can be found between the adult and the paediatric patient, such as the elevated prevalence of the higher risk HLA alleles in subjects with early onset. Second, the genetics of adult-onset type 1 diabetes patients has frequently been studied only in relation to genes that already showed association in paediatric patients. This approach precludes the possibility of discovering genes that could be associated exclusively to late-onset type 1 diabetes. The study of these two points is of great interest given that it could point to metabolic routes that take part in the acceleration of the disease and, therefore, genes in these routes would be excellent candidates for therapeutic strategies focused on the delay of the autoimmune β cell destruction.

In conclusion, we propose that type 1 diabetes, whether in its early or late-onset, is an autoimmune disease defined by a number of primary risk genes and a constellation of minor genetic modifiers that, together with environmental factors, define the pace of the autoimmune reaction that will determine the age at onset.

7. References

American Diabetes Association (2010) Diagnosis and classification of diabetes mellitus. *Diabetes Care 33 Suppl 1:*S62-69

Awata, T., Kawasaki, E., Tanaka, S., Ikegami, H., Maruyama, T., Shimada, A., Nakanishi, K., Kobayashi, T., Iizuka, H., Uga, M., Kawabata, Y., Kanazawa, Y., Kurihara, S., Osaki, M., and Katayama, S. (2009) Association of type 1 diabetes with two Loci on 12q13 and 16p13 and the influence coexisting thyroid autoimmunity in Japanese. *J Clin Endocrinol Metab 94*:231-235

Bailey, R., Cooper, J. D., Zeitels, L., Smyth, D. J., Yang, J. H., Walker, N. M., Hypponen, E., Dunger, D. B., Ramos-Lopez, E., Badenhoop, K., Nejentsev, S., and Todd, J. A. (2007) Association of the vitamin D metabolism gene CYP27B1 with type 1 diabetes. *Diabetes 56*:2616-2621

Barrett, J. C., Clayton, D. G., Concannon, P., Akolkar, B., Cooper, J. D., Erlich, H. A., Julier, C., Morahan, G., Nerup, J., Nierras, C., Plagnol, V., Pociot, F., Schuilenburg, H., Smyth, D. J., Stevens, H., Todd, J. A., Walker, N. M., and Rich, S. S. (2009) Genome-wide association study and meta-analysis find that over 40 loci affect risk of type 1 diabetes. *Nat Genet 41*:703-707

Bell, G. I., Horita, S., and Karam, J. H. (1984) A polymorphic locus near the human insulin gene is associated with insulin-dependent diabetes mellitus. *Diabetes 33*:176-183

Bottini, N., Musumeci, L., Alonso, A., Rahmouni, S., Nika, K., Rostamkhani, M., MacMurray, J., Meloni, G. F., Lucarelli, P., Pellecchia, M., Eisenbarth, G. S., Comings, D., and Mustelin, T. (2004) A functional variant of lymphoid tyrosine phosphatase is associated with type I diabetes. *Nat Genet 36*:337-338

Bottini, N., Vang, T., Cucca, F., and Mustelin, T. (2006) Role of PTPN22 in type 1 diabetes and other autoimmune diseases. *Semin Immunol 18*:207-213

Colli, M. L., Moore, F., Gurzov, E. N., Ortis, F., and Eizirik, D. L. (2010) MDA5 and PTPN2, two candidate genes for type 1 diabetes, modify pancreatic beta-cell responses to the viral by-product double-stranded RNA. *Hum Mol Genet 19*:135-146

Cooper, J. D., Smyth, D. J., Smiles, A. M., Plagnol, V., Walker, N. M., Allen, J. E., Downes, K., Barrett, J. C., Healy, B. C., Mychaleckyj, J. C., Warram, J. H., and Todd, J. A. (2008) Meta-analysis of genome-wide association study data identifies additional type 1 diabetes risk loci. *Nat Genet 40*:1399-1401

Duncan, G. E. (2006) Prevalence of diabetes and impaired fasting glucose levels among US adolescents: National Health and Nutrition Examination Survey, 1999-2002. *Arch Pediatr Adolesc Med 160*:523-528

Erlich, H., Valdes, A. M., Noble, J., Carlson, J. A., Varney, M., Concannon, P., Mychaleckyj, J. C., Todd, J. A., Bonella, P., Fear, A. L., Lavant, E., Louey, A., and Moonsamy, P. (2008) HLA DR-DQ haplotypes and genotypes and type 1 diabetes risk: analysis of the type 1 diabetes genetics consortium families. *Diabetes 57*:1084-1092

Espino-Paisan, L., de la Calle, H., Fernandez-Arquero, M., Figueredo, M. A., de la Concha, E. G., Urcelay, E., and Santiago, J. L. (2011a) A polymorphism in PTPN2 gene is associated with an earlier onset of type 1 diabetes. *Immunogenetics 63*:255-258

Espino-Paisan, L., de la Calle, H., Fernandez-Arquero, M., Figueredo, M. A., de la Concha, E. G., Urcelay, E., and Santiago, J. L. (2011b) Polymorphisms in chromosome region 12q13 and their influence on age at onset of type 1 diabetes. *Diabetologia.*

Espino-Paisan, L., de la Calle, H., Fernandez-Arquero, M., Figueredo, M. A., de la Concha, E. G., Urcelay, E., and Santiago, J. L. (2011c) Study of polymorphisms in 4q27, 10p15 and 22q13 regions in autoantibodies stratified type 1 diabetes patients. *Autoimmunity* (in press).

Fung, E. Y., Smyth, D. J., Howson, J. M., Cooper, J. D., Walker, N. M., Stevens, H., Wicker, L. S., and Todd, J. A. (2009) Analysis of 17 autoimmune disease-associated variants in type 1 diabetes identifies 6q23/TNFAIP3 as a susceptibility locus. *Genes Immun* 10:188-191

Hafler, D. A., Compston, A., Sawcer, S., Lander, E. S., Daly, M. J., De Jager, P. L., de Bakker, P. I., Gabriel, S. B., Mirel, D. B., Ivinson, A. J., Pericak-Vance, M. A., Gregory, S. G., Rioux, J. D., McCauley, J. L., Haines, J. L., Barcellos, L. F., Cree, B., Oksenberg, J. R., and Hauser, S. L. (2007) Risk alleles for multiple sclerosis identified by a genomewide study. *N Engl J Med* 357:851-862

Hakonarson, H., Grant, S. F., Bradfield, J. P., Marchand, L., Kim, C. E., Glessner, J. T., Grabs, R., Casalunovo, T., Taback, S. P., Frackelton, E. C., Lawson, M. L., Robinson, L. J., Skraban, R., Lu, Y., Chiavacci, R. M., Stanley, C. A., Kirsch, S. E., Rappaport, E. F., Orange, J. S., Monos, D. S., Devoto, M., Qu, H. Q., and Polychronakos, C. (2007) A genome-wide association study identifies KIAA0350 as a type 1 diabetes gene. *Nature* 448:591-594

Hakonarson, H., Qu, H. Q., Bradfield, J. P., Marchand, L., Kim, C. E., Glessner, J. T., Grabs, R., Casalunovo, T., Taback, S. P., Frackelton, E. C., Eckert, A. W., Annaiah, K., Lawson, M. L., Otieno, F. G., Santa, E., Shaner, J. L., Smith, R. M., Onyiah, C. C., Skraban, R., Chiavacci, R. M., Robinson, L. J., Stanley, C. A., Kirsch, S. E., Devoto, M., Monos, D. S., Grant, S. F., and Polychronakos, C. (2008) A novel susceptibility locus for type 1 diabetes on Chr12q13 identified by a genome-wide association study. *Diabetes* 57:1143-1146

Heinig, M., Petretto, E., Wallace, C., Bottolo, L., Rotival, M., Lu, H., Li, Y., Sarwar, R., Langley, S. R., Bauerfeind, A., Hummel, O., Lee, Y. A., Paskas, S., Rintisch, C., Saar, K., Cooper, J., Buchan, R., Gray, E. E., Cyster, J. G., Erdmann, J., Hengstenberg, C., Maouche, S., Ouwehand, W. H., Rice, C. M., Samani, N. J., Schunkert, H., Goodall, A. H., Schulz, H., Roider, H. G., Vingron, M., Blankenberg, S., Munzel, T., Zeller, T., Szymczak, S., Ziegler, A., Tiret, L., Smyth, D. J., Pravenec, M., Aitman, T. J., Cambien, F., Clayton, D., Todd, J. A., Hubner, N., and Cook, S. A. (2010) A trans-acting locus regulates an anti-viral expression network and type 1 diabetes risk. *Nature* 467:460-464

Hermann, R., Laine, A. P., Veijola, R., Vahlberg, T., Simell, S., Lahde, J., Simell, O., Knip, M., and Ilonen, J. (2005) The effect of HLA class II, insulin and CTLA4 gene regions on the development of humoral beta cell autoimmunity. *Diabetologia* 48:1766-1775

Hober, D. and Sauter, P. (2010) Pathogenesis of type 1 diabetes mellitus: interplay between enterovirus and host. *Nat Rev Endocrinol* 6:279-289

Hosszufalusi, N., Vatay, A., Rajczy, K., Prohaszka, Z., Pozsonyi, E., Horvath, L., Grosz, A., Gero, L., Madacsy, L., Romics, L., Karadi, I., Fust, G., and Panczel, P. (2003) Similar genetic features and different islet cell autoantibody pattern of latent autoimmune diabetes in adults (LADA) compared with adult-onset type 1 diabetes with rapid progression. *Diabetes Care* 26:452-457

Howson, J. M., Walker, N. M., Smyth, D. J., and Todd, J. A. (2009) Analysis of 19 genes for association with type I diabetes in the Type I Diabetes Genetics Consortium families. *Genes Immun* 10 Suppl 1:S74-84

Ikegami, H., Kawabata, Y., Noso, S., Fujisawa, T., and Ogihara, T. (2007) Genetics of type 1 diabetes in Asian and Caucasian populations. *Diabetes Res Clin Pract* 77 Suppl 1:S116-121

Johansson, S., Lie, B. A., Todd, J. A., Pociot, F., Nerup, J., Cambon-Thomsen, A., Kockum, I., Akselsen, H. E., Thorsby, E., and Undlien, D. E. (2003) Evidence of at least two type 1 diabetes susceptibility genes in the HLA complex distinct from HLA-DQB1, -DQA1 and -DRB1. *Genes Immun* 4:46-53

Klinker, M. W., Schiller, J. J., Magnuson, V. L., Wang, T., Basken, J., Veth, K., Pearce, K. I., Kinnunen, L., Harjutsalo, V., Wang, X., Tuomilehto, J., Sarti, C., and Ghosh, S. (2010) Single-nucleotide polymorphisms in the IL2RA gene are associated with age at diagnosis in late-onset Finnish type 1 diabetes subjects. *Immunogenetics* 62:101-107

Kordonouri, O., Hartmann, R., Badenhoop, K., Kahles, H., and Ilonen, J. (2010) PTPN22 1858T allele is associated with younger age at onset of type 1 diabetes and is not related to subsequent thyroid autoimmunity. *Hum Immunol* 71:731-732

Kurreeman, F. A., Goulielmos, G. N., Alizadeh, B. Z., Rueda, B., Houwing-Duistermaat, J., Sanchez, E., Bevova, M., Radstake, T. R., Vonk, M. C., Galanakis, E., Ortego, N., Verduyn, W., Zervou, M. I., Roep, B. O., Dema, B., Espino, L., Urcelay, E., Boumpas, D. T., van den Berg, L. H., Wijmenga, C., Koeleman, B. P., Huizinga, T. W., Toes, R. E., and Martin, J. (2010) The TRAF1-C5 region on chromosome 9q33 is associated with multiple autoimmune diseases. *Ann Rheum Dis* 69:696-699

Kurreeman, F. A., Padyukov, L., Marques, R. B., Schrodi, S. J., Seddighzadeh, M., Stoeken-Rijsbergen, G., van der Helm-van Mil, A. H., Allaart, C. F., Verduyn, W., Houwing-Duistermaat, J., Alfredsson, L., Begovich, A. B., Klareskog, L., Huizinga, T. W., and Toes, R. E. (2007) A candidate gene approach identifies the TRAF1/C5 region as a risk factor for rheumatoid arthritis. *PLoS Med* 4:e278

Lee, H. S., Park, H., Yang, S., Kim, D., and Park, Y. (2008) STAT4 polymorphism is associated with early-onset type 1 diabetes, but not with late-onset type 1 diabetes. *Ann N Y Acad Sci* 1150:93-98

Leslie, R. D., Williams, R., and Pozzilli, P. (2006) Clinical review: Type 1 diabetes and latent autoimmune diabetes in adults: one end of the rainbow. *J Clin Endocrinol Metab* 91:1654-1659

Liuwantara, D., Elliot, M., Smith, M. W., Yam, A. O., Walters, S. N., Marino, E., McShea, A., and Grey, S. T. (2006) Nuclear factor-kappaB regulates beta-cell death: a critical role for A20 in beta-cell protection. *Diabetes* 55:2491-2501

Lowe, C. E., Cooper, J. D., Brusko, T., Walker, N. M., Smyth, D. J., Bailey, R., Bourget, K., Plagnol, V., Field, S., Atkinson, M., Clayton, D. G., Wicker, L. S., and Todd, J. A. (2007) Large-scale genetic fine mapping and genotype-phenotype associations implicate polymorphism in the IL2RA region in type 1 diabetes. *Nat Genet* 39:1074-1082

Martinez, A., Perdigones, N., Cenit, M. C., Espino, L., Varade, J., Lamas, J. R., Santiago, J. L., Fernandez-Arquero, M., de la Calle, H., Arroyo, R., de la Concha, E. G., Fernandez-Gutierrez, B., and Urcelay, E. (2010) Chromosomal region 16p13: further evidence of increased predisposition to immune diseases. *Ann Rheum Dis* 69:309-311

Martinez, A., Varade, J., Marquez, A., Cenit, M. C., Espino, L., Perdigones, N., Santiago, J. L., Fernandez-Arquero, M., de la Calle, H., Arroyo, R., Mendoza, J. L., Fernandez-Gutierrez, B., de la Concha, E. G., and Urcelay, E. (2008) Association of the STAT4 gene with increased susceptibility for some immune-mediated diseases. *Arthritis Rheum* 58:2598-2602

McCarthy, M. I., Abecasis, G. R., Cardon, L. R., Goldstein, D. B., Little, J., Ioannidis, J. P., and Hirschhorn, J. N. (2008) Genome-wide association studies for complex traits: consensus, uncertainty and challenges. *Nat Rev Genet* 9:356-369

Nejentsev, S., Howson, J. M., Walker, N. M., Szeszko, J., Field, S. F., Stevens, H. E., Reynolds, P., Hardy, M., King, E., Masters, J., Hulme, J., Maier, L. M., Smyth, D., Bailey, R., Cooper, J. D., Ribas, G., Campbell, R. D., Clayton, D. G., and Todd, J. A. (2007) Localization of type 1 diabetes susceptibility to the MHC class I genes HLA-B and HLA-A. *Nature* 450:887-892

Nerup, J., Platz, P., Andersen, O. O., Christy, M., Lyngsoe, J., Poulsen, J. E., Ryder, L. P., Nielsen, L. S., Thomsen, M., and Svejgaard, A. (1974) HL-A antigens and diabetes mellitus. *Lancet* 2:864-866

Nistico, L., Buzzetti, R., Pritchard, L. E., Van der Auwera, B., Giovannini, C., Bosi, E., Larrad, M. T., Rios, M. S., Chow, C. C., Cockram, C. S., Jacobs, K., Mijovic, C., Bain, S. C., Barnett, A. H., Vandewalle, C. L., Schuit, F., Gorus, F. K., Tosi, R., Pozzilli, P., and Todd, J. A. (1996) The CTLA-4 gene region of chromosome 2q33 is linked to, and associated with, type 1 diabetes. Belgian Diabetes Registry. *Hum Mol Genet* 5:1075-1080

Ounissi-Benkalha, H. and Polychronakos, C. (2008) The molecular genetics of type 1 diabetes: new genes and emerging mechanisms. *Trends Mol Med* 14:268-275

Palmer, J. P., Hampe, C. S., Chiu, H., Goel, A., and Brooks-Worrell, B. M. (2005) Is latent autoimmune diabetes in adults distinct from type 1 diabetes or just type 1 diabetes at an older age? *Diabetes* 54 Suppl 2:S62-67

Pociot, F., Akolkar, B., Concannon, P., Erlich, H. A., Julier, C., Morahan, G., Nierras, C. R., Todd, J. A., Rich, S. S., and Nerup, J. (2010) Genetics of type 1 diabetes: what's next? *Diabetes* 59:1561-1571

Pugliese, A., Zeller, M., Fernandez, A., Jr., Zalcberg, L. J., Bartlett, R. J., Ricordi, C., Pietropaolo, M., Eisenbarth, G. S., Bennett, S. T., and Patel, D. D. (1997) The insulin gene is transcribed in the human thymus and transcription levels correlated with allelic variation at the INS VNTR-IDDM2 susceptibility locus for type 1 diabetes. *Nat Genet* 15:293-297

Qu, H. Q., Bradfield, J. P., Grant, S. F., Hakonarson, H., and Polychronakos, C. (2009) Remapping the type I diabetes association of the CTLA4 locus. *Genes Immun* 10 Suppl 1:S27-32

Raz, I., Eldor, R., and Naparstek, Y. (2005) Immune modulation for prevention of type 1 diabetes mellitus. *Trends Biotechnol* 23:128-134

Redondo, M. J., Fain, P. R., and Eisenbarth, G. S. (2001a) Genetics of type 1A diabetes. *Recent Prog Horm Res* 56:69-89

Redondo, M. J., Yu, L., Hawa, M., Mackenzie, T., Pyke, D. A., Eisenbarth, G. S., and Leslie, R. D. (2001b) Heterogeneity of type I diabetes: analysis of monozygotic twins in Great Britain and the United States. *Diabetologia* 44:354-362

Remmers, E. F., Plenge, R. M., Lee, A. T., Graham, R. R., Hom, G., Behrens, T. W., de Bakker, P. I., Le, J. M., Lee, H. S., Batliwalla, F., Li, W., Masters, S. L., Booty, M. G., Carulli, J. P., Padyukov, L., Alfredsson, L., Klareskog, L., Chen, W. V., Amos, C. I., Criswell, L. A., Seldin, M. F., Kastner, D. L., and Gregersen, P. K. (2007) STAT4 and the risk of rheumatoid arthritis and systemic lupus erythematosus. *N Engl J Med* 357:977-986

Santiago, J. L., Alizadeh, B. Z., Martinez, A., Espino, L., de la Calle, H., Fernandez-Arquero, M., Figueredo, M. A., de la Concha, E. G., Roep, B. O., Koeleman, B. P., and Urcelay, E. (2008) Study of the association between the CAPSL-IL7R locus and type 1 diabetes. *Diabetologia 51*:1653-1658

Sarkar, S. A., Kutlu, B., Velmurugan, K., Kizaka-Kondoh, S., Lee, C. E., Wong, R., Valentine, A., Davidson, H. W., Hutton, J. C., and Pugazhenthi, S. (2009) Cytokine-mediated induction of anti-apoptotic genes that are linked to nuclear factor kappa-B (NF-kappaB) signalling in human islets and in a mouse beta cell line. *Diabetologia 52*:1092-1101

Smyth, D. J., Cooper, J. D., Bailey, R., Field, S., Burren, O., Smink, L. J., Guja, C., Ionescu-Tirgoviste, C., Widmer, B., Dunger, D. B., Savage, D. A., Walker, N. M., Clayton, D. G., and Todd, J. A. (2006) A genome-wide association study of nonsynonymous SNPs identifies a type 1 diabetes locus in the interferon-induced helicase (IFIH1) region. *Nat Genet 38*:617-619

Smyth, D. J., Plagnol, V., Walker, N. M., Cooper, J. D., Downes, K., Yang, J. H., Howson, J. M., Stevens, H., McManus, R., Wijmenga, C., Heap, G. A., Dubois, P. C., Clayton, D. G., Hunt, K. A., van Heel, D. A., and Todd, J. A. (2008) Shared and distinct genetic variants in type 1 diabetes and celiac disease. *N Engl J Med 359*:2767-2777

Steck, A. K. and Eisenbarth, G. S. (2008) Genetic similarities between latent autoimmune diabetes and type 1 and type 2 diabetes. *Diabetes 57*:1160-1162

Steck, A. K. and Rewers, M. J. (2011) Genetics of Type 1 Diabetes. *Clin Chem 57*: 176-185

Todd, J. A., Walker, N. M., Cooper, J. D., Smyth, D. J., Downes, K., Plagnol, V., Bailey, R., Nejentsev, S., Field, S. F., Payne, F., Lowe, C. E., Szeszko, J. S., Hafler, J. P., Zeitels, L., Yang, J. H., Vella, A., Nutland, S., Stevens, H. E., Schuilenburg, H., Coleman, G., Maisuria, M., Meadows, W., Smink, L. J., Healy, B., Burren, O. S., Lam, A. A., Ovington, N. R., Allen, J., Adlem, E., Leung, H. T., Wallace, C., Howson, J. M., Guja, C., Ionescu-Tirgoviste, C., Simmonds, M. J., Heward, J. M., Gough, S. C., Dunger, D. B., Wicker, L. S., and Clayton, D. G. (2007) Robust associations of four new chromosome regions from genome-wide analyses of type 1 diabetes. *Nat Genet 39*:857-864

Ueda, H., Howson, J. M., Esposito, L., Heward, J., Snook, H., Chamberlain, G., Rainbow, D. B., Hunter, K. M., Smith, A. N., Di Genova, G., Herr, M. H., Dahlman, I., Payne, F., Smyth, D., Lowe, C., Twells, R. C., Howlett, S., Healy, B., Nutland, S., Rance, H. E., Everett, V., Smink, L. J., Lam, A. C., Cordell, H. J., Walker, N. M., Bordin, C., Hulme, J., Motzo, C., Cucca, F., Hess, J. F., Metzker, M. L., Rogers, J., Gregory, S., Allahabadia, A., Nithiyananthan, R., Tuomilehto-Wolf, E., Tuomilehto, J., Bingley, P., Gillespie, K. M., Undlien, D. E., Ronningen, K. S., Guja, C., Ionescu-Tirgoviste, C., Savage, D. A., Maxwell, A. P., Carson, D. J., Patterson, C. C., Franklyn, J. A., Clayton, D. G., Peterson, L. B., Wicker, L. S., Todd, J. A., and Gough, S. C. (2003) Association of the T-cell regulatory gene CTLA4 with susceptibility to autoimmune disease. *Nature 423*:506-511

Urcelay, E., Santiago, J. L., de la Calle, H., Martinez, A., Mendez, J., Ibarra, J. M., Maluenda, C., Fernandez-Arquero, M., and de la Concha, E. G. (2005) Type 1 diabetes in the Spanish population: additional factors to class II HLA-DR3 and -DR4. *BMC Genomics 6*:56

Vafiadis, P., Bennett, S. T., Todd, J. A., Nadeau, J., Grabs, R., Goodyer, C. G., Wickramasinghe, S., Colle, E., and Polychronakos, C. (1997) Insulin expression in human thymus is modulated by INS VNTR alleles at the IDDM2 locus. *Nat Genet* 15:289-292

Valdes, A. M., Erlich, H. A., and Noble, J. A. (2005) Human leukocyte antigen class I B and C loci contribute to Type 1 Diabetes (T1D) susceptibility and age at T1D onset. *Hum Immunol 66:*301-313

Vella, A., Cooper, J. D., Lowe, C. E., Walker, N., Nutland, S., Widmer, B., Jones, R., Ring, S. M., McArdle, W., Pembrey, M. E., Strachan, D. P., Dunger, D. B., Twells, R. C., Clayton, D. G., and Todd, J. A. (2005) Localization of a type 1 diabetes locus in the IL2RA/CD25 region by use of tag single-nucleotide polymorphisms. *Am J Hum Genet 76:*773-779

Wallace, C., Smyth, D. J., Maisuria-Armer, M., Walker, N. M., Todd, J. A., and Clayton, D. G. (2009) The imprinted DLK1-MEG3 gene region on chromosome 14q32.2 alters susceptibility to type 1 diabetes. *Nat Genet 42:*68-71

Wang, H., Jin, Y., Reddy, M. V., Podolsky, R., Liu, S., Yang, P., Bode, B., Reed, J. C., Steed, R. D., Anderson, S. W., Steed, L., Hopkins, D., Huang, Y., and She, J. X. (2010) Genetically dependent ERBB3 expression modulates antigen presenting cell function and type 1 diabetes risk. *PLoS One 5:*e11789

The Wellcome Trust Case-Control Consortium (2007) Genome-wide association study of 14,000 cases of seven common diseases and 3,000 shared controls. *Nature 447:*661-678

Windsor, L., Morahan, G., Huang, D., McCann, V., Jones, T., James, I., Christiansen, F. T., and Price, P. (2004) Alleles of the IL12B 3'UTR associate with late onset of type 1 diabetes. *Hum Immunol 65:*1432-1436

Wong, F. S., Hu, C., Xiang, Y., and Wen, L. (2010) To B or not to B-pathogenic and regulatory B cells in autoimmune diabetes. *Curr Opin Immunol 22:*723-731

Genetic Determinants of Microvascular Complications in Type 1 Diabetes

Constantina Heltianu[1], Cristian Guja[2] and Simona-Adriana Manea[1]
[1]Institute of Cellular Biology and Pathology "N. Simionescu", Bucharest,
[2]Institute of Diabetes, Nutrition and Metabolic Diseases "Prof. NC Paulescu", Bucharest,
Romania

1. Introduction

Diabetes mellitus is one of the most prevalent chronic diseases of modern societies and a major health problem in nearly all countries. Its prevalence has risen sharply worldwide during the past few decades (Amos et al., 1997; Shaw et al., 2010). Moreover, predictions show that diabetes prevalence will continue to rise, reaching epidemic proportions by 2030: 7.7% of world population, representing 439 million adults worldwide (Shaw et al., 2010). This increase is largely due to the epidemic of obesity and consequent type 2 diabetes (T2DM). However, the incidence of type 1 diabetes (T1DM) is also rising all over the world (DiaMond Project Group, 2006; Maahs et al., 2010). Recent data for Europe (Patterson et al., 2009) predict the doubling of new cases of T1DM between 2005 and 2020 in children younger than 5 years and an increase of 70% in children younger than 15 years, old.

Despite major progresses in T1DM treatment during the past decades, mortality in T1DM patients continues to be much higher than in general population, with wide variations in mortality rates between countries. In Europe, these variations are not explained by the country T1DM incidence rate or its gross domestic product, but are greatly influenced by the presence of its chronic complications, especially diabetic renal disease (Groop et al., 2009; Patterson et al., 2007). In fact, much of the health burden related to T1DM is created by its chronic vascular complications, involving both large (macrovascular) and small (microvascular) blood vessels.

Many genetic, metabolic and hemodynamic factors are involved in the genesis of diabetic vascular complications. However, major epidemiological and interventional studies showed that chronic hyperglycemia is the main contributor to diabetic tissue damage (DCCT Research Group, 1993). If the degree of metabolic control remains the main risk factor for the development of diabetic chronic complications, an important contribution can be attributed to genetic risk factors, some of them common for all microvascular complications (diabetic retinopathy, neuropathy, and renal disease) and some specific for each of them (Cimponeriu et al., 2010). Additional factors are represented by some accelerators such as hypertension and dyslipidemia.

In the following pages, we present briefly the pathogenesis type 1 diabetes and its chronic microvascular complications. The main information of the genetic background in T1DM with particular focus on gene variants having strong impact on endothelial dysfunction as the key factor in the development of microvascular disorders are also summarized.

2. Type 1 diabetes mellitus

T1DM is a common, chronic, autoimmune disease characterized by the selective destruction of the insulin secreting pancreatic beta cells, destruction mediated mainly by the T lymphocytes (Eisenbarth, 1986). The destruction of the insulin secreting pancreatic beta cells is progressive, leading to an absolute insulin deficiency and the need for exogenous insulin treatment for survival. The pathogenic factors that trigger anti beta cell autoimmunity in genetically predisposed subjects are not yet fully elucidated, but there is clear evidence that it appears consequently to an alteration of the immune regulation. The destruction of the beta cells in T1DM is massive and specific and it is associated with some local (Gepts, 1965) or systemic (Bottazzo et al., 1978) evidence of anti-islet autoimmunity.

It is currently considered that, on the "background" of genetic predisposition, some putative environmental trigger factors will initiate the autoimmune process that will finally lead to T1DM. Identifying these triggers proved to be difficult, mainly due to a long period of time elapses between the intervention of the putative environmental trigger and the clinical onset of overt diabetes. The most important factors seem to be non-genetic external (environmental) ones. However, from environmental factors repeatedly associated with T1DM, the most important were viral infections, dietary and nutritional factors, nitrates and nitrosamines, etc. (Akerblom et al., 2002).

Genetic factors in the pathogenesis of T1DM in humans. T1DM is a common, complex, polygenic disease, with many predisposing or protective gene variants, interacting with each other in generating the global genetic disease risk (Todd, 1991). The study of candidate genes identified several susceptible genes for T1DM (Concannon et al., 2009): IDDM1 encoded in the HLA region of the major histocompatibility complex (MHC) genes on chromosome 6p21 and genes mapped to the *DRB1, DQB1* and *DQA1* loci , IDDM2 encoded by the insulin gene on chromosome 11p15.5 and mapped to the *VNTR* 5' region, IDDM12 encoded by the cytotoxic T lymphocyte associated antigen 4 (*CTLA4*) gene on chromosome 2q33, the lymphoid tyrosine phosphatase 22 (*PTPN22*) gene on chromosome 1p13 and the *IL2RA/CD25* gene on chromosome 10p15. The genome wide linkage (GWL) analysis strategies (Morahan et al., 2011) or genome wide association (GWA) techniques (Todd et al., 2007) led to the identification of other T1DM associated loci, for most of which the causal genes are still not elucidated.

3. Chronic complications in T1DM

T1DM is characterized by the slow progression towards the generation of some specific lesions of the blood vessels walls, affecting both small arterioles and capillaries (microangiopathy) and large arteries (macroangiopathy). The "classical" diabetes microvascular complications are represented by *diabetic retinopathy* (DR) the main cause of blindness, *diabetic nephropathy* (DN) also known as renal disease, the main cause of renal substitution therapy (dialysis or renal transplantation) in developed countries, and *diabetic neuropathy* (DPN) as reported (IDF, 2009). As we already mentioned, chronic hyperglycemia represents the key determinant in the development of T1DM chronic microvascular complications. Meanwhile, considerable biochemical and clinical evidence (Hadi & Suwaidi, 2007) indicated that endothelial dysfunction is a critical part of the pathogenesis of vascular complications both in T1DM and T2DM.

Several mechanisms explain the contribution of chronic hyperglycemia to the development of endothelial dysfunction and chronic diabetes complications. An unifying mechanism was proposed by Michael Brownlee, suggesting that overproduction of superoxide anion (O_2^-) by the mitochondrial electron transport chain might be the key element (Brownlee, 2005). According to this theory, hyperglycemia determines increased mitochondrial production of reactive oxygen species (ROS). Increased oxidative stress induces nuclear DNA strand breaks that, in turn, activate the enzyme poly ADN-ribose polymerase (PARP) leading to a cascade process that finally activates the four major pathways of diabetic complications: (1) *Increased aldose reductase* activity and activation of the *polyol pathway* lead to increased sorbitol accumulation with osmotic effects, NADPH depletion and decreased bioavailability of nitric oxide (NO). (2) *Activation of protein kinase C* with subsequent activation of NF-kB pathway and superoxide-producing enzymes. (3) *Advanced glycation end-products* (AGEs) generation with alteration in the structure and function of both intracellular and plasma proteins. (4) *Activation of the hexosamine pathway* leads to a decrease in endothelial NO synthase (NOS3) activity as well as an increase in the transcription of the transforming growth factor (TGF-β) and the plasminogen activator inhibitor-1 (PAI-1) as reported (Brownlee, 2005).

In Europe, the prevalence of DN was estimated at 31%, DR was diagnosed in 35.9% of patients while proliferative DR in 10.3%. Apart hyperglycemia, the most important risk factor was the duration of the disease. Thus, the prevalence of proliferative DR is null before 10 years diabetes duration but 40% after 30 years duration while the prevalence of DN is null before 5 years diabetes duration but reaches 40% after 15 years of diabetes (EURODIAB IDDM Complications Study Group, 1994). Similar data were provided by the diabetes control and complications trial (DCCT) study in USA. Thus, after 30 years of diabetes, the cumulative incidence of proliferative DR and DN was 50% and 25%, respectively, in the DCCT conventional treatment group (DCCT/EDIC Research Group et al., 2009).

3.1 Diabetic nephropathy

DN in T1DM can be defined by the presence of increased urinary albumin excretion rate (UAER) on at least two distinct occasions separated by 3–6 months (Mogensen, 2000). DN is usually accompanied by hypertension, progressive rise in proteinuria, and decline in renal function. According to several guidelines, normal UAER is defined as an excretion rate below 30 mg/24 h; microalbuminuria represents an UAER between 30-300 mg/24 h while more than 300 mg/24 h defines overt proteinuria. In T1DM, five DN stages have been proposed (Mogensen, 2000). Stage 1 is characterized by renal hypertrophy and hyperfiltration, being frequently reversible with good metabolic control. Stage 2 is typically asymptomatic and lasts for an average of 10 years. Typical histological abnormalities include diffuse thickening of the glomerular and tubular basement membranes as well as glomerular hypertrophy. About 30% of subjects will progress towards microalbuminuria. Stage 3 (incipient DN) develops 10 years after the onset of diabetes. Microalbuminuria, the earliest clinically detectable sign, is well correlated with histological findings of nodular glomerulosclerosis. About 80% of subjects will progress to overt proteinuria. This proportion may decrease with tight glycemic control, hypoproteic diet and early treatment with angiotensin I-converting enzyme (ACE) inhibitors or angiotensin II receptor (Ang II R) blockers. Stage 4 (clinical or late DN) occurs on average 15–20 years after diabetes onset and is characterized by macroalbuminuria. The glomerular filtration rate (GFR) declines progressively, UAER increases usually to more than 500 mg/day and blood pressure starts to rise. Histologically, mesangial expansion develops, renal fibrosis becomes more evident and leads to diffuse and nodular glomerulosclerosis. Stage 5 (end-stage renal disease) occurs on average 7 years after the development of persistent proteinuria. GFR decreases below 40 ml/min and an advanced destruction of all renal structures is observed.

DN pathogenesis is very complex and comprises both metabolic and haemodynamic factors in the renal microcirculation (Stehouwer, 2000). The glucose dependent pathways were presented briefly above. Haemodynamic factors mediate renal injury via effects on systemic hypertension, intraglomerular haemodynamics or via direct effects on renal production of cytokines, such as TGFβ and vascular endothelial growth factor (VEGF), or hormones such as angiotensin II or endothelin (ET) as reported (Schrijvers et al., 2004). In addition to the diabetes duration reflected by the level of glycated hemoglobin (HbA1c), the specific risk factors for DN are the blood pressure, older age, male sex, smoking status, and ethnic background.

Despite clear evidence for the role of genetic factors in DN, success in identifying the responsible genetic variants has been limited due to both objective and subjective difficulties, the main being represented by the small size of the DNA collections available to individual research groups (Pezzolesi et al., 2009). Strategies for the genetic investigation of DN included the analysis of candidate gene polymorphisms in case-control settings (hypothesis driven approach) as well as the GWL or GWA strategies with DN (hypothesis free approach). Numerous candidate genes were tested explaining the complexity of the diabetic renal disease pathogenesis (Cimponeriu et al., 2010; Mooyaart et al., 2011) but just few of them were reconfirmed in multiple, independent, studies. We give a list of the stronger associations in Table 1.

Gene	Chromosome	SNP	Allele	No. studies	Case/ Control	OR
ACE	17q23	rs179975	D	14	2215/2685	1.13
AKR1B1	7q35	(AC)n repeat	Z-2	10	1380/1308	1.12
		(AC)n repeat	Z+2	10	1380/1308	0.79
		rs759853	T	4	636/537	1.58
APOC1	19q13.2	rs4420638	G	2	857/935	1.54
APOE	19q13.2	E2/E3/E4	E2	6	889/803	1.48
EPO	7q21	rs1617640	T	2	1244/715	0.67
GREM1	15q13-q15	rs1129456	T	2	859/940	1.53
HSPG2	1p36.1	rs3767140	G	2	417/240	0.64
NOS3	7q36	rs3138808	a-del 393 bp	3	679/657	1.45
		rs2070744	C	2	273/450	1.39
UNC13B	9	rs13293564	T	4	1572/1910	1.23
VEGFA	6p12	rs833061	C	2	242/301	0.48

Table 1. Gene variants associated with DN in T1DM subjects. Identified by candidate gene study and confirmed after meta-analysis of at least 2 studies (adapted from a recent report, Mooyaart et al., 2011). I-converting *ACE*, angiotensin I-converting enzyme; *AKR1B1*, aldose reductase; *APOC1*, apoprotein C1; *APOE*, apoprotein E; *EPO*, erythropoietin; *GREM1*, gremlin 1 homolog; *HSPG2*, heparan sulfate proteoglycan; *NOS3*, endothelial nitric oxide synthase; *UNC13B*, presynaptic protein; *VEGFA*, vascular endotehlial growth factor A.

3.2 Diabetic retinopathy

DR is one of the most severe diabetes complications, potentially leading to severe sight decrease or even blindness. The first clinical signs of DR (incipient, non-proliferative DN) are retinal microaneurysms, dot intraretinal hemorrhages and hard exudates (Frank, 2004). The most severe stage, proliferative DR, is characterized by retinal haemorrhages from fragile neo-vessels and, in advanced eye disease by vitreous hemorrhages and tractional detachments of the retina, both resulting in visual loss. Histologically, DR is characterized by a selective loss of pericytes from the retinal capillaries followed by the loss of capillary endothelial cells (Frank, 2004). DR pathogenesis is complex, involving both metabolic and haemodynamic factors. The most important DR specific pathways seem to be the local production of several polypeptide growth factors, including VEGF, pigment-epithelium–derived factor (PEDF), growth hormone and insulin-like growth factor-1 , as well as cytokines and inflammatory mediators such as TNFα, TNFβ, TGFβ and NO (Frank, 2004). Genetic factors appear also to have an important role in generating the DR risk in T1DM subjects with similar degrees of metabolic control and disease duration (Keenan et al., 2007). The most often studied DR candidate genes include blood pressure regulators (RAS), metabolism factors (AKR1B1, AGER, GLUT1), growth factors (VEGF, PEDF), NOS2A, NOS3, TNFα, TGFβ, ET-1 and its receptors, etc. (Cimponeriu et al., 2010; Ng, 2010). As for all diabetes chronic complications, the studies of candidate genes were more often underpowered to detect true associations, and most often the results were not reconfirmed by additional, independent studies. However, published meta-analyses suggest a real role in DR for at least four genes (Abhary et al., 2009a; Cimponeriu et al., 2010; Ng, 2010).

Similar with DN, *ACE* gene was the most studied for DR in T1DM and data regarding its involvement will be presented further (see subchapter 6.1). *VEGFA* gene on chromosome 6p12-p21 was also intensively studied and a recent large study (including both T1DM and T2DM cases) suggested a possible effect of two gene variants (*rs699946* and *rs833068*) on DR risk in T1DM subjects (Abhary et al., 2009b). Among the candidate genes from the oxidative stress/increased ROS pathway, *NOS3* gene was intensively studied in DR and data will be presented in subchapter 4.3. Finally, maybe the strongest evidence for a role in the genetic risk for DR is provided by the analysis of *AKR1B1* gene on chromosome 7q35, encoding the rate-limiting enzyme of the polyol pathway. The most intensively studied polymorphism was the *(AC)n* microsatellite located at 2.1 kb upstream of the transcription start site (Z-2, Z and Z+2 alleles). A recent meta-analysis (Abhary et al., 2009a) showed that the Z-2 allele of the *(CA)n* microsatellite is significantly associated with DR risk in both T1DM and T2DM subjects. In addition, the *T* allele of *rs759853* in the *AKR1B1* promoter   seems to be protective. To our best knowledge, no attempts for both GWL and GWA for identification of DR genes in T1DM were reported so far.

3.3 Diabetic polyneuropathy

DPN is a chronic microvascular complication affecting both somatic and autonomic peripheral nerves. It may be defined as the presence of symptoms and/or signs of peripheral nerve dysfunction in people with diabetes, after the exclusion of other causes of neuropathy. Many neuropathic patients have signs of neurological dysfunction upon clinical examination, but have no symptoms at all (negative symptoms neuropathy). On the contrary, some patients have positive symptoms (burning, itching, freezing, sometimes intense pain and often with nocturnal exacerbations), usually with distal onset and proximal progression. This form is designated as painful DPN. Correct estimates regarding the prevalence of DPN are hard to obtain since the diagnosis of the "negative symptom patients" can be made only by active screening, usually with complex investigations such as nerve conduction velocity.

It is generally accepted that DPN results from the micro-angiopathy damage of the *vasa nervorum* (responsible for the microcirculation of neural tissue) associated with the direct damage of neuronal components induced by various metabolic factors, the most important being chronic hyperglycemia (Kempler, 2002). The vascular and metabolic mechanisms act simultaneously and have an additive effect. The most important links between the two are represented by the local NO depletion and failure of antioxidant protection, both resulting in increased oxidative stress. Apart the unquestionable role of chronic hyperglycemia (diabetes duration and level of metabolic control), other risk factors for DPN are increasing age, cigarette smoking, alcohol or other drug abuse, hypertension and hypercholesterolemia.

Data regarding the genetic background of DPN are rather scarce. To our best knowledge, no GWL or GWA were performed for the identification of DPN genes in T1DM. Several data regarding the effect of some candidate genes were published, but these included usually only small number of patients/controls and few were replicated in other, independent datasets. Maybe the most significant effect on DPN genetic risk in T1DM is conferred by variants of the *AKR1B1* gene. Other significant but not reconfirmed associations with the risk for DPN were reported for variants of *PARP-1*, *NOS2A*, *NOS3*, uncoupling protein *UCP2* and *UCP3*, genes encoding the antioxidant proteins, catalase and the superoxide dismutase, and the gene encoding the neuronal Na^+/K^+-ATPase (Cimponeriu et al., 2010).

In conclusion, during the past two decades we have witnessed an explosion of studies regarding the genetic background of diabetes microvascular complications, both in T1DM and T2DM. These efforts, mainly focusing on candidate genes and often using study groups underpowered to detect genuine associations, have contributed to the identification of a few credible predisposing gene variants (Doria, 2010). In order to make significant progresses in elucidating the genetics of microvascular complications, there is an urgent need for assembling large population collections of different backgrounds for both GWA scanning and candidate gene association studies.

4. Nitric oxide synthase genes

NO is one of the vasodilatory substances released by the endothelium and has the crucial role in vascular physiopathology including regulation of vascular tone and blood pressure, hemostasis of fibrinolysis, and proliferation of vascular smooth muscle cells (SMC). In T1DM, NO has an increased stimulatory effect on the released insulin from β cells, mostly to the early phase of the effect of glucose upon insulin secretion. Abnormality in its production and action can cause endothelial dysfunction leading to increased susceptibility to hypertension, hypercholesterolemia, diabetes mellitus, thrombosis and cerebrovascular disease. Serum nitrite and nitrate (NOx) concentrations assessed as an index of NO production was used as a marker for endothelial function.

In DN, the NO production was significantly higher. A strong link between circulating NO, glomerular hyperfiltration, and microalbuminuria in young T1DM patients with early nephropathy was reported (Chiarelli et al., 2000). It has been postulated that in diabetic kidney there is increased NO synthase (NOS) activity, and the excessive NO production can induce the renal hyperfiltration and hyperperfusion and by its perturbing effect contributes to the DN appearance (Bazzaz et al., 2010). In early diabetes, the retinal circulation devoided of any extrinsic innervation and depending entirely on endothelium-mediated autoregulation, is dramatically affected by the ECs dysfunction due to the lack of the local NO, a state seen in DR (Qidwai & Jamal, 2010).

In active progressive DR, aqueous NO levels are significantly high, while plasma NO levels remained at the level of diabetics without DR (Yilmaz et al., 2000). Raised plasma NO levels in T1DM patients were reported (Heltianu et al., 2008) indicating that pathogenesis of diabetic-associated vascular complications is connected with a generalized increased synthesis of NO throughout the body. This phenomenon occurs early in the natural course of diabetes and independently of the presence of microvascular complications. So, we suggest that the high NO levels found in diabetic patients (including those without any clinically manifested microangiopaties) might represent an overproduction of NO that is associated with diffuse endothelial dysfunction (Heltianu et al., 2008).

There is a family of NOS enzymes which produces NO. The two constitutive isoforms NOS1 (neuronal) and NOS3 (endothelial) as well as the inducible isoform NOS2 have similar enzymatic mechanisms but are encoded on separate chromosomes by different genes. The NOS1 gene is located on chromosome 12q24.2-24.31, has 29 exons, spaning a region greater than 240 kb and encodes a protein of ~161 kDa. The NOS2A gene is on chromosome 17q11.2–12 having 27 exons, spaning 37 kb and encodes a protein of ~131 kDA (Li et al., 2007). NOS3 gene is on chromosome 7q35-36, includes 26 exons, having a genomic size of 21 kb, and encodes a protein of ~133 kDa (Chen et al., 2007; http://www.genecards.org, version 3).

4.1 *NOS1* gene

The NOS1-derived NO is implicated in local regulation of vascular tone and blood flow using different mechanisms. This process appears to be independent of central NOS1 action on autonomic function (Melikian et al., 2009). In the early stages of diabetes, the NOS1 expression in the nitrergic axons decreases and its level in the cell bodies is unaffected probably due to a defect in axonal transport. Insulin treatment is able to reverse NOS1 decrease. With the progression of diabetes, NOS1 accumulates in the cell bodies due to an affected transport down to the axons, and the degenerative changes become irreversible without any response to insulin treatment (Cellek, 2004). The NOS1 gene has 12 different potential first exons (*1A–1L*) and as consequence the NOS1 protein is expressed as a very complex enzyme (Wang et al., 1999). The NOS1B is expressed in renal microvasculature (Freedman et al., 2000). To our knowledge, there are only two reports in which NOS1 polymorphisms were analyzed for the relationship with diabetic microvascular disorders. Microsatellite markers in NOS1B were assessed in T2DM and an association with ESDR for alleles 7 and 9 was reported (Freedman et al., 2000). The CA repeat in the 3'-UTR region (exon 29) of NOS1 was found not to be a risk for DPN (Zotova et al., 2005).

4.2 *NOS2A* gene

NOS2A gene has the transcription start site in exon 2 and the stop codon in exon 27. This gene encodes NOS2 protein which has two different functional catalytic enzyme domains, the oxygenase domain encoded by 1 to 13 exons, and reductase domain by 14 to 27 exons. The NOS2 differs from the constitutive forms (NOS1 and NOS3) being Ca^{2+} independent.

Due to strong binding of calmodulin to NOS2, this is insensitive to changes in calcium ion concentrations (Jonannesen et al., 2001; Qidwai & Jamal, 2010). Under normal conditions, NOS2 is not expressed. Exposure to high ambient glucose or cytokines, the upregulation of NOS2 occurs in a variety of cell type and tissues. As a consequence, a sudden burst of NO synthesis occurs leading to severe vasodilation and circulatory collapse. In diabetic milieu as long as NOS3 expression is low, the induction of NOS2 expression may occur in an attempt to achieve homeostasis, being crucial in preventing or delaying pathological alterations in the microcirculation (Warpeha & Chakravarthy 2003). In studies of diabetic complications, as DR and DN, influenced by vascular functional disturbances, the increased NO formation via NOS2 expression has been reported (Johannesen et al., 2000a).

In human *NOS2A* gene has been identified a large number of polymorphisms. In the promoter region there are single nucleotide polymorphisms (*-954G/C*, *-1173C/T*, *-1659 A/T*) and two microsatellite repeats, the biallelic *(TAAA)*n, and the *(CCTTT)*n with nine alleles, which might affect the *NOS2* transcription. Explanations for this modulation was proposed for *-1173C/T* polymorphism, when the *C* to *T* change predicts the formation of a new sequence recognition site for the GATA-1 or GATA-2 transcription factors, which further bind to specific DNA sequences and potentially increase the degree of mRNA transcription (Qidwai & Jamal, 2010). The gene variants in the coding region might alter the activity of *NOS2* with subsequence variability in the NO levels which might be responsible for the susceptibility or/and severity of the disease. Other polymorphisms in exons and introns were reported, *rs16966563* (exon 4, *Pro68Pro*), *rs1137933* (exon 10, *Asp385Asp*), *rs2297518* (exon 16, *Leu608Ser*), *rs3794763* (intron 5, *G>A*), *rs17718148* (intron 11, *C>T*), *rs2314809* (intron 17, *T>C*), and *rs2297512* (intron 20, *A>G*).

In T1DM, the *NOS2A* polymorphisms in the promoter region [*-954G/C*, *(TAAA)*n and *(CCTTT)*n] and exons (*Asp346Asp* and *Leu608Ser*) were analyzed and the results showed that none of them has a role in the development of the disease (Johannesen et al., 2000a). Using the transmission disequilibrium test, it was found in Caucasian population that there is an increased risk for T1DM among *HLA DR3/4*-positive individuals with a *T* in position 150 in exon 16 (*Leu608Ser*) of *NOS2A*. This finding suggests an interaction between the *NOS2A* locus and the HLA region and a role for *NOS2A* in the pathogenesis of human T1DM (Johannesen et al., 2001).

Assessement of polymorphisms in T1DM for the prevalence of DR showed that the *14-repeat* allele of *(CCTTT)*n *repeat* polymorphism in *NOS2A* was significantly associated with the absence of the disease. A person with diabetes carrying this allele has 0.21-fold chance of developing retinopathy as compared to those not carrying the allele, suggesting that the carriage of the *14-repeat* allele is not a feature of diabetes itself, but is specific to DR development (Warpeha et al., 1999; Warpeha & Chakravarthy, 2003). In addition, the same *NOS2A* variant, the *14-repeat* allele, was found to represent a low risk for DN (Johannesen et al., 2000b), and other report indicated that carriers of this allele have the low risk of DPN in T1DM (Nosikov, 2004; Zotova et al., 2005).

4.3 *NOS3* gene

NOS3 is the most relevant and frequent isoform   studied to assess the role of genetic issues in the development of angiopathic disease in T1DM. This enzyme is a constitutively expressed in vascular endothelial cells, and the protein expression depends on Ca^{2+} and calmodulin. It was suggested a possible dual functionality of NO. Excessive production of

NO, in DN, induces the renal hyperfiltration and hyperperfusion and contributes to the vascular disorder. More often, reduced NO production or availability was reported in other vascular pathologies. The effect of NO on the endothelial modulation is influenced by the duration of diabetes; so, at early stages of diabetes the endothelial function is enhanced, and with the progression of diabetic duration the endothelial dysfunction is accelerated (Bazzaz et al., 2010; Chen et al., 2007; Mamoulakis et al., 2009).

Several polymorphisms have been reported in NOS3 promoter, exon and intron regions (Table 2). The most studied variant from the promoter region was the single nucleotide polymorphism at position -786 where there is a base substitution from T to C (*rs2070744*). In previous studies it was shown that individuals with *−786C* allele had a reduced activity of the *NOS3* gene promoter (Taverna et al., 2005), explained by the fact that DNA binding protein (replication protein A1) has the ability to bind only to the *−786C* allele resulting a ~50% reduced *NOS3* transcription, with the subsequent decrease in both protein expression and serum NOx levels (Erbs et al., 2003). The interrelationships among *rs2070744* genotypes, NOS3 (mRNA, protein levels, and enzymatic activity), and plasma NOx levels have never been linear.

NOS3 polymorphism in intron 4 (*4a/4b*) is based on a variable 27-base pair tandem repeat four (allele *4a*), five (allele *4b*) or six (allele *4c*) repeats. Previous studies have suggested that deletion of one of the five nucleotide repeats in intron 4 could affect the rates of *NOS3* transcription and processing rate, thus resulting the modulation of NOS3 enzymatic activity and, apparently, affecting the plasma NOx concentrations (Zanchi et al., 2000), with the potentiality of this genotype to have an effect on microangiopathy later on in diabetic life (Mamoulakis et al., 2009).

SNP ID	Chromosome position	Location type	Alleles
		intron 4	4b/4ba
743507	150707488	intron	A/G
1799983	150696111	exon	G/T
1800783	150689397	intron	T/A
2070744	150690079	the 5' promoter region	T/C
2373929	150345745	the 3' region	G/A
2373961	150312143	the 5' promoter region	C/T
3138808		Del/Ins 393 bp	D/I
3918188	150702781	intron	A/C/T
12703107	150314562	the 5' region	G/T
41322052	150690106	intron	C/T

Table 2. *NOS3* gene polymorphisms. Source, http://www.genecards.org; version 3

Carriers of the *4a* allele were found exhibiting ~20% lower NOx levels that appearing in *4b/4b* homozygous subjects. The regulation of *NOS3* expression is more complicated considering the strong linked of *4a/4b* variant with *rs2373961* and *rs2070744* when the *b/b* genotype might acts independently and in coordination with the other variants (Chen et al., 2007; Zintzaras et al., 2009). Among polymorphisms found in exons of *NOS3*, the G to T polymorphism at position 894 in exon 7 (*rs1799983*) was most studied. It was reported that this variant changes the NOS3 protein sequence, probable resulting an alteration of enzyme activity (Costacou et al., 2006), and control the NOS3 intracellular distribution interacting with proteins of degradating process (Brouet et al., 2001).

From many polymorphisms of the *NOS3* gene some of them are associated with the development of diabetic microvascular complications while others indicated their protective role (Freedman et al., 2007; Heltianu et al., 2009). A recent study of *rs2070744* in Caucasian T1DM reported a positive association with diabetes *per se* as well as DR and two possible explanations were found; either *NOS3* is a candidate gene for the microvascular disease, or there is a linkage disequilibrium between *NOS3* and the neighbouring genes. It is known that in the same position (7q35) to *NOS3* gene the AKR1B1 and T-cell receptor beta-chain (TCRBC) genes in the 7q34 position are located (Bazzaz et al., 2010). In a hyperglycaemic milieu, the retinal NO bioavailability due to the presence of C-786 mutant allele of rs2070744 is decreased, and therefore the lack of NO stimulates aldose reductase, known to be implicated in the development of diabetes complications (Chandra et al., 2002). Other report showed that the onset pattern of severe DR in longstanding C-peptide-negative T1DM is affected by *NOS3 rs2070744* and *C774T* polymorphisms (Taverna et al., 2005). In the case of *C774T NOS3* polymorphism, the association with severe DR was related to the influence of the DN presence, which is a well-known strong risk factor for DR (Cimponeriu et al., 2010). Oppose, the rare allele *4a* of *4b/4a* variant of *NOS3* was found to be related to absent or non-severe DR in T1DM Caucasians patients, suggesting a protective role. Although the *4b* allele was more frequent among patients with severe DR, a modest effect on the microvascular disorder was evaluated from the broad confidence interval (Cheng et al., 2007). Recent reports and our studies showed that there were no relationships between *4b/4a* variant of NOS3 and DR or other microangiopathic complications. Similar results for *rs1799983* in relation with DR were also reported (Heltianu et al., 2009; Mamulakis et al., 2009). In a meta-analysis of genetic association studies for DR in T1DM, from the three *NOS3* polymorphisms (*rs1799983*, *rs3138808* and *rs41322052*) included in the sub analysis for Caucasian subjects, none of them were found to be significantly associated with any form of DN (Abhary et al., 2009a)

The progression of renal disease was associated with the *NOS3 rs2070744* variant (Freedman et al., 2007; Zanchi et al., 2000), a result confirm recently by meta-analysis (Mooyaart et al., 2011; Ned et al., 2010). Contradictory results were obtained for the relationship of *NOS3 4b/4a* polymorphism with DN. Some reports showed no association (Degen et al., 2001; Heltianu et al., 2009) and others indicated that the *4a* allele represents an excess risk for advanced DN (Nosikov, 2004; Zanchi et al., 2000; Zinzaras et al., 2009). It was hypothesized that the *NOS3 4b/4a* itself plays a role in tissue-specific regulation of *NOS3* expression, a mechanism related to the importance of intron structure in the splicing of immature to mature RNA or to the presence of enhancer sequences within the intron 4. On the other hand, both *rs2070744* and *4b/4a* polymorphisms were specifically associated with advanced DN, and the *-786C/4a* haplotype was reported to be transmitted from heterozygous parents to siblings with advanced DN, suggesting that the *4a* allele is coupled almost exclusively with the *-786C* allele of *rs2070744* (Zanchi et al., 2000). The *NOS3 rs1799983* was analyzed in T1DM Caucazians from different countries and some reports showed no association with DN (Heltianu et al., 2009; Möllsten et al., 2009; Nosikov, 2004) and others found a marginal relationship (Ned et al., 2010) or strong association with increased risk of DN (Zintzaras et al., 2009). The *-786C/894T* haplotype of *NOS3* was found to be significantly associated with albuminuria, suggesting a strong implication of this gene in the susceptibility to kidney damage (Ned et al., 2010). The *rs3138808* variant of *NOS3* was also analyzed in a meta-analysis and was found to be associated with DN (Mooyaart et al., 2011).

There are only few reports which analyze the influence of *NOS3* polymorphisms on DPN in T1DM. Data from Caucasian patients genotyped for *rs1799983* and *4b/4a* variants showed that both polymorphisms were not associated with DPN (Nosikov, 2004; Zotova et al., 2005). Our findings showed that only *NOS3 4b/4a* was not associated with DPN (Heltianu et al., 2009). In T1DM subjects with the lowest incidence of confirmed DPN, it was reported that the *894G* carriers of *rs1799983* variant had fivefold increased risk for DPN, suggesting that despite low risk for the disease in these individuals, there is a genetic predisposition to develop diabetes-related complication (Costacou et al., 2006). In agreement with this report we found a prevalence of DPN among the *894GG* as compared with *894TT* homozygotes in diabetic patients with normal kidney function, suggesting that *894GG* genotype might be a risk factor for T1DM-related microvascular disease. This subgroup of DPN patients with *894GG* had over 42% DR as an additional vascular complication, and the presence or absence of DR did not modify the significance of the relationship between the *rs1799983* polymorphism and DPN. In addition, these subjects were recorded with high systolic blood pressure and raised levels of NOx, indicating a possible endothelial dysfunction, as well as with high levels of triglycerides, suggesting that additional high risk lipid profile contribute to the aggravation of the microvascular disorder. We presume that the rare-type *894T* allele might have a protective role against the development of DPN and a tendency to counterbalance increased NO production due to both chronic hyperglycemia and hypoxic effect at the microvascular level, by a not yet elucidated, compensatory-type mechanism (Heltianu et al., 2009).

Taken together, these results indicate that in T1DM, from various *NOS3* polymorphisms the most studied were *rs2070744*, *rs1799983* and *4b/4a* variants. Even in Caucasians there are differences among populations for the effects of gene polymorphisms on the microvascular complications. Diverse factors contribute to the variations between studies, analysis of early or late microvascular complication, incidence of the studied disorder in subjects with other confirmed disease, small sample size, the lack of haplotype analysis. Further studies on larger numbers of samples and on different populations are required to confirm these results.

5. Endothelin genes

The family of endothelins (ET) is represented by three peptides (1 to 3) and two receptors (ETRA and ETRB), which are widely distributed, in different proportions, being mostly abundant in vascular endothelial cells (EC). Their ET-1 and ET-2 are strong vasoconstrictors, whereas ET-3 is a potentially weaker vasoconstrictor compared to the other two isoforms. The ET-1 which is the most potent vasoconstrictor peptide acts as a paracrine or autocrine factor and its effects are ~10 times higher that of angiotensin II. The ET-1 has a variety of functions including its significant contribution to the maintenance of basal vascular tone, modulation of vascular permeability for proinflammatory mediators and proliferation of SMC. Having a long half-life, only a slight activation of its receptors into the signaling pathways might contribute to progressive disturbances, as hypertension and diabetic microvascular disorders (Cimponeriu et al., 2010). From the two receptors, the ETRA, expressed in SMC, has the highest affinity for ET-1, and is involved in the short term regulation of SMC and in the long term control of cell growth, adhesion and migration in the vasculature. The ETRB, expressed on both EC and SMC, has a dual function and can cause both vasoconstriction on SMC and vasodilation by the release of endothelial NO (Kalani, 2008; Potenza et al., 2009). The components of ET family are encoded by different genes (Table 3) with a generic name *EDN* (*EDN1, EDN2, EDN3, EDNRA,* and *EDNRB*). All three *EDN* genes (1 to 3) translate a respective amino acid prepropeptide, which is cleaved by one or more dibasic pair-specific endopeptidases to yield big ET. For ET-1, the large precursor is then converted into the mature and active ET-1 by a putative converting enzyme (ECE-1) encoded by the *ECE1* gene.

In diabetes, the secreted ET-1 by kidney cells activates its receptors and leads to constriction of renal vessels, inhibition of salt and water reabsorption, and enhanced glomerular proliferation. Correlations between plasma or urinary levels of ET-1 and signs of DN at different stages, as well as a close association between systemic endothelial dysfunction and microalbuminuria have been reported. Elevated ET-1 levels are present before the onset of microalbuminuria in T1DM, and worsen in association with it. In DR, the increased ET-1 levels strongly correlate with the enhanced endothelial permeability and loss of endothelial-mediated vasodilation in the retinal microvasculature (Kalani, 2008; Kankova et al., 2001). In DNP, the ET-1 is a potent vasoconstrictor of vasa nervorum and contributes to the EC abnormalities, when the balance of vasodilatation and vasoconstriction is in the favor of the latter. Moreover, ETA receptors contribute to the development of peripheral neuropathy, while ETB receptors have a protective role (Kalani, 2008; Lam, 2001). Most of the reported findings were for T2DM. A difference in the ET-1 involvement in the development of microvascular disorders in T1DM can not be excluded, knowing that differences in the pathogenesis of microangiopathy between type 1 and type 2 diabetes might exist.

Gene		Protein			
Name	Location	Name	Size		Subcellular location
			a.a.	kDa	
EDN1	6p24.1	ET-1	212	24.43	secreted
EDN2	1p34.2	ET-2	178	19.96	secreted
EDN3	20q13.2-13.3	ET-3	238	25.45	secreted
ECE1	1p36.1	ECE1	770	87.16	cell membrane
EDNRA	4q31.22	ETA receptor	427	48.72	cell membrane
EDNRB	13q22	ETB receptor	442	49.64	cell membrane

Table 3. The endothelin family. Source, http://www.genecards.org; a.a., amino acids; kDa, kiloDalton

The *EDN1* gene has different polymorphisms including the *-3A/-4A*, a *−138* insertion/deletion and the *CA/CT* dinucleotide repeat in promoter, the *C8002T* or TaqI variant in intron 4, and the *Lys198Asn*, a *G/T* polymorphism in exon 5. In *EDNRA* gene were reported the *−231 A/G* and *C1363T* variants, while in *EDNRB* gene the *A30G* polymorphism. Assessments of relationship between variability of plasma concentrations of ET-1 (and big ET-1) and *EDN1* polymorphisms (*G8002A* and *−3A/−4A*) in patients with chronic heart failure indicated that there was no significant association, suggesting that the genetic variants are not risk factors, but plasma ET-1 level influences more the disease severity (Spinarová et al., 2008).

Insufficient data exists regarding the influence of *EDN1* polymorphisms on the development of microvascular disorders. In a previous review was shown that *EDN1* gene was directly involved in hypertension and polymorphisms in *EDNRA* were associated with essential hypertension testifying the necessity of a balance within the endothelin system for normal functioning in vascular tissues. Although the importance of ET-1 expression in retinal microvasculature in high glucose was incontrovertible, it appears to be a lack of association between *EDN1* and *ECE1* polymorphisms and DR (Warpeha & Chakravarthy, 2003). Interestigly, in T2DM the *TT* genotype of *EDN1 G/T* polymorphism was associated with reduce risk of DN (Li et al., 2008).

6. Genes of renin – Angiotensin system

Renin-angiotensin system plays a central role in blood pressure regulation and fluid electrolyte balance, being a modulator of vascular tone and structure. RAS components are produced by different organs and are delivered to their site of action by the bloodstream. Angiotensinogen (ANGT) is synthesized primarily by the liver and the released hormone precursor is cleaved by renin enzyme and aspartyl proteinase, to generate angiotensin I (Ang I). The key enzyme of RAS is angiotensin I-converting enzyme (ACE) which converts Ang I to angiotensin II (Ang II) by the release of the terminal His-Leu, when an increase of the vasoconstrictor activity of angiotensin occurs. The Ang II acts through two main receptors, the type 1 Ang II receptor and the type 2 Ang II receptor (Table 4). It is generally believed that type I Ang II receptor is the dominant one in the cardiovascular system, being expressed in different organs including the brain, kidney, heart, skeletal muscle (Abdollahi et al., 2005).

Gene		Protein			
Name	Location	Name	Size		Subcellular location
			a.a.	kDa	
ACE	17q23.3	ACE	1306	149.72	secreted and cell membrane
ACE2	Xp22	ACE2	805	92.46	secreted and cell membrane
AGT	1q42-q43	ANGT	485	53.15	secreted
AGTR1	3q24	Type 1 Ang II receptor	359	41.06	cell membrane
AGTR2	Xq22-q23	Type 2 Ang II receptor	363	41.18	cell membrane

Table 4. Renin-angiotensin system. Source, http://www.genecards.org; a. a., amino acids; kDa, kiloDalton

The RAS effects are primarily mediated by Ang II, a trophic hormone, which acts either directly on tissues, including vascular remodeling and inflammation or indirectly on NO bioavailability and its consequences (Chung et al., 2010; Ringel et al., 1997). In distinct local organs (brain, kidney, eye, vessel wall, heart) RAS regulatory mechanisms and function are different, so the Ang II actions may be modulated by a specific physiological process of a given tissue system. A variety of stimuli, including hyperglycemia, hypertension, sodium intake, inflammation modulate the expression of the tissue RAS components in pathophysiological states, and chronic production of Ang II may proceed remodeling and restructuring in various cardiovascular organs (Conen et al., 2008).

Discovery of ACE homologue, angiotensin I-converting enzyme 2 (ACE2) increased the complexity of RAS. ACE2 is predominantly expressed in endothelium of different tissues (i.e. kidney), although its distribution is much less widespread than ACE. The enzyme hydrolyses different peptides, including Ang I and Ang II, and is implicated in hypertension, diabetic nephropathy, and cardiovascular disease (Fröjdö et al., 2005). ACE2 seems to act as a negative regulator of the RAS, counterbalancing the function of ACE thus promoting vasodilation (Giunti et al., 2006).

RAS is a causative factor in diabetic microvascular complications inducing a variety of tissue responses including vasoconstriction, inflammation, oxidative stress, cell hypertrophy and proliferation, angiogenesis and fibrosis. Most of previous reports showed the RAS role in the initiation and progression of diabetic nephropathy. In the kidney, Ang II affects renal hemodynamics, tubular transport and stimulates growth and proto-oncogenes in various renal cell types. Increased production of angiotensin II within nephrons and their vasculature could participate in the local renal injury through both hemodynamic and nonhemodynamic actions and is a well-established factor promoting renal damage (Gumprecht et al., 2000). Because the low conversion of Ang I in the kidney, it has been proposed that the plasma ACE circulating through the kidney is an important contributor but yet a limiting factor in angiotensin II production within the renal circulation (Marre et al., 1997).

On the other hand, ACE2 which has a similar distribution to ACE, being largely localized in renal tubules, when is downregulated, as in diabetes-associated kidney disease, leads to an increase of tubular Ang II, which, in turn, may promote tubulointerstitial fibrosis. In early phases of diabetes in the absence of renal injury, it was suggested that ACE2 expression is increased, and in compensation the ACE was inhibited preventing the diabetes associated renal disease. These findings suggest that ACE inhibition may confer a renoprotective effect (Giunti et al., 2006). In diabetes, damage to the retina occurs in the vasculature, neurons and glia resulting in pathological angiogenesis, vascular leakage and a loss in retinal function. All components of RAS have been identified in the retina and iris and it is likely that the local rather than systemic RAS is involved in ocular neovascularization. It was reported that the RAS components were upregulated in DR.

6.1 *ACE* gene

ACE, the main enzyme of RAS, is encoding by the *ACE* gene, composed of 26 exons, and span a total of 21 kb (Table 4). The genetic structure is made up of three ancestral regions, and two intragenic ancestral recombination breakpoints flank the gene region (Boright et al., 2005). Several polymorphisms have been reported in *ACE* gene. The two biallelic SNPs within and flanking the gene are in strong linkage disequilibrium with each other (Boright et al., 2005). The most extensively studied polymorphism was insertion/deletion of a *287-bp Alu* repeat in intron 16 (*rs179975; Ins/Del; I/D*) being considered a "reference" polymorphism (Hadjadj et al., 2007; Mooyaart et al., 2011). ACE activity is significantly connected with genetic variations at the *ACE* gene. The *rs179975* accounts for 44% of the interindividual variability of plasma ACE levels, and high ACE values were found among subjects with *DD* genotype. Other report showed that about 24% of the variance in the ACE activity was attributed to other *ACE* polymorphisms *rs4343, rs495828* and *rs8176746* (Chung et al., 2010).

Some reports indicated in Caucasian T1DM patients that *ACE I/D* was not associated with the development of persistent microalbuminuria, or overt DN (Möllsten et al., 2008; Ringel et al., 1997; Tarnow et al., 2000). A protective role to the homozygosity for the insertion (*I/I*) of *ACE* gene in the DN development was attributed. With the increase of duration of diabetes it seems that the *ACE I/I* genotype is associated with longevity and survival in T1DM patients but not particularly in DN subjects (Boright et al., 2005). Other reports indicated that the *ACE D/D* genotype was more frequent in patients with DN and the presence of the *ACE D/D* or *I/D* genotypes was associated with a faster rate of the decline of the renal function, suggesting that the *ACE D* allele represents an increased risk for both the onset and the progression of DN (Costacou et al., 2006; Gumprecht et al., 2000; Ng et al., 2005; Nosikov, 2004).

From other *ACE* polymorphisms studied for the association with DN, it was reported that the *G7831A* (Nosikov, 2004), *rs4293* and *rs4309* (Currie et al., 2010) were not associate, while *rs1800764* and *rs9896208* (Boright et al., 2005) were associate with the disease. Regarding the *rs1800764 (T/C)* variant, patients who carried the wild-type *T* allele were at lower risk for persistent microalbuminuria or severe DN, while heterozygous patients *(T/C)* had a higher risk for severe nephropathy, suggesting a genotype rather than an allele effect (Hadjadj et al., 2007). The reported haplotypic structure of *ACE* was considered to contain four polymorphisms *rs4311, rs4366, rs1244978* and *rs1800764* (Hadjadj et al., 2007). Interestingly, the homozygosity for the common haplotype that carries the *ACE I* allele, as *TIC* haplotype, corresponding to the wild type alleles of *rs1800764, I/D* and *rs9896208*, respectively was associated with lower risk for development of severe DN. This finding provides a strong evidence that genetic variation at the *ACE* gene is associated with the development of DN (Boright et al., 2005). On the other hand it was reported that a haplotype containing the rare allele the *D* of *I/D* variant, *G* of *rs4366* and *G* of *rs12449782* was associated with a higher risk for DN (Hadjadj et al., 2007).

Diabetic nephropathy is rarely diagnosed using invasive kidney biopsies and generally in genetic studies DN patients were those who presented albuminuria. Conflicting results of the gene association with the disease might occur, in addition, from the fact that a substantial number of subjects were classified as having DN but actually have nondiabetic kidney disease instead. Certain investigators have proposed that DN cases should be required to have diabetic retinopathy as well. From 1994 up to 2006 there were numbers of reports analyzing T1DM patients with DN having in addition various proportion of DR (Ng et al., 2008). The relationship between *ACE* polymorphisms and DR was less studied. Most reports found no association of *ACE I/D* with the development of any form of DR in adult or younger Type 1 diabetic patients (Abhary et al., 2009a; Zhou & Yang, 2010). Other data showed that in patients with DR, the severity of DR was associated with *ACE I/D* polymorphism (Marre et al., 1997). While nearly all T1DM individuals can develop DR or DPN, only a fraction of the subjects develops DN. So, it is hard to determine whether any observed association between *ACE I/D* and DN or DR or combined DN/DR truly exists. Including DR in the identification of potential genetic factors for the microvascular disorders might help, considering that some patients manifest a joint retinal-renal phenotype (Ng et al., 2008).

Taken together, these data indicate that the *I/D* variant of *ACE* gene, considered a "reference" polymorphism, responsible, at least in part, for the interindividual variability of plasma ACE levels, is associated with the faster rate decline of renal function, particularly in patients with a less than 10 years of diabetes duration, and the *ACE D* allele represents an increased risk for both the onset and the progression of DN. These findings were confirmed by multiple, independent studies. This potential genetic factor for DN development might be correlated also with DR, suggesting its involvement in the diabetic complex phenotype.

6.2 Other RAS genes

ACE2 has approximately 40% homology with ACE sharing 42% identity with the catalytic domain of somatic ACE, and promotes vasodilatation counterbalancing the ACE effect. The ACE2 gene consists of 18 exons is stable and conserved, indicating, that the genetic effect is small, and it intertwines and functions in concert with many other genes, suggesting the presence of epistatic effects (Fröjdö et al., 2005; Zhou & Yang, 2010). Data of genes for other RAS components are presented in Table 4. From the variants (rs714205; rs879922; rs1978124; rs2023802; rs2048684; rs2074192; rs2285666; rs4646188; rs5978731) reported few studies implied genomic analyses of diabetes microvascular disorders. None of the studied polymorphisms were associated with DR (Currie et al., 2010; Fröjdö et al., 2005). An increased in ACE2 expression in early phases of diabetes in the absence of renal injury was reported (Giunti et al., 2006).

Angiotensinogen gene has more than 30 genetic polymorphisms as reported in different studies, M24686, C1015T (T174M; rs4762; Thr/Met), T1198C (M235T; rs699; Met/Thr), A1237G (Tyr/Cys), A1204C (A-20C; rs5050), G1218A (G-6A; rs5051). The most studied polymorphism in relation with diabetic microvascular disorders was rs699 in exon 2 when a T to C base substitution at position 702 take place, with the consequent replacement of methionine 235 with threonine. A relationship between the T allele of rs699 and increased plasma Ang II levels was reported only in male subjects and may account for no more than 5% of ANGT variability (Marre et al., 1997, Ruggenenti et al., 2008). Reports on the association of AGT rs699 and the development of DN in adults with T1DM showed conflicting results; some finding indicated no association (Chowdhury et al., 1996; Currie et al., 2010; Hadjadj et al., 2001; Möllsten et al., 2008; Nosikov, 2004; Ringel et al., 1997; Tarnow et al., 2000), and others suggested that this variant contribute to the increased risk for chronic renal failure (Gumprecht et al., 2000). In young T1DM subjects, the TT genotype of AGT rs699 had a fourfold increased risk for persistent microalbuminuria, suggesting that this variant is a strong predictor for early stage of DN (Gallego et al., 2008). One report analyzed AGT T174M in relation with DN, and the findings indicated no association with the disease (Nosikov, 2004). There were no reports indicated a significant relationship between AGT rs699 and DR, but in patients with incipient diabetic renal failure the T allele of AGT rs699 was associated with DR. In these patients interaction between the D allele of ACE I/D and the T allele of AGT rs699 tended towards protection against DN (Van Ittersum et al., 2000). Oppose, other study indicated that the same interaction increases risk for DN in patients cu DR (Marre et al., 1997). All these data suggest that extensive studies has to be done in large number of T1DM patients with combined DN and DR vs only one microvascular disorder for the epistatic interactions between ACE and AGT polymorphisms and their relationship of the disease.

In AGTR1 gene were identify a variety of polymorphisms AF245699, A49954G (rs5183; A1878G; Pro/Pro), A50058C (rs5186; A1166C), T4955A (rs275651), T5052G (rs275652), C5245T (rs1492078), A1062G, T573C, G1517T (Ruggenenti et al., 2008). Reports on the relationship of AGTR1 polymorphisms with DN showed that the AA genotype of rs5186 was independently associated with overt DN, being with a threefold increase in the risk for the disease compared to *AC* and *CC* genotypes (Möllsten et al., 2008). The treatment with renoprotective antihypertensive (losartan) for slowing down the progression of diabetic glomerulopathy reduced significantly albuminuria, systolic and diastolic blood pressure in the *A* allele vs *C* allele carriers of *rs5186* polymorphism (Dragović et al., 2010). Oppose, the rs5186 of *AGTR1* was found not associated with DN in other reports (Gallego et al., 2008; Nosikov, 2004; Tarnow et al., 2000). There are no data on the influence of *AGTR1* gene polymorphism on the development of DR or DPN. For *AGTR2* gene have been identified few variants, *U20860* (*T3786C*; *rs5192*; *Ala/Ala*), *G1675A* (*rs1403543*), *G4297T* (*rs5193*), *A4303G* (*rs5194*) but there are no reports showing the involvement of one polymorphism with T1DM microvascular disorders.

Although the prognosis of patients with DN has improved, the decline in the GFR still varies among T1DM patients. The nongenetic risk factors (elevated blood pressure, albuminuria, and HbA$_{1c}$) for excessive loss of GFR, explain only approximately 30 to 50% of the decrease, and the epistatic interactions between *ACE*, *ACE2*, *AGT*, *AGTR1* or *AGTR2* polymorphisms in the RAS, a concept previously suggested (Jacobsen et al., 2003) might represent a risk factor for DN. It was reported that despite the non-significant effects of a single-gene on DN progression, a combined genetic variable including the potential "bad" alleles (*D* of *ACE I/D*, *M* of *AGT rs699*, and *A* of *AGTR1 rs5186*) represent a risk factor for the disease (Jacobsen et al., 2003). These data suggest that in some conditions a single gene variant may cause appreciable phenotypic changes only upon combination with other polymorphisms, having additional or synergistic effects on the same metabolic pathways (Ruggenenti et al., 2008). Oppose, other data showed that DN was not influenced by the epistatic interactions between the polymorphisms of the RAS genes. (Gallego et al., 2008; Tarnow et al., 2000)

7. Conclusion

All over the world, the incidence of type 1 diabetes continue to be much higher than in general population. Despite major progresses done in the recent years to identify candidate genes involved in the development of diabetic microvascular complications, there are still controversial results and insufficient knowledge in the literature, although a variety of genomic strategies were applied. While the degree of metabolic control remains the main risk factor for the development of diabetic chronic complications, the genetic risk factors, common for retinopathy, neuropathy, and renal disease, or specific for each of them, are important contributors to the disease severity. Discrepancies between reported data are due to differences in the genetic background between studied populations, small sample sizes, insufficient phenotype description, genotyping procedures, individual gene polymorphism assessment, few numbers of loci included in the studies, and requirement of interaction analysis between gene-gene variants. Genetic prediction and use of individual aetiological processes, as well as the translation of recent molecular knowledge into potential therapeutic agents will contribute selectively to the preventive and therapeutic interventions in this complex disease.

8. Acknowledgment

This work was financially supported by grants from the Romanian Academy, Ministry of Education and Research and by an EFSD New Horizons Grant.

9. References

Abdollahi, MR., Gaunt, TR., Syddall, HE., Cooper, C., Phillips, DIW., Ye, S. & Day, INM. (2005) Angiotensin II type I receptor gene polymorphism: anthropometric and metabolic syndrome traits. *Journal Medical Genetics*, Vol. 42, No. 5, (May), pp. 396–401, ISSN 0022-2593.

Abhary, S., Hewitt, A., Burdon, K. & Craig, J. (2009a). A systematic meta-analysis of genetic association studies for diabetic retinopathy. *Diabetes*, Vol. 58, No. 9, (September), pp. 2137-2147, ISSN 0012-1797.

Abhary, S., Burdon, KP., Gupta, A., Lake, S., Selva, D., Petrovsky, N. & Craig, JE. (2009b) Common sequence variation in the VEGFA gene predicts risk of diabetic retinopathy. *Investigative Ophthalmology & Vissual Science*, Vol. 50, No. 12, (December), pp. 5552-5558, ISSN 0146-0404.

Akerblom, HK., Vaarala, O., Hyöty, H., Ilonen, J. & Knip, M. (2002) Environmental factors in the etiology of type 1 diabetes. *American Journal of Medical Genetics*, Part A, Vol. 115, No. 1, (March), pp. 18-29, ISSN 0148-7299.

Amos, A., McCarty, D. & Zimmet, P. (1997) The rising global burden of diabetes and its complications: estimates and projections to the year 2010. *Diabetic Medicine*, Vol. 14, Suppl. 5, (December), pp. S1–S85, ISSN 0742-3071.

Bazzaz, JT., Amoli, MM., Pravica, V., Chandrasecaran, R., Boulton, AJ., Larijani, B. & Hutchinson, IV. (2010) eNOS gene polymorphism association with retinopathy in type 1 diabetes. *Ophthalmic Genetics*, Vol. 31, No. 3, (September), pp. 103-107, ISSN 1381-6810.

Boright, AP., Paterson, AD., Mirea, L., Bull, SB., Mowjoodi, A., Scherer, SW., Zinman, B. & the DCCT/EDIC Research Group. (2005) Genetic variation at the ACE gene is associated with persistent microalbuminuria and severe nephropathy in type 1 diabetes. The DCCT/EDIC Genetics Study. *Diabetes*, Vol. 54, No. 6, (June), pp. 1238-1244, ISSN 0012-1797.

Bottazzo, GF., Mann, JI., Thorogood, M., Baum, JD. & Doniach, D. (1978) Autoimmunity in juvenile diabetics and their families. *British Medical Journal*, Vol. 2, No. 6131, (July), pp. 165–168, ISSN 0007-1447.

Brouet, A., Sonveaux, P., Dessy, C., Balligand, JL. & Feron, O. (2001) Hsp90 ensures the transition from the early Ca2+-dependent to the late phosphorylation-dependent activation of the endothelial nitricoxide synthase in vascular endothelial growth factor-exposed endothelial cells. *The Journal of Biological Chemistry*, Vol. 276, No. 35, (August), pp. 32663–32669, ISSN 0021-9258.

Brownlee, M. (2005) The pathobiology of diabetic complications. A unifying mechanism. *Diabetes*, Vol. 54, No. 6, (June), pp. 1615-1625, ISSN 0012-1797.

Cellek, S. (2004) Point of NO return for nitrergic nerves in diabetes: a new insight into diabetic complications. *Current Pharmaceutical Design*, Vol. 10, No. 29, pp. 3683-3695, ISSN 1381-6128.

Chandra, D., Jackson, EB., Ramana, KV., Kelley, R., Srivastava, SK. & Bhatnagar, A. (2002) Nitric oxide prevents aldose reductase activation and sorbitol accumulation during diabetes. *Diabetes*, Vol. 51, No. 10, (October), pp. 3095–3101, ISSN 0012-1797.

Chen, Y., Huang, H., Zhou, J., Doumatey, A., Lashley, K., Chen, G., Agyenim-Boateng, K., Eghan, BA., Acheampong, J., Fasanmade, O., Johnson, T., Akinsola, FB., Okafor, G.,

Oli, J., Ezepue, F., Amoah, A., Akafo, S., Adeyemo, A. & Rotimi CN. (2007) Polymorphism of the endothelial nitric oxide synthase gene is associated with diabetic retinopathy in a cohort of West Africans. *Molecular Vision*, Vol. 13, (16 November), pp. 2142-2147, ISSN 1090-0535.

Chiarelli, F., Cipollone, F., Romano, F., Tumini, S., Costantini, F., di Ricco, L., Pomilio, M., Pierdomenico, SD., Marini, M., Cuccurullo, F. & Mezzetti, A. (2000) Increased circulating nitric oxide in young patients with type 1 diabetes and persistent microalbuminuria: relation to glomerular hyperfiltration. *Diabetes*, Vol. 49, No. 7, (July), pp. 1258-1263, ISSN 0012-1797.

Chowdhury, TA., Dronsfield, MJ., Kumar, S., Gough, SLC., Gibson, SP., Khatoon, A., MacDonald, F., Rowe, BR., Dunger DB. & Dean, JD. (1996) Examination of two genetic polymorphisms within the renin–angiotensin system: no evidence for an association with nephropathy in IDDM. *Diabetologia*, Vol. 39, No. 9, (September), pp. 1108–1114, ISSN0012-186X.

Chung, C-M., Wang, R-Y., Chen, J-W., Fann, CSJ., Leu, H-B., Ho, H-Y., Ting, C-T., Lin, T-H., Sheu, S-H., Tsai, W-C., Chen, J-H., Jong, Y-S., Lin, S-J., Chen, Y-T. & Pan, W-H. (2010) A genome-wide association study identifies new loci for ACE activity: potential implications for response to ACE inhibitor. *The Pharmacogenomics Journal*, Vol. 10, No. 6, (December), pp. 537–544, ISSN 1470-269X/10.

Cimponeriu, D., Crăciun, A-M., Apostol, P., Radu, I., Guja, C. & Cheţa, D. (2010) The genetic background of diabetes chronic complications. In: *Genetics of diabetes. The Truth Unveiled*, D. Cheţa (Ed), 193-334, Academia Romana & S. Karger AG, ISBN 978-973-27-1901-5, Bucharest/Basel, Romania.

Concannon, P., Rich, SS. & Nepom, GT. (2009) Genetics of type 1A diabetes. *The New England Journal of Medicine*, Vol. 360, No. 16, (April), pp. 1646-1654, ISSN 0028-4793.

Conen, D., Glynn, RJ., Buring, JE., Ridker, PM. & Zee, RYL. (2008) Association of renin-angiotensin and endothelial nitric oxide synthase gene polymorphisms with blood pressure progression and incident hypertension: prospective cohort study. *Journal of Hypertension*, Vol. 26, No. 9, (September), pp. 1780–1786, ISSN 0263-6352.

Costacou, T., Chang, Y., Ferrell, RE. & Orchard, TJ. (2006) Identifying genetic susceptibilities to diabetes-related complications among individuals at low risk of complications: An application of tree-structured survival analysis. *American Journal of Epidemiology*, Vol. 164, No. 9, (November), pp. 862–872, ISSN 0002-9262.

Currie, D., McKnight, AJ., Patterson, CC., Sadlier, DM. & Maxwell, AP. (2010) The UK Warren/GoKinD study group investigation of ACE, ACE2 and AGTR1 genes for association with nephropathy in Type 1 diabetes mellitus. *Diabetic Medicine*, Vol. 27, No. 10, (October), pp. 1188–1194, ISSN 0742-3071.

DCCT Research Group. (1993) The effect of intensive treatment of diabetes on the development and progression of long-term complications in insulin-dependent diabetes mellitus. The Diabetes Control and Complications Trial Research Group. *The New England Journal of Medicine*, Vol. 329, No. 14, (September), pp. 977-986, ISSN 0028-4793.

DCCT/EDIC Research Group, Nathan, DM., Zinman, B., Cleary, PA., Backlund, JY., Genuth, S., Miller, R. & Orchard, TJ. (2009) Modern-day clinical course of type 1 diabetes mellitus after 30 years' duration: the diabetes control and complications trial/epidemiology of diabetes interventions and complications and Pittsburgh epidemiology of diabetes complications experience (1983-2005). *Archives of Internal Medicine*, Vol. 169, No. 14, (July), pp. 1307-1316, ISSN 0003-9926.

Degen, B., Schmidt, S. & Ritz, E. (2001) A polymorphism in the gene for the endothelial nitric oxide synthase and diabetic nephropathy. *Nephrology Dialysis Transplantation*, Vol. 16, No. 1, (January), pp. 185-198, ISSN 0931-0509.

DIAMOND Project Group. (2006) Incidence and trends of childhood Type 1 diabetes worldwide 1990-1999. *Diabetic Medicine*, Vol. 23, No. 8, (August), pp. 857-866, ISSN 0742-3071.

Doria, A. (2010) Genetics of diabetes complications. *Current Diabetes Reports*, Vol. 10, No. 6, (December), pp. 467-475, ISSN 1534-4827.

Dragović, T., Ajdinović, B., Hrvacević, R., Ilić, V., Magić, Z., Andelković, Z. & Kocev, N. (2010) Angiotensin II type 1 receptor gene polymorphism could influence renoprotective response to losartan treatment in type 1 diabetic patients with high urinary albumin excretion rate. *Vojnosanitetski pregled. Military-medical and pharmaceutical review*, Vol. 67, No. 4, (May), pp. 273-278, ISSN 0042-8450.

Eisenbarth, GS. (1986) Type 1 diabetes: a chronic autoimmune disease. *The New England Journal of Medicine*, Vol. 314, No. 21, (May), pp. 1360-1368, ISSN 0028-4793.

Erbs, S., Baither, Y., Linke, A., Adams, V., Shu, Y., Lenk, K., Gielen, S., Dilz, R., Schuler, G. & Hambrecht, R. (2003) Promoter but not exon 7 polymorphism of endothelial nitric oxide synthase a Vects training induced correction of endothelial dysfunction. *Arteriosclerosis, Thrombosis, and Vascular Biology*, Vol. 23, No. 10, (October), pp. 1814–1819, ISSN 1079-5642.

EURODIAB IDDM Complications Study Group. (1994) Microvascular and acute complications in insulin dependent diabetes mellitus: the EURODIAB IDDM Complications Study. *Diabetologia*, Vol. 37, No. 11, (November), pp. 278-285, ISSN 0012-186X.

Frank, RN. (2004) Diabetic retinopathy. *The New England Journal of Medicine*, Vol. 350, No. 1, (January), pp. 48-58, ISSN 0028-4793.

Freedman, BI., Yu, H., Anderson, PJ., Roh, BH., Rich, SS. & Bowden, DW. (2000) Genetic analysis of nitric oxide and endothelin in end-stage renal disease. *Nephrology Dialysis Transplantation*, Vol. 15, No. 11, (November), pp.1794-800, ISSN 0931-0509.

Freedman, BI., Bostrom, M., Daeihagh, P. & Bowden, DW. (2007) Genetic factors in diabetic nephropathy. *Clinical Journal of the American Society of Nephrology*, Vol. 2, No. 6, (November), pp. 1306-1316, ISSN 1555-9041.

Fröjdö, S., Sjölind, L., Parkkonen, M., Mäkinen, V-P., Kilpikari, R., Pettersson-Fernholm, K., Forsblom, C., Fagerudd, J., Tikellis, C., Cooper, ME., Wessman, M., Groop, P-H. & FinnDiane Study Group. (2005) Polymorphisms in the gene encoding angiotensin I converting enzyme 2 and diabetic nephropathy. *Diabetologia*, Vol. 48, No. 11, (November), pp. 2278–2281, ISSN 0012-186X.

Gallego, PH., Shephard, N., Bulsara, MK., van Bockxmeere, FM., Powell, BL., Beilby, JP., Arscott, G., Le Page, M., Palmer, LJ., Davis, EA., Jones, TW. & Choong, CSY. (2008) Angiotensinogen gene T235 variant: a marker for the development of persistent microalbuminuria in children and adolescents with type 1 diabetes mellitus. *Journal of Diabetes and Its Complications*, Vol. 22, (May – June), pp. 191– 198, ISSN 1056-8727.

Gepts, W. (1965) Pathologic anatomy of the pancreas in juvenile diabetes mellitus. *Diabetes*, Vol. 14, No. 10, (October), pp. 619–633, ISSN 0012-1797.

Groop, PH., Thomas, MC., Moran, JL., Wadèn, J., Thorn, LM., Mäkinen, VP., Rosengård-Bärlund, M., Saraheimo, M., Hietala, K., Heikkilä, O., Forsblom, C. & FinnDiane Study Group. (2009) The presence and severity of chronic kidney disease predicts all-cause mortality in type 1 diabetes. *Diabetes*, Vol. 58, No. 7, (July), pp. 1651-1658, ISSN 0012-1797.

Gumprecht, J., Zychma, MJ., Grzeszczak, W., Zukowska-Szczechowska, E. & End-Stage Renal Disease study group. (2000) Angiotensin I-converting enzyme gene insertion/deletion and angiotensinogen M235T polymorphisms: Risk of chronic renal failure. *Kidney International*, Vol. 58, No. 2, (August), pp. 513–519, ISSN 0085-2538.

Giunti, S., Barit, D. & Cooper, ME. (2006) Mechanisms of diabetic nephropathy: Role of hypertension. *Hypertension*, Vol. 48, No. 4, (October), pp. 519-526, ISSN 0194-911X.

Hadi, HA. & Suwaidi, JA. (2007) Endothelial dysfunction in diabetes mellitus. *Vascular Health and Risk Management*, Vol. 3, No. 6, (December), pp. 853-876, ISSN 1176-6344.

Hadjadj, S., Belloum, R., Bouhanick, B., Gallois, Y., Guilloteau, G., Chatellier, G., Alhenc-Gelas, F. & Marre, M. (2001) Prognostic value of angiotensin-I converting enzyme I/D polymorphism for nephropathy in type 1 diabetes mellitus: A prospective study. *Journal of American Society of Nephrology*, Vol. 12, No. 3, (March), pp. 541–549, ISSN 1046-6673.

Hadjadj, S., Tarnow, L., Forsblom, C., Kazeem, G., Marre, M., Groop, PH., Parving, HH., Cambien, F., Tregouet, DA., Gut, IG., Theva, A., Gauguier, D., Farrall, M., Cox, R., Matsuda, F., Lathrop, M. & Hager-Vionnet, N. (2007) Association between angiotensin-converting enzyme gene polymorphisms and diabetic nephropathy: Case-control, haplotype, and family-based study in three European populations. *Journal of American Society of Nephrology*, Vol. 18, No. 4, (April), pp. 1284–1291, ISSN 1046-6673.

Heltianu, C., Manea, SA., Guja, C., Mihai, C. & Ionescu-Tirgoviste, C. (2008). Correlation of low molecular weight advanced glycation end products and nitric oxide metabolites with chronic complications in type 1 diabetic patients. *Central European Journal of Biology*, Vol. 3, No. 3, (September), pp. 243-249, ISSN 1895-104X.

Heltianu, C., Manea, SA., Guja, C., Robciuc, A. & Ionescu-Tirgoviste, C. (2009) Polymorphism in exon 7 of the endothelial nitric oxide synthase gene is associated with low incidence of microvascular damage in type 1 diabetic neuropathy. *Central European Journal of Biology*, Vol. 4, No. 4, (December), pp. 521-5273, ISSN 1895-104X.

International Diabetes Federation. (2009). *IDF Diabetes Atlas* (4th), (May), International Diabetes Federation, ISBN 13: 978-2-930229-71-3, Brussels, Belgium.

Jacobsen, P., Tarnow, L., Carstensen, B., Hovind, P., Poirier, O. & Parving, H-H. (2003) Genetic variation in the renin-angiotensin system and progression of diabetic nephropathy. *Journal of American Society of Nephrology*, Vol. 14, No. 11, (November), pp. 2843-2850, ISSN 1533-3450.

Johannesen, J., Pociot, F., Kristiansen, OP., Karlsen, AE., Nerup, J., DIEGG. & DSGD. (2000a) No evidence for linkage in the promoter region of the inducible nitric oxide synthase gene (NOS2) in a Danish type 1 diabetes population. *Genes and Immunity*, Vol. 1, No. 6, (August), pp. 362–366, ISSN 1466-4879.

Johannesen, J., Tarnow, L., Parving, HH., Nerup, J. & Pociot, F. (2000b)   CCTTT-repeat polymorphism in the human NOS2-promoter confers low risk of diabetic nephropathy in type 1 diabetic patients. *Diabetes Care*, Vol. 23, No. 4, (April), pp. 560-562, ISSN 0149-5992 .

Johannesen, J., Pie, A., Pociot, F., Kristiansen, OP., Karlsen, AE. & Nerup, J. (2001) Linkage of the human inducible nitric oxide synthase gene to type 1 diabetes. *The Journal Clinical Endocrinology and Metabolism*,   Vol. 86, No. 6, (June), pp. 2792–2796, ISSN 0021-972X.

Kalani, M. (2008) The importance of endothelin-1 for microvascular dysfunction in diabetes. *Vascular Health and Risk Management*, Vol. 4, No. 5, (May),   pp. 1061–1068,   ISSN 1178-2048.

Kankova, K., Muzik, J., Karaskova, J., Beranek, M., Hajek, D., Znojil, V., Vlkova, E. & Vacha, J. (2001) Duration of non-insulin-dependent diabetes mellitus and the TNF-ß NcoI genotype as predictive factors in proliferative diabetic retinopathy. *Ophthalmologica*, Vol. 215, No. 4, (July – August), pp. 294–298, ISSN 0030-3755.

Keenan, HA., Costacou, T., Sun, JK., Doria, A., Cavellerano, J., Coney, J., Orchard, TJ., Aiello, LP. & King, GL. (2007) Clinical factors associated with resistance to microvascular complications in diabetic patients of extreme disease duration: the 50-year medalist study. *Diabetes Care*, Vol. 30, No. 8, (August), pp. 1995–1997, ISSN 0149-5992.

Kempler, P. (2002) Pathomorphology and pathomechanism. In: *Neuropathies. Pathomechanism, clinical presentation, diagnosis, therapy.* P. Kempler (Ed.), 21-39, Springer Scientific Publisher, ISBN 963-699-166-9, Budapest, Hungary.

Lam, H-C. (2001) Role of endothelin in diabetic vascular complications. *Endocrine*, Vol. 14, No. 3, (April), pp. 277–284, ISSN 0969-711X.

Li, C., Hu, Z., Liu, Z., Wang, L-E., Gershenwald, JE., Lee, JE., Prieto, VG., Duvic, M., Grimm, EA. & Wei, Q. (2007) Polymorphisms of the neuronal and inducible nitric oxide synthase genes and the risk of cutaneous melanoma.   *Cancer*, Vol. 109, No. 8, (April), pp. 1570–1578, ISSN 0008-543X.

Li, H., Louey, JWC., Choy, KW, Liu, DTL., Chan, WM., Chan, YM., Fung, NSK., Fan, BJ., Baum, L., Chan, JCN., Lam, DSC. & Pang, CP. (2008) *EDN1* Lys198Asn is associated with diabetic retinopathy in type 2 diabetes. *Molecular Vision*, Vol. 14, (15 September), pp. 1698-1704, ISSN 1090-0535.

Maahs, DM., West, NA., Lawrence, JM. & Mayer-Davis, EJ. (2010) Epidemiology of type 1 diabetes. *Endocrinology Metabolism Clinics of North America*, Vol. 39, No. 3, (September), pp. 481-497, ISSN 0889-8529.

Mamoulakis, D., Bitsori, M., Galanakis, E., Vazgiourakis, V., Panierakis, C. & Goulielmos, GN. (2009) Intron 4 polymorphism of the endothelial nitric oxide synthase eNOS gene and early microangiopathy in type 1 diabetes. *International Journal of Immunogenetics*, Vol. 36, No. 3, (June), pp. 153-157, ISSN 1744-3121.

Marre, M., Jeunemaitre, X., Gallois, Y., Rodier, M., Chatellier, G., Sert, C., Dusselier, L., Kahal, Z., Chaillous, L., Halimi, S., Muller, A., Sackmann, H., Bauduceau, B., Bled, F., Passa, P. & Alhenc-Gelas, F. (1997) Contribution of genetic polymorphism in the renin–angiotensin system to the development of renal complications in insulin-dependent diabetes. Génétique de la néphropathie diabétique (GENEDIAB) study group. *The Journal of Clinical Investigation*, Vol. 99, No. 7, (April), pp. 1585–1595, ISSN 0021-9738.

Melikian, N., Seddon, MD., Casadei, B., Chowienczyk, PJ. & Shah, AM. (2009) Neuronal nitric oxide synthase and human vascular regulation. *Trends in Cardiovascular Medicine*, Vol. 19, No. 8, (November), pp. 256–262, ISSN 1050-1738.

Mogensen, CE. (2000) Definition of diabetic renal disease in insulin dependent diabetes mellitus, based on renal function tests. In: *The Kidney and Hypertension in Diabetes Mellitus*. CE. Mogensen (Ed), 13-29, Kluwer Academic Publishers, ISBN 9780792379010, ISBN 0792379012, Boston, USA.

Möllsten, A., Kockum, I., Svensson, M., Rudberg, S., Ugarph-Morawski, A., Brismar, K., Eriksson, JW. & Dahlquist, G. (2008) The effect of polymorphisms in the renin–angiotensin–aldosterone system on diabetic nephropathy risk. *Journal of Diabetes and Its Complications*, Vol. 22, No. 6, (November – December) , pp. 377– 383, ISSN 1056-8727.

Möllsten, A., Lajer, M., Jorsal, A. & Tarnow, L. (2009) The endothelial nitric oxide synthase gene and risk of diabetic nephropathy and development of cardiovascular disease in type 1 diabetes. *Molecular Genetics and Metabolism*, Vol. 97, No. 1, (May), pp. 80–84, ISSN 1096-7192.

Mooyaart, AL., Valk, EJJ., van Es, LA., Bruijn, JA., de Heer, E., Freedman, BI., Dekkers, OM. & Baelde, HJ. (2011) Genetic associations in diabetic nephropathy: a meta-analysis. *Diabetologia*, Vol. 54, No. 3, (March), pp. 544-553, ISSN 0012-186X.

Morahan, G., Mehta, M., James, I., Chen, WM., Akolkar, B., Erlich, HA., Hilner, JE., Julier, C., Nerup, J., Nierras, C., Pociot, F., Todd, JA., Rich, SS. & Type 1 Diabetes Genetics Consortium. (2011) Tests for genetic interactions in type 1 diabetes: Linkage and stratification analyses of 4,422 affected sib-pairs. *Diabetes*, Vol. 60, No. 3, (March), pp. 1030-1040, ISSN 0012-1797.

Ned, RM., Yesupriya, A., Imperatore, G., Smelser, DT., Moonesinghe, R., Chang, M-H. & Dowling, NF. (2010) Inflammation gene variants and susceptibility to albuminuria in the U.S. population: analysis in the Third National Health and Nutrition Examination Survey (NHANES III), 1991-1994. *BMC Medical Genetics*, Vol. 11, (5 November), pp. 155-170, ISSN 1471-2350.

Ng, DPK., Tai, BC., Koh, D., Tan, KW.& Chia, KS. (2005) Angiotensin-I converting enzyme insertion/deletion polymorphism and its association with diabetic nephropathy: a meta-analysis of studies reported between 1994 and 2004 and comprising 14,727 subjects. *Diabetologia*, Vol. 48, No. 5, (May), pp. 1008–1016, ISSN 0012-186X.

Ng, DPK., Tai, BC. & Lim, X-L. (2008) Is the presence of retinopathy of practical value in defining cases of diabetic nephropathy in genetic association studies? The experience with the *ACE* I/D polymorphism in 53 studies comprising 17,791 subjects. *Diabetes*, Vol. 57, No. 9, (September), pp. 2541-2546, ISSN 0012-1797.

Ng, DPK. (2010) Human genetics of diabetic retinopathy: current perspectives. *Journal of Ophthalmology*, Vol. 2010, Article ID 172593, pp. 1-6, ISSN 2090-004X.

Nosikov, VV. (2004) Genomics of type 1 diabetes mellitus and its late complications. *Molecular Biology (Mosk)*, Vol. 38, No. 1, (January – February), pp. 150-164, ISSN 0026-8933.

Patterson, CC., Dahlquist, G., Harjutsalo, V., Joner, G., Feltbower, RG., Svensson, J., Schober, E., Gyürüs, E., Castell, C., Urbonaité, B., Rosenbauer, J., Iotova, V., Thorsson, AV. & Soltész, G. (2007) Early mortality in EURODIAB population-based cohorts of type 1 diabetes diagnosed in childhood since 1989. *Diabetologia*, Vol. 50, No. 12, (December), pp. 2439-2442, ISSN 0012-186X.

Patterson, CC., Dahlquist, GG., Gyürüs, E., Green, A., Soltész, G. & EURODIAB Study Group. (2009) Incidence trends for childhood type 1 diabetes in Europe during 1989-2003 and predicted new cases 2005-20: A multicentre prospective registration study. *The Lancet*, Vol. 373, No. 9680, (13 June), pp 2027-2033, ISSN 0140-6736.

Pezzolesi, MG., Poznik, GD., Mychaleckyj, JC., Paterson, AD., Barati, MT., Klein, JB., Ng, DP., Placha, G., Canani, LH., Bochenski, J., Waggott, D., Merchant, ML., Krolewski, B., Mirea, L., Wanic, K., Katavetin, P., Kure, M., Wolkow, P., Dunn, JS., Smiles, A., Walker, WH., Boright, AP., Bull, SB., DCCT/EDIC Research Group, Doria, A., Rogus, JJ., Rich, SS., Warram, JH. & Krolewski, AS. (2009) Genome-wide association scan for diabetic nephropathy susceptibility genes in type 1 diabetes. *Diabetes*, Vol. 58, No. 6, (June), pp. 1403-1410, ISSN 0012-1797.

Potenza, MA, Gagliardi, S., Nacci, C., Carratu, MR. & Montagnani, M. (2009) Endothelial dysfunction in diabetes: from mechanisms to therapeutic targets. *Current Medicinal Chemistry*, Vol. 16, No. 6, pp. 94-112, ISSN 0929-8673.

Qidwai, T. & Jamal, F. (2010) Inducible nitric oxide synthase (iNOS) gene polymorphism and disease prevalence. *Scandinavian Journal of Immunology*, Vol. 72, No. 5, (November), pp. 375–387, ISSN 1365-3083.

Ringel, J., Beige, J., Kunz, R., Distler, A. & Sharma, AM. (1997) Genetic variants of the renin-angiotensin system, diabetic nephropathy and hypertension. *Diabetologia*, Vol. 40, No. 2, (January), pp. 193–199, ISSN 0012-186X.

Ruggenenti, P., Bettinaglio, P., Pinares, F. & Remuzzi, G. (2008) Angiotensin converting enzyme insertion/deletion polymorphism and renoprotection in diabetic and nondiabetic nephropathies. *Clinical Journal American Society of Nephrology*, Vol. 3, No. 5, (September), pp. 1511–1525, ISSN 1555-9041.

Schrijvers, BF., De Vriese, AS. & Flyvbjerg, A. (2004) From hyperglycemia to diabetic kidney disease: the role of metabolic, hemodynamic, intracellular factors and growth factors/cytokines. *Endocrine Reviews*, Vol. 25, No. 6, (December), pp. 971-1010, ISSN 0163-769X.

Shaw, JE., Sicree, RA. & Zimmet, PZ. (2010) Global estimates of the prevalence of diabetes for 2010 and 2030. *Diabetes Research and Clinical Practice*, Vol. 87, No. 1, (January), pp. 4-14, ISSN 0168-8227.

Spinarová, L., Spinar, J., Vasku, A., Pávková-Goldbergová, M., Ludka, O., Tomandl, J. & Vítovec, J. (2008) Genetics of humoral and cytokine activation in heart failure and its importance for risk stratification of patients. *Experimental and Molecular Pathology*, Vol. 84, No. 3, (June), pp. 251-255, ISSN 0014-4800.

Stehouwer, CDA. (2000) Dysfunction of the vascular endothelium and the development of renal and vascular complications in diabetes. In: *The Kidney and Hypertension in Diabetes Mellitus*, E. Mogensen (Ed), 179-192, Kluwer Academic Publishers, ISBN 9780792379010, Boston, USA.

Tarnow, L., Kjeld, T., Knudsen, E., Major-Pedersen, A. & Parving, H-H. (2000) Lack of synergism between long-term poor glycaemic control and three gene polymorphisms of the renin angiotensin system on risk of developing diabetic nephropathy in Type I diabetic patients. *Diabetologia*, Vol. 43, No. 6, (June), pp. 794-799, ISSN 0012-186X.

Taverna, MJ., Elgrably, F., Selmi, H., Selam, JL. & Slama, G. (2005) The T-786C and C774T endothelial nitric oxide synthase gene polymorphisms independently affect the onset pattern of severe diabetic retinopathy. *Nitric Oxide*, Vol. 13, No. 1, (August), pp. 88-92, ISSN 1089-8603.

Todd, JA. (1991) A protective role of the environment in the development of type 1 diabetes? *Diabetic Medicine*, Vol. 8, No. 10, (December), pp. 906-910, ISSN 0742-3071.

Todd, JA., Walker, NM., Cooper, JD., Smyth, DJ., Downes, K., Plagnol, V., Bailey, R., Nejentsev, S., Field, SF., Payne, F., Lowe, CE., Szeszko, JS., Hafler, JP., Zeitels, L., Yang, JHM., Vella, A., Nutland, S., Stevens, HE., Schuilenburg, H., Coleman, G., Maisuria, M., Meadows, W., Smink, LJ., Healy, B., Burren, OS., Lam, AAC., Ovington, NR., Allen, J., Adlem, E., Leung, H-T., Wallace, C., Howson, JMM., Guja, C., Ionescu-Tîrgovişte, C., Genetics of Type 1 Diabetes in Finland, Simmonds, MJ., Heward, JM., Gough, SCL., Dunger , DB., the Wellcome Trust Case Control Consortium, Wicker, LS. & Clayton, DG. (2007) Robust associations of four new chromosome regions from genome-wide analyses of type 1 diabetes. *Nature Genetics*, Vol. 39, No. 7, (July), pp. 857–864, ISSN 1061-4036.

Van Ittersum, FJ., de Man, AME., Thijssen, S., de Knijff, P., Slagboom, E., Smulders, Y., Tarnow, L., Donker AJM., Bilo, HJG. & Stehouwer, CDA. (2000) Genetic polymorphisms of the renine-angiotensin system and complications of insulin-dependent diabetes mellitus. *Nephrology Dialysis Transplantation*, Vol.15, No. 7, (July), pp.1000-1007, ISSN 0931-0509.

Zanchi, A., Moczulski, DK., Hanna, LS., Wantman, M., Warram, JH. & Krolewski, AS. (2000) Risk of advanced diabetic nephropathy in type 1 diabetes is associated with endothelial nitric oxide synthase gene polymorphism. *Kidney International*, Vol. 57, No. 2, (February), pp. 405–413, ISSN 0085-2538.

Zhou, JB. & Yang, JK. (2010) Angiotensin-converting enzyme gene polymorphism is associated with proliferative diabetic retinopathy: a meta-analysis. *Acta Diabetologica*, Vol. 47, Suppl. 1, (December), pp. 187-193, ISSN 0940-5429.

Zintzaras, E., Papathanasiou, AA. & Stefanidis, I. (2009) Endothelial nitric oxide synthase gene polymorphisms and diabetic nephropathy: a HuGE review and meta-analysis. *Genetics in Medicine*, Vol. 11, No. 10, (October), pp. 695-706, ISSN 1098-3600.

Zotova, EV., Voron'ko, OE., Bursa, TR., Galeev, IV., Strokov, IA. & Nosikov, VV. (2005) Polymorphic markers of the NO synthase genes and genetic predisposition to diabetic polyneuropathy in patients with type 1 diabetes mellitus. *Molecular Biology (Mosk)*, Vol. 39, No. 2, (March – April), pp. 224-229, ISSN 0026-8933.

Yilmaz, G., Esser, P., Kociok, N., Aydin, P. & Heimann, K. (2000) Elevated vitreous nitric oxide levels in patients with proliferative diabetic retinopathy. *American Journal of Ophthalmology*, Vol. 130, No. 1, (July), pp. 87–90, ISSN 0002-9394.

Wang, Y., Newton, DC. & Marsden, PA. (1999) Neuronal NOS: gene structure, mRNA
        diversity, and functional relevance. *Critique Review Neurobiology*, Vol. 13, No. 1, pp.
        21-43, ISSN 0892-0915.
Warpeha, KM., Xu, W., Liu, L., Charles, IG., Patterson, CC., Ah-Fat, F., Harding, S., Hart,
        PM., Chakravarthy, U. & Hughes, AE. (1999) Genotyping and functional analysis
        of a polymorphic (CCTTT)(n) repeat of NOS2A in diabetic retinopathy. *FASEB
        Journal*, Vol. 13, No. 13, (October), pp. 1825-1832, ISSN 0892-6638.
Warpeha, KM. & Chakravarthy, U. (2003) Molecular genetics of microvascular disease in
        diabetic retinopathy. *Eye (London)*, Vol. 17, No. 3, (April), pp. 305-311, ISSN 0950-
        222X.

3

Islet Endothelium: Role in Type 1 Diabetes and in Coxsackievirus Infections

Enrica Favaro, Ilaria Miceli, Elisa Camussi and Maria M. Zanone
Department of Internal Medicine, University of Turin,
Italy

1. Introduction

The heterogeneity of microvascular endothelial cells derived from different organs, suggests that these cells have specialised functions at different anatomical sites. The microvasculature is, in fact, a key interface between blood and tissues and participates in numerous pathophysiological processes. Pancreatic islet microcirculation exhibits distinctive features, in an interdependent physical and functional relationship with β cells, from organogenesis to adult life. The islet microendothelium behaves as an active "gatekeeper" in the control of leukocyte recruitment into the islets during autoimmune insulitis in type 1 diabetes.

Furthermore, microvascular endothelial cells, forming the key lining between the vascular space and organ parenchyma, have been shown to influence organ and tissue specific susceptibility to viral infection, and to modulate the pathological expression of virus-induced diseases, which potentially includes type 1 diabetes. Endothelial cells expressing appropriate receptors would fail to act as effective barrier to infections, allowing viral particles to pass through, and replicate in, the vascular endothelium. Human Enteroviruses (EV), especially those of the Coxsackievirus B (CVB) group, are associated with a wide variety of clinical syndromes and have long been considered possible culprits of inflammatory conditions and immune-mediated pathological processes, such as chronic dilated cardiomyopathy, chronic myositis and type 1 diabetes mellitus (Rose et al., 1993; Luppi et al., 1998; Hyöty & Taylor, 2002). Several mechanisms, including molecular mimicry, bystander activation of autoreactive T cells, superantigenic activity of viral proteins, not mutually exclusive, have been proposed to explain the relationship between EV infections and induction of autoimmune diseases (Varela-Calvino & Peakman, 2003; Horwitz et al., 1998; Wucherpfennig, 2001). Evidences of a link between viral infections and initiation or acceleration of pancreatic islet autoimmunity have been under investigation for almost 30 years, and EVs, especially those of the Coxsackievirus B (CVB) group, are historically the prime suspects as important aetiological determinants in type 1 diabetes (Hyöty & Taylor, 2002; Varela-Calvino & Peakman, 2003). Endothelial cells derived from different organs show distinct susceptibility to CVB infections, and the behaviour against a viral challenge of endothelial cells in large vessels and microvessels may differ (Friedman et al. 1981; Huber et al., 1990; Conaldi et al. 1997; Zanone et al., 2003; Saijets et al., 2003).

2. Pancreatic islet microvasculature: Structure and specialised functions

It is widely accepted that remarkable heterogeneity of endothelial phenotype and function exists amongst different vascular beds (Kubota et al., 1988; Charo etal., 1984; Swerlick et al., 1991; Swerlick et al., 1992; Fujimoto & Singer, 1988; Lidington et al., 1999), in particular between cells derived from large versus small vessels, supporting the notion that tissue-specific vascular beds have specialised functions. These diversities include morphology, growth requirement in vitro (Kubota et al., 1988; Charo et al., 1984; Swerlick et al., 1991; Swerlick et al., 1992; Fujimoto & Singer, 1988; Lidington et al., 1999, Folkman et al., 1979) prostaglandin secretory profile (Charo etal., 1984), immunologic phenotype (Swerlick et al., 1992) and amounts and regulation of cell adhesion molecules (Swerlick et al., 1992; Fujimoto & Singer, 1988; Petzelbauer et al., 1993; Swerlick A.R., et al., 1992; Lee et al., 1992). At a functional level, differential and sequential expression of adhesion molecules mediates trafficking of leukocytes to specific lymphoid and non-lymphoid tissues.

Endothelium heterogeneity is the result of microenvironmental signals, in particular those induced by the family of vascular endothelial growth factor (VEGF) proteins (D'Amore & Ng, 2002). VEGF is a major stimulator of neovascularisation by inducing proliferation and migration of endothelial cells and tube formation. Pancreatic islets are one of the most vascularised organs, having a blood perfusion of about 10% of that of the whole pancreas, despite representing only 1% of the gland; this reflects high exchange demand with the endocrine cells and high metabolic supply (Figure 1). Deletion studies indicate that VEGF-A is responsible for this dense islet vascularisation, being more expressed in the endocrine than the exocrine pancreas (Lammert et al., 2003). Endothelial cells migrate to the source of VEGF-A, the neighboring β cells, proliferate and form blood vessels, organised in a network of sinusoidal capillaries reminiscent of those present in the renal glomerulus, with a five times higher density and ten times more fenestrations than in the exocrine tissue.

Islets receive blood from 1 to 3 arterioles and drain into collecting venules forming a network covering the islet surface, and an insulo-acinar portal system connects the islet capillaries with capillaries of the exocrine pancreas. The pattern of blood flow within the islet is still a matter of debate, with the β cell-rich islet core possibly perfused before the non-β cells in the periphery of the islet (Brunicardi et al., 1996).

Specific markers of islet microvasculature have been identified. These include the α-1 proteinase inhibitor (Api, α-1 antitrypsin), a major proteinase inhibitor with immuno-regulatory properties, and nephrin (Favaro et al., 2005), a highly specific barrier protein, known to be located in the renal glomerular ultrathin filter membrane "slit diaphragm" (Ruotsalainen et al., 1999; Tryggvason & Wartiovaara, 2001) (Figure 2). The nephrin expressed in islet microendothelial cells has functional characteristics that are highly reminiscent of the same protein expressed by podocytes in the renal glomeruli, in that in both cell types treatment with TNF-α acts on the cell cytoskeleton to induce a marked re-distribution of nephrin expression. Nephrin is a cell adhesion transmembrane protein of the immunoglobulin superfamily, which has a pivotal role in the regulation of renal glomerular selective permeability (Henderson & Moss, 1985; Bonner-Weir, 1993; Konstantinova & Lammert, 2004; Bonner-Weir & Orci, 1982). Islet endothelial expression of this protein is consistent with the ultrastructural features of these cells in the islets, which form a microvasculature that is characterized by a glomerulus-like network of fenestrated capillaries.

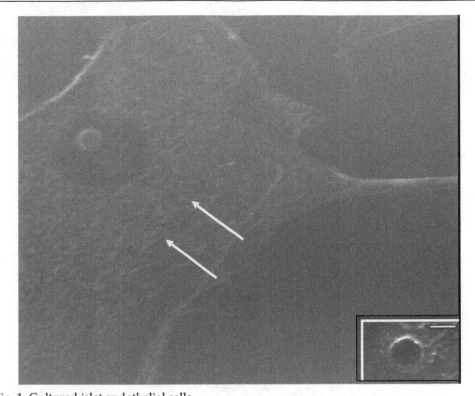

Fig. 1. Cultured islet endothelial cells.
Representative micrograph of scanning electron microscopy of primary islet MECs. The arrows show typical cellular fenestrations (original magnification 1500X). Inset: representative magnification of a cellular fenestra (original magnification 15,000X). Bar: 0.1 µm.

Nephrin appears to be more than just a structural component, as it is an adhesion and signalling molecule that can activate mitogen-activated protein kinase cascades, modulating a variety of cellular programs, including proliferation, differentiation and apoptosis (Karin et al., 1997; Flickinger & Olson, 1999). It has been shown that nephrin, once phosphorylated associates with PI3K and itself stimulates the Akt-dependent signaling pathway (Huber et al., 2003) that plays a pivotal role in preventing apoptosis in a variety of settings (Datta et al., 1999). In particular, Akt activation is crucial for the ability of factors such as insulin, IGF-I and VEGF to inhibit apoptosis in cultured endothelium (Jung et al., 2000). Recent data highlight the Akt role also in insulin-mediated glucose transport and pancreatic β cell mass and function (Bernal-Mizrachi et al., 2004; Elghazi et al., 2006).
Islet endothelium is crucially involved in fine-tuning blood glucose sensing and regulation (Lammert et al., 2003). Besides providing oxygen and nutrients to the endocrine cells, islet endothelium is in fact involved in the trans-endothelial rapid passage of secreted insulin into the circulation. In perfusion experiments with horseradish peroxidase it has been demonstrated that the endothelial fenestrae are sites through which proteins quickly permeate (Takahashi et al., 2002). Thus the islet fenestrae allow the fastest way for insulin to enter the circulation. Studies in mice with pancreatic VEGF-A deletion, showed that these

mice not only displayed loss of endothelial fenestrations and thicker endothelial cell body but also defective blood glucose levels on glucose tolerance test, pointing to a possible defect in the release of insulin (Lammert et al., 2003). A more recent study indicated that mice with β cell reduced VEGF-A expression show impaired glucose-stimulated insulin secretion, related to vascular alterations of the islets (Brissova et al., 2006).

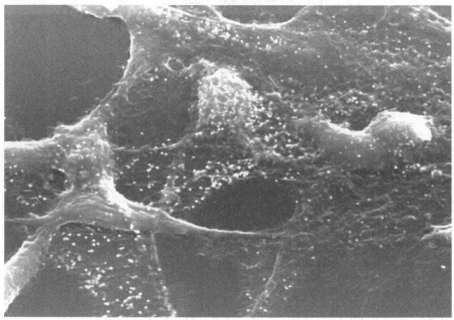

Fig. 2. Nephrin is expressed by islet endothelial cells.
Representative immunogold labelling micrograph of islet MECs stained with anti-nephrin Abs. By immunogold staining, nephrin appears distributed on the surface of islet MECs, without accumulation at cell-to-cell junctions (original magnification 1000X).

The microvasculature participates in sensing the environment of the islets and generates signals to affect adult islet endocrine function, being accepted that post-natal β cell mass is dynamic and can increase in function and mass to compensate for added demand (Bonner-Weir & Sharma, 2006). In an in vitro system, purified islet endothelial cells have been shown to stimulate β cell proliferation, through secretion of hepatocyte growth factor (HGF) (Suschek et al., 1994). VEGF-A and insulin are the islet-derived factor that induce HGF secretion. In vivo experiments, using pancreas of pregnant rats in which a high physiological proliferation of β cell occurs, showed prominent expression of HGF, coinciding with the peak of β cell proliferation.
Islet endothelium exhibits a unique phenotype also in the activities of the constitutive and cytokine-inducible endothelial nitric oxide (NO) synthases, forming the vasoactive mediator NO, since these enzymes are specifically regulated by the glucose level (Kolb & Kolb-Bachofen, 1992). This indicates an organ-specific control of NO production, whose role in islet cytotoxicity is well established (Kroncke et al., 1993; Steiner et al., 1997; Southern et al., 1990; Schmidt et al., 1992). The role of NO in the physiology of insulin release instead

remains controversial (Welsh & Sandler, 1992; Corbett et al., 1993; Henningsson et al., 2002; von Andrian & Mackay CR, 2000; Ostermann et al., 2002).

Immunohistochemical studies have shown that the expression of Platelet-activating factor (PAF) receptor (PAF-r) within the islet, is restricted to endothelial cells, providing potential target for therapeutic intervention (Biancone et al., 2006). PAF, is a phospholipid with diverse physiological effects that mediates a host of biochemical activities, including angiogenesis and inflammation. Islet endothelial cells have also been shown to rapidly produce PAF under stimulation with trombin, and PAF accelerated angiogenesis (Mattsson et al., 2006). These data suggest that intra-islet production of PAF, induced by inflammatory mediators, may contribute to the neovascularisation of transplanted islets.

Lastly, islet endothelial cells express genes encoding for a number of other factors involved in angiogenesis, including potent pro-angiogenic factors, such as VEGF, and angiostatic factors, such as endostatin and pigment epithelial-derived factor (Lammert et al., 2001).

2.1 Endothelial signalling during development and interplay between endothelial and β cells

Elegant experiments on early pancreatic development demonstrated that blood vessel endothelium in the dorsal aorta provides inductive signals for the differentiation of the primitive endoderm into islet cells (Lammert et al., 2001; Yoshitomi & Zaret, 2004). *In vivo* embryonic manipulation of frog embryos to block the formation of the dorsal aorta endothelium, leads to failure of pancreatic gene and insulin expression. To assay blood vessel-pancreas interactions later in development, VEGF-A was overexpressed in transgenic mice using the pancreatic promoter, *Pdx1*; this leads to hypervascularisation of the pancreas and hyperplasia of the pancreatic islets (threefold increase in islet area), at the expense of acinar cell types. Further, coculture experiments with endoderm and dorsal aortic endothelium from early mouse embryos, result in pancreatic gene *Pdx1* induction and insulin expression, indicating that endothelial signals are sufficient for the pancreatic organogenesis program. A successive study on pancreatic organogenesis, has shown that aortal endothelial cells induce in the dorsal pancreatic endoderm the crucial pancreatic transcription factor Ptf1a, that has been shown to be necessary for the development of endocrine and duct cell lineages.

A two sep-model for islet development has been proposed (Konstantinova & Lammert, 2004): the first step involves signals from the endothelium to the pancreatic epithelium, the second involves signals in the opposite direction, with islets expressing VEGF-A at later stages of their development to attract capillaries. As for the molecular basis for such signals, recent studies indicate that β cells, by using VEGF-A attract endothelial cells, which form capillaries with a vascular basement membrane next to the β cells. In turn, laminins, amongst other vascular basement membrane proteins, regulate insulin gene expression and β cell proliferation; these effects require β_1 integrin on β cells (Nikolova et al., 2006).

Studies on β cell proliferation in humans are limited, but there is evidence that this process occurs at relatively high levels in the first 2 years of life, declining thereafter, with the possibility, at least in animals, of re-induction under conditions of insulin-resistance, such as pregnancy or obesity (Meier et al., 2008; Cnop et al., 2010). This suggests that β cell may retain an intrinsic capacity to replicate, and an increase of the islet vasculature has been observed in association with conditions of expanded islet mass (Mizuno et al., 1999; Like

1970; Predescu et al., 1998). Islet endothelium-derived hepatocyte growth factor (HGF) is one of the factors potentially involved in the stimulation of β cell proliferation (Suschek et al., 1994).

Also collagen IV and other basement membrane proteins, laminins, could potentiate insulin secretion, promote insulin gene expression and proliferation in β cells, via interaction with integrin $α_1β_1$ on β cell (Treutelaar et al., 2003; Kroncke et al., 1991).

These studies confirm the existence of an endothelial-endocrine axis within adult pancreatic islets.

3. Islet endothelium and type 1 diabetes

Islet endothelium forms the barrier across which autoreactive T cells transmigrate during the development of islet inflammation in autoimmune diabetes. Transendothelial migration and recruitment of autoreactive T cells into the pancreatic islets is a critical event during the development of chronic insulitis in type 1 diabetes. Transmigration is a complex, multistep process involving first selectins and their counter ligands that induce rolling of cells along the luminal surface of endothelial cells, followed by firm adhesion between cells and endothelium, and diapedesis (von Andrian & Mackay, 2000).

Several human and murine studies indicate that during autoimmune insulitis, the endothelial cells surrounding the inflamed islets adopt an activated phenotype, upregulate a variety of adhesion molecules, and are likely to be involved in regulating mononuclear cell accumulation (transmigration and homing) in the islets (Hanafusa et al., 1990; Hanninen et al., 1992; Hanninen et al., 1993; Itoh et al., 1993; Somoza et al.,1994). Activation of the islet endothelium may either initiate or enhance subsequent leukocyte infiltration of the islets. The islet endothelium is able to hyperexpress adhesion molecules, to secrete numerous cytochines and chemokines, and to hyperexpress class I and class II HLA molecules (Itoh et al., 1993; Somoza et al.,1994; Alejandro et al., 1982). Endothelial cells participate also in presentation of cognate antigens to T cells, which has potent effects on their migration in vitro and in vivo (Epperson & Pober, 1994; Marelli-Berg et al., 1999; Marelli-Berg et al., 2004; Pober et al., 2001) .

In particular, in humans, immunohistological studies of islets obtained near to the time of type 1 diabetes diagnosis, show abundant adhesion molecule expression on vessel and immune cells. In particular, bioptic studies showed that infiltrating mononuclear cells consisted of CD4[+] T, predominant CD8[+] T and B lymphocytes and macrophages, accompanied by increased expression class I and class II HLA antigens in endothelial cells (Itoh et al.,1993; Greening et al., 2003; Lozanoska-Ochser & Peakman, 2005). Pancreatic islet endothelial MHC class I hyperexpression has been observed also in NOD mice and the bio-breeding rat model of autoimmune diabetes (Kay et al., 1991; Ono et al., 1988), and represents a mechanism through which tissue-specific migration of T cells is refined and promoted.

In support to this, human islet endothelial cells have been shown *in vitro* to be capable of internalizing, processing and presenting to autoreactive CD4 T cell clones, disease-relevant epitopes of the islet autoantigen GAD65 (Greening et al., 2003; Di Lorenzo et al., 2007). This resulted in markedly enhanced transmigration.

Islet endothelial cells have also been shown to possess the necessary repertoire of the costimulatory molecules for adequate T cell activation. In vitro studies on the molecular interactions between generated human islet endothelial cells and autoreactive T cells, indicate that islet endothelial cells constitutively express the CD86 (B7-2) and ICOS-L, but not CD80 (B7-1) and CD40 costimulatory molecules. Such co-stimulatory molecules are capable of functionally co-stimulating CD4+ T cell activation, and to help activated memory (CD45R0+) CD4 T cells to migrate across the endothelial barrier (Lozanoska et al., 2008). These studies provide strong indication that islet endothelium actively participates in the recruitment of recently activated lymph node migrant autoreactive T cells. Blockade of the costimulation may represent a mode of *in vivo* action of intervention therapies that interfere with costimulation, such as CTLA-4 Ig (abatacept). Furthermore, analysis of the immunophenotype of endothelial cells, focusing on endothelial MHC class I molecule expression, in a range of different tissues and mouse strain, including the NOD mice, shows that MHC levels have a profound effect on activation, adhesion and transmigration of pathogenic, islet autoreactive CD8 T cells (Lozanoska-Ochser & Peakman, 2009). These finding have a direct relevance to the pathogenesis of autoimmune diabetes in the MOD mouse, and are in concert with those with Savinov et al. (Savinov et al., 2001) who demonstrated that homing of a diabetogenic insulin-specific CD8+ T cell clone was severely impaired when clone cells were infused in IFN-γ knock-out mice, despite normal adhesion to the microvasculature. More recently, the same authors showed that islet-specific homing of the same diabetogenic clone depends in part upon recognition of the cognate MHC/peptide complexes presented by pancreatic islet endothelial cells, which are presumed to acquire insulin from adjacent β cells (Savinov et al., 2003).

Based on these observations, it is proposed the model in which, during islet inflammation due to as-yet non-defined environmental insult (possibly a viral infection), cytokines and other inflammatory mediators, such as IFN-γ, are released and elicit activation of vascular endothelium. Endothelial activation leads to increased adhesion and extravasation of leukocytes. Further, insulin, to high level of which endothelial cells are chronically exposed, and islet antigens released by damaged β cells, may be taken up by activated endothelial cells, processed and presented to autoreactive T cells.

Furthermore, sustained and intermitted hyperglycemia has been shown to affect endothelial cellular survival and proliferation, including islet microendothelium (Favaro et al., 2008). Several metabolic mechanisms are involved, including oxidative stress, increased intracellular Ca^{++}, mitochondrial dysfunction, changes in intracellular fatty-acid metabolism, impaired tyrosine phosphorylation and activation of PI3K/Akt and ERK1/2 pathways and reduced intracellular cAMP and its target, the cAMP-dependent PKA pathways (Datta et al., 1999; Favaro et al., 2010). These multifunctional pathways transmit signals that result in prevention of apoptosis or induction of cell cycle progression, depending on the cell type and can cross-regulate one another (Stork & Schmitt, 2002). Akt signaling cascade has also a role in insulin-mediated glucose transport and pancreatic β-cell mass and function (Bernal-Mizrachi et al., 2004; Elghazi et al., 2006). Pro-survival Bcl-2 protein, which stabilizes the mitochondrial membrane and prevents the release of cytocrome c from the mitochondria and the activation of caspases (Choy et al., 2001), is also found to be down-regulated by high glucose in human islet microendothelial cells. In contrast, the pro-apoptotic member Bax, which antagonizes Bcl-2, is up-regulated (Favaro et al., 2010). It is noteworthy that over-expression of Bcl-2 in endothelial cells has been described to decrease T cell cytotoxicity, suggesting that this protein may also protect endothelial cells from apoptosis resulting from an immunological insult (Zheng et al., 2000).

Due to the established interdependent physical and functional relationship between islet endothelium and β cells, from pancreatic organogenesis to adult life (Zanone et al., 2008), and the notion that post-natal β -cell mass is dynamic and can increase in function and mass for added demand by replication or neogenesis, possibly through endothelial inductive signals (Nikolova et al., 2006; Johansson et al., 2006; Bonner-Weir & Sharma, 2002; Dor et al., 2004), these high glucose-induced changes in islet endothelium carry relevant consequences on β cells. In fact, production of the vasoactive mediator NO (Meier, 2008; Favaro et al., 2008) to upregulate CD40L expression in human islet microendetelial cells *in vitro* (Favaro et al., 2010). Functional CD40L is expressed on vascular endothelium (Mach et al., 1997) and contributes to B cell activation, isotype switching, costimulation in T cell mediated immunity, activation of extravasating monocytes (Yang & Wilson, 1996; Wagner et al., 2004), with an impact in atherosclerosis and in chronic inflammatory and autoimmune diseases. Blockers of the CD40L have been strikingly effective in animal models of autoimmune diseases, such as systemic lupus erythematosus and type 1 diabetes (Homann et al., 2002). Therefore, high glucose-induced overexpression of CD40L on islet endothelial cells might accelerate the targeting and loss of the remaining β-cell capacity during ongoing autoimmune insulitis.

In fact, production of the vasoactive mediator NO by islet endothelium (Meier, 2008; Favaro et al., 2008) is increased in hyperglycaemic conditions and has an established direct cytotoxicity on islets and potentially impairs insulin release (Corbett JA et al., 1993). Islet microendothelial cells also are source of the proinflammatory cytokine IL-1β under hyperglycaemic conditions, independently of any viral or immune-mediated process. IL-1β impairs insulin release in human islet, induces Fas expression enabling Fas-mediated apoptosis and it is implicated as a mediator of glucotoxicity (Maedler K, et al. 2002). The high glucose condition is also reported to upregulate CD40L expression in human islet microendothelial cells in vitro (Favaro E et al., 2010).

4. Enteroviruses and type 1 diabetes

Viral infection has been long implicated in the development of type 1 diabetes and evidences of a link between viral infections and initiation or acceleration of pancreatic islet autoimmunity have been under investigation for more than 30 years. Rubella virus (Karvonen et al., 1993), mumps virus (Hyoty et al., 1988), cytomegalovirus (Ward et a., 1979), rotavirus (Honeyman et al., 2000) and enteroviruses (EV) (Lonnrot et al., 2000; Stene et al., 2010) have all been suggested as environmental factors contributing to type 1 diabetes. EV, especially those of the Coxsackievirus B (CVB) group (Hyöty et al., 1988; Varela-Calvino & Peakman , 2003; Green et al., 2004), are historically the prime suspects as important aetiological determinants and seroepidemiological, histopathological, animal studies, and *in vitro* experiments have provided the strongest overall evidence for these viruses. The EV genus of the Picornaviridae family is a large group of human pathogens traditionally divided into polioviruses, coxsackieviruses, echoviruses and the new EV, and each group contains a range of serotypes (King et al., 2000; Roivainen, 2006). Human EV are the most common cause of viral infection in humans, are associated with a wide variety of clinical syndromes and have long been considered possible culprits of inflammatory conditions and immune-mediated pathological processes, such as chronic myocarditis, dilated cardiomyopathy and chronic myositis (Tam, 2006; Luppi et al., 2000). In the cardiac context, injury is caused by a direct cytopathic effect of the virus, an immune response to viral infection or autoimmunity triggered by the viral infection (Huber, 2006).

Several mechanisms, including molecular mimicry, bystander activation of autoreactive T cells, superantigenic activity of viral proteins, viral infection and persistence, not mutually exclusive, have been proposed to explain the relationship between EV infections and induction of autoimmune diseases (extensively reviewed in Varela-Calvino & Peakman, 2003; Ercolini & Miller, 2009).

As for a role in type 1 diabetes, results have been somewhat conflicting and not conclusive (von Herrath, 2009; Tauriainen et al., 2010). Autoantibodies to islet autoantigens are detected years prior to diagnosis of type 1 diabetes and prospective studies evaluating whether EV could predict islet autoimmunity have yielded conflicting results, with positive associations in the Finnish studies (Lönnrot et al., 2000; Salminen et al., 2003; Sadeharju et al., 2003), and no association in other reports (Graves et al., 2003; Füchtenbusch et al., 2001). Discrepancies could be related to the fact that in most studies the determination of EV infection was carried out indirectly through the determination of IgM and IgG anti-EV antibodies, while studies using multiple approaches to identify EV infection (serology, RT-PCR, faeces analysis) appear more likely to report an association with type 1 diabetes or islet autoimmunity. A higher frequency of EV RNA has been consistently shown in the serum of patients with diabetes compared to healthy control subjects, demonstrating a recent or a persistent infection (Lönnrot, M., Salminen, K., et al., 2000; Lönnrot, M., Korpela, K., et al., 2000), and in some of the cases the detection of EV RNA preceded the synthesis of islet cell autoantibodies. In most studies viruses of the CVB group, usually CVB3 and CVB4 were identified (Clements et al., 1995; Andréoletti et al., 1997; Chehadeh et al., 2000), in agreement with serological studies.

As for T cell responses to EV, studies are inconclusive. However, it has been shown that CD4 T cells from newly diagnosed patients up-regulate CD69 early activation marker after exposure to CVB4-infected lysates (Varela-Calvino et al., 2001) and produce more IFN-γ a pro-inflammatory cytokine generated by effector memory CD4 T cells, but show less T cell proliferation (Varela-Calvino & Peakman, 2003). Proliferation is dependent upon IL-2 secretion associated with central memory T cells. This implies that anti-CVB4 effector cells are mobilized from the central memory pool, which may be depleted. Response to CVB4 antigens at diabetes diagnosis appears thus to be active, indicating recent or prolonged exposure.

Results from animal models indicate that viral infections *per se* usually cannot initiate the autoimmune disease process leading to diabetes, but may accelerate an already ongoing disease process. Studies in various NOD mice strains show that EV infections may accelerate the progression to diabetes only if they occur after autoreactive T cells have been accumulated in the islets (Hiltunen et al.,1997; Lönnrot et al., 1998; Lönnrot et al., 2000; Otonkoski et al., 2000). CVB infection appears to accelerate the development of the disease via bystander activation of autoreactive T cells, due to inflammation of the pancreas, tissue damage, release of sequestered autoantigens in concert with production of pro-inflammatory cytokines, all leading to activation of autoreactive T cells, but apparently only when a certain threshold of these autoreactive T cells have already accumulated in the pancreas. Timing of a CVB infection, rather than its simple presence or absence, may thus have etiological implications for the development of type 1 diabetes.

A recent report evaluating whether such a general model of disease progression rather than initiation by EV applies to human type 1 diabetes (Stene et al., 2010), suggests that progression from islet autoimmunity to type 1 diabetes in high-risk individuals may increase after an EV infection characterised by the presence of viral RNA in blood. Indeed, most EV are avid triggers of production of pro-inflammatory cytokines by human leukocytes (Vreugdenhil et al., 2000), notably type I interferons, and it is noteworthy that increased levels of IFN-γ have been detected in the blood of newly diagnosed patients (Chehadeh et al., 2000), and EV RNA was detected in half of the IFN-α positive patients. These data are consistent with a recent EV infection.

4.1 Enteroviruses and pancreatic islets

Major determinants of the different clinicopathological manifestations of EV infections, ranging from silent infections to autoimmune diseases, are represented by the viral variants, the nature of the infection, acute, chronic or re-infection, and the distinct tissue tropism of the viral strain, modulated by the local expression of appropriate cellular receptors and coreceptors. The first step in viral infection is the attachment of the virus to its receptor, a cell surface molecule which viruses have adapted to use for their entry into the cells. These include the Coxsackie-Adenovirus receptor (CAR), integrin VLA-2, $\alpha_v\beta_3$, $\alpha_v\beta_5$, ICAM-1 and decay-accelerating factor (DAF) (Bergelson et al., 1997; Noutsias et al., 2001; Shafren, 1998). In cultured cells, CVB have been found to interact with at least three receptors. CAR is a 46kD adhesion molecule and all tested clinical and laboratory isolates bind to this receptor (Bergelson, 2002; Kallewaard et al., 2009). A large subset of CVB isolates also binds to DAF, a complement regulatory protein (Coyne & Bergelson, 2006) which appears to act as a receptor for cell attachment (Shafren et al., 1995), and some CVB3 isolates have been shown to use a third receptor, heparan sulfate, to infect CAR-deficient cells *in vitro* (Zautner et al., 2003).

These receptor molecules do not simply bind viruses, but may activate a series of events influencing the organ-specific outcome of disease (Ito et al., 2000; Selinka et al., 2004). CAR expression, for instance, is positively related to the extent of inflammation in the cardiac myosin-induced myocarditis model (Ito et al., 2000), and knockout of MyD88, an adaptor involved in toll-like receptor signaling, causes reduced cardiac expression of CAR and pro-inflammatory cytokines (Fuse et al., 2005) or TGF-β reduced CAR levels inhibit CVB3 infection of cardiac myocytes (Shi et al., 2010). CAR appears as the major receptor mediating CVB infection also in the pancreas *in vitro* and *in vivo*, since tissue-specific CAR gene deletion generated a 1000-fold reduction in virus titres within the pancreas during infection, and a significant reduction in virus-induced pancreatic tissue damage and inflammation (Kallewaard et al., 2009).

While acute infection in the pancreas has been clearly detected among the cells of the exocrine tissue, β cell infection by EV has been extensively studied and the issue of whether microvariants of EV can directly infect, replicate and persist in, and cause damage of β cells remains controversial (Flodstrom et al., 2002). More than three decade ago Yoon et al. showed that CVB4 is capable of replicating in cultured human islets (Yoon et al., 1978). Other works suggested that the CVB group has variants that can replicate in islet cells (Harting et al., 1983; Chatterjee et al.,1988), and by growing viruses on islets of Langerhans it is possible to isolate strains that can induce insulitis experimentally in animals and replicate in islet cells *in vivo*. Prototype CVB3, CVB4 and CVB5 as wells as CVA9 can replicate *in vitro* in purified insulin-producing β cells, and infection may result in functional impairment or cytolytic death of the β cells, but it may also have no apparent adverse effect (Roivainen et al., 2000; Roivainen et al., 2002). It appears that the consequences of the virus replication on β cell survival and function are not entirely dependent on the serotype but on a as-yet unidentified characteristics of the virus strain. For instance, between the diabetogenic strain E2 of CVB4 and the prototype CVB4, a 111 amino acid difference has been identified, and amino acids or nucleotides potentially most critical for the pathogenesis of type 1 diabetes have to be identified amongst the microvariants of relevant virus strains.

Another work (Chehadeh et al., 2000) indicates that the CVB group is capable to replicate at a low level in human islet cells *in vitro,* persisting without cytolytic effect. This replication is associated with chronic synthesis of IFN-α by the islet cells. Neutralization of the IFN-α leads to a rise in viral replication and rapid islet destruction.

Type I interferons induce an anti-viral state in infected cells, providing an early defense against viral infections (Stark et al., 1998), and it appears that β cells may depend on interferons to lower their permissiveness to CVB4 infection, thus regulating the susceptibility to virus-induced diabetes (Flodstrom et a., 2002; Flodstrom et al., 2003). In this model, NOD mice that expressed the suppressor of cytokine signalling 1 (SOCS-1) in β cells developed diabetes, due to the replication of the virus in the β cells. A critical link between the target β cell antiviral responses and susceptibility to disease is thus established.

Furthermore, due to its immunoregulatory properties, IFN-α represents a link between the innate and the adaptive immunity: a pathological event may commence with activation of the innate immune system in order to avoid cytolytic destruction, followed by T cell activation and expansion, including autoreactive T cells. Viral expansion of non–specific T cell responses has been shown to be mimicked by injection of IFN-α (Tough & Sprent, 1996), or IFN-α expression by pancreatic β cells (Stewart et al., 1993; Chakrabarti et al., 1996). In humans, IFN-α has been detected in β cells (Foulis et al., 1987; Huang et al., 1995) and in blood of type 1 diabetic patients (Chehadeh et al., 2000).

A very recent report, indicates that rare genetic variations occurring in the gene IFIH1 and affecting the expression and structure of its protein product IFIH, lower the risk of developing type 1 diabetes (Nejentsev et al., 2009). IFIH1 triggers the secretion of interferons. Another study showed that IFIH1 expression in peripheral blood cells is associated with type 1 diabetes (Liu et al., 2009). These data allows to speculate that, on viral infection, interferon-response genes are activated in insulin-producing cells, leading to increased levels of interferons. Interferons inhibit viral replication, but also enhance the expression of surface MHC-I molecules. Cytotoxic CD8 T cells recognize infected β cells, through the MHC-I molecules, damaging and eventually killing them. Thus, viral infection can contribute to the development of type 1 diabetes.

As for *in vivo* studies in humans, the isolation of an EV has been documented only few times. Historically, CVB4 was successfully cultured from the pancreas of a diabetic child at disease onset and it induced diabetes in susceptible animals, more than 30 years ago (Yoon et al., 1979). The diabetogenic E2 strain was likewise obtained by plaque purification of the human isolate Edwards of CVB4, that was isolated from a child with widespread CVB4 infection, presenting with acute myocarditis and pancreatitis (Chatterjee et al., 1988).

In contrast with the apparent success in the detection of EV mRNA from blood, no EV genome could be detected when pancreas from cases of type 1 diabetes were analysed post-mortem during the first year after diagnosis (Foulis et al., 1997). However, in the same study EV genome could be detected in the pancreas of children who died of acute myocarditis in which the heart was EV positive. These discrepancies may be explained with the argument that there is a critical window for virus detection in the pancreas, and this is only potentially achieved when there is an acute presentation of viral illness, as in the case of myocarditis. By *in situ* hybridisation studies on post-mortem pancreatic tissues of several type 1 diabetic patients, EV RNA positive cells were for the first time detected, and exclusively in islets (Ylipaasto et al., 2004).

In recent years, other studies have eventually indicated the presence of EV in pancreatic tissue in a sizable proportion of patients dying soon after diabetes onset (Tauriainen et al., 2009; Dotta et al., 2007; Richardson et al., 2009; Ylipaasto et al., 2004). A β cell infectious CVB4 was isolated in the pancreas of three patients at disease onset, by immunohistochemical, electron microscopy, genome nucleotide sequencing, cell culture and immunological studies (Dotta et al., 2007). Infection was specific to β cells, which showed islet inflammation mediated mainly by natural killer cells, reduced insulin secretion. The virus was also able to infect β cells from human islets of non diabetic donors.

A strain of echovirus 3 was isolated from an individual currently with appearance of islet cell and IA-2 autoantibodies (Williams at al., 2006). Richardson et al (Richardson et al., 2009) identified EV VP1 capsid protein in islets of 44 out of 72 recent-onset type 1 diabetic patients, and the staining was restricted to β cells. A recent report suggests that the virus is present in the intestinal mucosa of diabetic patients (Oikarinen et al., 2008).

These detection reports strengthen the case for a viral role in the pathogenesis of type 1 diabetes.

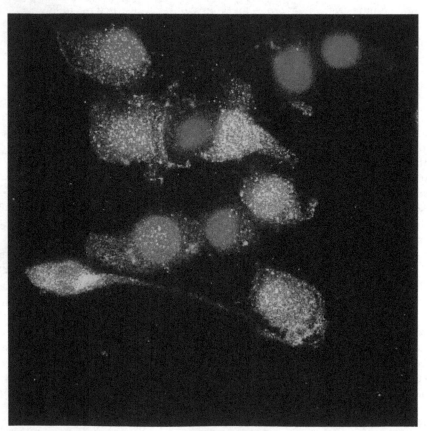

Fig. 3. Representative confocal immunofluorescence micrographs of islet MECs, stained with polyclonal anti-HCAR Ab, showing a diffuse expression in a fine punctate pattern in islet MECs (original magnification 630X, nuclei stained in blue with DAPI).

4.2 Coxsackievirus infection and endothelial cells

The host factors modulating viral infections include not only the host immune response, but also types and characteristics of cells that become infected in different tissues. Parenchymal cells of an organ are rarely in direct contact with the circulatory system, and viruses in the circulation must either circumvent or infect vascular endothelial cells to reach secondary organs. Vascular endothelial cells act in fact as important interface between the vascular space and the organ parenchyma, and, as previously stated, endothelial cells in different organs exhibit diverse structural and functional characteristics that can influence biological and pathological functions. Amongst these, vascular endothelial cells have an established role as mediators of tissue tropism and access for virus, influencing organ and tissue specific susceptibility to viral infection. Therefore, they can modulate the pathological expression of virus-induced diseases (Friedman et al., 1981; Huber et al., 1990; Conaldi et al., 1997; Zanone et al., 2003). For instance, in murine studies on CVB infectivity of different organs, CVB3 isolates from the heart showed greater infectivity and replication in heart endothelial cells than endothelial cells derived from liver or lung (Huber et al., 1990), thus confirming the essential role of host factors in developing specific diseases.

In line with this scenario, it is essential that, to gain access to secondary organs, viruses pass through the vascular endothelium by transcytosis or infection, or via infected circulating cells migrating into the target tissues. Endothelial cells derived from different organs show distinct susceptibility to CVB infections, and the behaviour against a viral challenge of endothelial cells in large vessels and microvessels may differ (Friedman et al., 1981; Huber et al., 1990; Conaldi et al., 1997; Zanone et al., 2003; Saijets et al., 2003). Endothelial cells expressing appropriate receptors would fail to act as effective barrier to infections, allowing viral particles to pass through, and replicate in, the vascular endothelium.

Human umbilical vein-derived endothelial cells have been shown to be persistently infected by different CVB strains (Flodstrom et al., 2000; Huber et al., 1990; Conaldi et al., 1997).

However, physiological and pathological events take place mainly at the level of the microvasculature. Using a dermal microvascular endothelial cell line, we have provided evidence that small vessel endothelial cells can harbour a persistent CVB viral infection (Zanone et al., 2003). All 3 CVB tested productively infected microvascular endothelial cells for up to 3 months without obvious cytolysis. A small proportion of the cells, approximately 10%, appeared to be involved in viral replication during chronic infection, suggesting that persistence is probably established through a mechanism of carrier-state culture, as proposed to explain CVB persistence in other cell types (Flodstrom et al., 2002; Greening et al., 2003). In addition, the infection increased production of proinflammatory cytokines IL-6 and IL-8, indicating endothelial cell activation by virus, and induced quantitative modification of adhesion molecule expression (ICAM-1, VCAM-1). These upregulation may influence the pattern of migration and extravasation of leucocytes in inflammation and immunity. These data add weight to the view that common CV infections are able to trigger complex pathophysiological processes, rather than simple cell lysis, as is becoming increasingly evident in clinical and experimental settings. These viruses can in fact persist for a considerable time in infected patients and cause chronic pathology or trigger immunopathological damage to infected and uninfected tissues (Muir et al., 1989; Stone, 1994). Furthermore, chronic infection of endothelial cells *in vivo* could provide better viral access to tissues underlying the endothelial layer and subsequent parenchymal cell infection.

The mechanisms of CVB persistence is not clear. It is possible that the infected cells undergo cytolysis and release virions to infect more cells, thus maintaining a chronic infection of the culture without massive cell destruction. Alternatively, it could be hypothesized that the cells can cure themselves of viruses, e.g. by limiting production of cell host products required for viral replication, or by production of anti-viral mediators. Stability of the cell membrane could also be another important factor in the ability of infected cells to survive infection, without lysis. In previous studies, the distinct susceptibility of different cell types to long-term infection has been related to the production of interferons (Conaldi et al., 1997; Heim et al., 1992).

It has also been suggested that the persistent infection of cultured HUVEC may be due to down-regulation of viral receptors in infected cells. However, a study indicates that the expression of the specific CVB receptor, CAR, in these cells was not quantitatively altered by infection with CVB but rather by culture confluence (Huber et al., 1990).

Human islet endothelial cells have been more recently shown to express the specific human Coxsackievirus and Adenovirus receptor (HCAR) (Figure 3) and CVB co-receptors, such as DAF, integrins and ICAM-1, that have differentiated functions on virus attachment and entry into target cells (Zanone et al., 2007). Islet endothelial cells can harbour a persistent, low level infection by CVB, assessed as detection of VP1 capsid protein and release of infectious particles. The infection has no obvious effects on cell morphology or viability and can provide better viral access to the underlying islet tissue. Under experimental conditions to avoid massive cytolysis and possibly to mimic silent *in vivo* infection, as EV infections can cause little or no clinical symptoms, only a proportion of cells appeared to be involved in viral replication, suggesting a mechanism of carrier-state culture (Conaldi et al., 1997; Zanone et al., 2003).

Notably, the infection of islet enodothelial cells upregulates the expression of DAF, HCAR and integrin $\alpha_v\beta_3$, in contrast to the behaviour of other macro- and microvascular endothelial cells lines, i.e. HUVEC, HMEC-1 and human aortic ECs. In fact, it has been shown that CVB infection downregulates DAF on HUVEC and HMEC-1 (Zanone et al., 2003), leaves HCAR expression unchanged on HUVEC (Carson et al., 1999), and downregulates HCAR expression and upregulates DAF expression on human aortic endothelial cells (Zanone et al., 2007).

This differential behaviour underlines the widely accepted heterogeneity of phenotype and function amongst endothelial cells derived from different vascular beds (Swerlick et al., 1992; Lidington et al., 1999), and may be relevant for the pathological sequelae of the infection. Despite detailed knowledge of the molecular structure and virus interaction of HCAR, its biological and possible pathogenic relevance are uncertain. HCAR belongs to the immunoglobulin superfamily and appears to have signalling functions (Bergelson et al., 1997; Noutsias et al., 2001; Fechner et al., 2003). Remarkably, CAR has been shown to be upregulated on affected cardiomyocytes in a rat model of experimental autoimmune myocarditis (Ito et al., 2000) and in human idiopatic dilated cardiomyopathy (Noutsias et al., 2001), for which EVs are the most frequently implicated pathogens (Feldman, 2000). CAR expression could therefore represent a key determinant of cardiac susceptibility to viral infections and have a pathogenic relevance in chronic cardiomyopathies. It has also been suggested that cell-to-cell contact modulates CAR-to-CAR interaction-based signals (Carson et al., 1999; Fechner et al., 2003).

The CVB infection upregulates in islet endothelial cells the expression of adhesion molecules and increases the production of proinflammatory cytokines and chemokines such as IL-1β, IL-6, IL-8 as well as IFN-α, once again pointing to endothelial cell activation (Zanone et al., 2007), in line with studies that suggest that a low-grade inflammation may cause profound impairments of endothelial function (Hingonari et al., 2000; Charakida et al., 2005).

In time course analyses, infected cells transiently upregulated expression of two major adhesion molecules, which may have *in vivo* functional consequences, enhancing cellular recruitment and leading to persistent tissue inflammation.

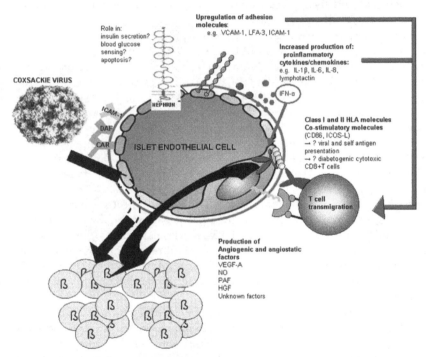

Fig. 4. Schematic representation of the relationship between Coxsackievirus infection, islet endothelial cells and β cells.

The highly fenestrated endothelial cells exhibit expression of classical endothelial markers, adhesion and co-stimulatory molecules, with the potential of being involved in autoreactive T cell adhesion, activation and transmigration in type 1 diabetes. They express specific markers, such as nephrin, whose functions at this site remain to be unravelled. Human islet endothelial cells express receptors and coreceptors for Coxsackievirus (such as HCAR, DAF, integrin and ICAM-1). These cells are potential target of an acute or persistent CVB infection, that activates the endothelium, upregulates expression of adhesion molecules, increases the production of proinflammatory cytokines and chemokines, and provides better viral access to tissues underlying the endothelial layer. Moreover, the increased production of IFN-α may enhance the expression of surface class I and II HLA molecules involved in viral and self antigen presentation, with selective recruitment and expansion of cytotoxic CD8+ T cells, which recognize infected endothelial and β cells, eventually damaging and killing them.

Infection also increased the production of pro-inflammatory cytokines, IL-1β, IL-6 and IL-8, further contributing to viral pathogenetic sequelae and to an indirect amplification of virus specific and non-specific responses. In this scenario, an exacerbated local inflammatory response secondary to viral infection represents an attempt to restrict virus replication, but it could promote chemoattraction and homing of circulating viral or, in susceptible individuals, islet antigen-specific T cells, in a bystander activation model (Horwitz et al., 1998). Cytokines may also be directly toxic to β cells, leading to release of sequestered antigens, presentation by professional dendritic cells, and activation of autoantigen-specific T cells. Endothelial cells themselves may serve as antigen-presenting cells (Greening et al., 2003; Savinov et al., 2003).

The infection was also accompanied by increased production of IFN-α, that has a role in initiation and maintenance of chronic CVB infection, as shown for other infected cell lines including islet β cells, and in line with the extensive studies documenting abnormal localization of IFN-α in the pancreas of type 1 diabetic patients (Chehadeh et al., 2000, Huber et al., 1990, Conaldi et al., 1997; Heim et al., 1992). As stated above, IFN-α may be responsible for a viral expansion of non–specific T cell responses, including autoreactive T cells.

Again, in dilated cardiomyopathy inflammatory endothelial activation is present, and endothelial CAM expression correlates with the intramyocardial counterreceptor-bearing lymphocyte infiltrates (Noutsias et al., 1999; Seko et al., 1993). In this model, it is likely that endothelial cells are infected before cardiotropic viruses invade the myocardium (Klingel et al., 1992).

An increased production of lymphotactin RNA by the infected cells is also reported. Lymphotactin is a chemokine with the ability to chemoattract highly specifically CD4+ and CD8+ T cells and NK cells (Kennedy et al., 1995; Hedrick et al., 1997), with possible anti-viral and anti-tumor effects. An inappropriate T cell infiltration, drawn by lymphotactin, is present in other inflammatory conditions (Middel et al., 2001; Blaschke et al., 2003), and lymphotactin exposed on infected islet endothelial cells could, therefore, play a role in islet infiltration by T cells.

The endothelium infection may thus contribute to selective recruitment and expansion of subsets of leukocytes during inflammatory immune responses in type 1 diabetes. These findings add to a body of work that highlights the possible role of human EVs as environmental triggers that are capable of influencing the incidence of type 1 diabetes, the susceptibility of which to environmental influences is well established.

5. Conclusion

There is a body of work that highlights the possible role of human EVs as environmental triggers that are capable of influencing the incidence of type 1 diabetes, the susceptibility of which to environmental influences is well established (Hyöty & Taylor, 2002; Varela-Calvino & Peakman, 2003). Vascular endothelial cells have a major role in viral tropism and disease pathogenesis. Islet endothelium appears to be endowed of distinctive structural and functional features, and is acquiring a role in type 1 and type 2 diabetes (Figure 4). An interaction between islet endothelium and an EV, CVB in particular, infection might trigger a series of pro-inflammatory events that could be important in islet inflammation and possibly influence the development of autoimmune diabetes, through the initiation or acceleration of islet autoimmunity in susceptible individuals.

6. References

Alejandro, R., Shienvold, F.L., Hajek, S.V., Ryan, U., Miller, J., & Mintz, D.H. (1982). Immunocytochemical localization of HLA-DR in human islets of Langerhans. *Diabetes*, Vol. 31 Suppl 4, pp 17-22, ISSN 1939-327X

Andréoletti, L., Hober, D., Hober-Vandenberghe, C., Belaich, S., Vantyghem, M.C., Lefebvre, J., & Wattré, P. (1997). Detection of coxsackie B virus RNA sequences in whole blood samples from adult patients at the onset of type I diabetes mellitus. *J Med Virol*, Vol. 52, pp 121-127, ISSN 1096-9071

Bergelson, J. M.,Cunningham, J. A., Droguett, G., Kurt-Jones, E. A., Krithivas, A., Hong, J. S., Horwitz, M. S., Crowell, R. L., & Finberg, R. W. (1997). Isolation of a common receptor for Coxsackie B viruses and Adenoviruses 2 and 5. *Science*, Vol. 275, pp 1320-1323, ISSN 1095-9203

Bernal-Mizrachi, E., Fatrai, S., Johnson, J.D., Ohsugi, M., Otani, K., Han, Z., Polonsky, K.S., & Permutt, M.A. (2004). Defective insulin secretion and increased susceptibility to experimental diabetes are induced by reduced Akt activity in pancreatic islet beta cells. *J Clin Invest*, Vol. 114, pp 928–936, ISSN 1558-8238

Bergelson, J.M. (2002). Receptors for coxsackieviruses and echoviruses. In: *Molecular Biology of Picornaviruses. Washington, DC: ASM Press*, Semler BL, Wimmer E, editors. pp 107–113, ISBN 1-55581-210-4

Biancone, L., Cantaluppi, V., Romanazzi, G.M., Russo, S., Figliolini, F., Beltramo, S., Scalabrino, E., Deregibus, M.C., Romagnoli, R., Franchello, A., Salizzoni, M., Perin, P.C., Ricordi, C., Segoloni, G.P., & Camussi, G. (2006). Platelet-activating factor synthesis and response on pancreatic islet endothelial cells: relevance for islet transplantation. *Transplantation*, Vol. 81, pp 511-518, ISSN 1534-0608

Blaschke, S., Middel, P., Dorner, B. G., Blaschke, V., Hummel, K. M., Kroczek, R. A., Reich, K. P., Benoehr, M., Koziolek, M., & Muller, G. A. (2003). Expression of activation-induced, T cell-derived, and chemokine-related cytokine/lymphotactin and its functional role in rheumatoid arthritis. *Arthritis Rheum.*, Vol. 48, pp 1858-1872, ISSN 1529-0131

Bonner-Weir, S., & Orci, L. (1982). New perspectives on the microvasculature of the islets of Langerhans in the rat. *Diabetes*, Vol. 31, pp 883-889, ISSN 1939-327X

Bonner-Weir, S. (2000). Perspective: Postnatal pancreatic beta cell growth. *Endocrinology*, Vol. 141, pp 1926-1929, ISSN 1945-7170

Bonner-Weir S, & Sharma A. (2002). Pancreatic stem cells. *J Pathol*, Vol. 197, pp 519–526, ISSN 0022-3417

Bonner-Weir, S., & Sharma, A. (2006). Are there pancreatic progenitor cells from which new islets form after birth? *Nat Clin Pract Endocrinol Metab.*, Vol. 2, pp 240-241, ISSN 1759-5029

Bonner-Weir, S. (1993) *The pancreas. Biology, pathobiology and disease. The microvasculature of the pancreas, with special emphasis on that of the islets of Langerhans. Anatomy and functional implications*, Go V.L.W., Dimagno E.P., Gardner J.D., Lebenthal E., Reber H.A., Scheele G.A., (Ed.), pp 759−768. Raven Press, New York.

Brissova, M., Shostak, A., Shiota, M., Wiebe, P.O., Poffenberger, G., Kantz, J., Chen, Z., Carr, C., Jerome, W.G., Chen, J., Baldwin, H., Nicholson, W. Bader, D., Jetton, T., Gannon, M., & Powers, A.C. (2006) Pancreatic islet production of vascular endothelial growth factor--a is essential for islet vascularization, revascularization, and function. Diabetes. Vol. 55, pp 2974-85, ISSN 1939-327X

Brunicardi, F.C., Stagner, J., Bonner-Weir, S., Wayland, H., Kleinman, R., Livingston, E., Guth, P., Menger, M., McCuskey, R., Intaglietta, M., Charles, A., Ashley, S., Cheung, A., Ipp, E., Gilman, S., Howard, T., & Passaro E. Jr. (1996). Microcirculation of the islets of Langerhans. *Diabetes*, Vol. 45, pp 385-392, ISSN 1939-327X

Carson, S. D., Hobbs, J. T., Tracy, S. M., & Chapman, N. M. (1999). Expression of the coxsackievirus and adenovirus receptor in cultured human umbilical vein endothelial cells: regulation in response to cell density. *J. Virol.*, Vol. 73, pp 7077-7079, ISSN 1098-5514

Chakrabarti, D., Hultgren, B., & Stewart, T. A. (1996). IFN-alpha induces autoimmune T cells through the induction of intracellular adhesion molecule-1 and B7.2. *J. Immunol*, Vol. 157, pp 522-528, ISSN 1550- 6606

Charakida, M., Donald, A. E., Terese, M., Leary, S., Halcox, J. P., Ness, A., Smith, G. D., Golding, J., Friberg, P., Klein, N. K., & Deanfield JE; ALSPAC (Avon Longitudinal Study of Parents and Children) Study Team. (2005). Endothelial dysfunction in childhood infection. *Circulation*, Vol. 111, pp 1660-1665, ISSN 0009-7322

Charo, I.F., Shak, S., Karasek, M.A., Davison, P., & Goldstein, I.M. (1984). Prostaglandin I2 is not a major metabolite of arachidonic acid in cultured endothelial cells from human foreskin microvessels. *J Clin Invest*, Vol. 7, pp 914–919, ISSN 1558-8238

Chatterjee, N.K., Nejman, C., & Gerling, I.. (1988). Purification and characterization of a strain of coxsackievirus B4 of human origin that induces diabetes in mice. *J Med Virol*, Vol. 26, pp 57-69, ISSN 1096-9071

Chehadeh, W., Kerr-Conte, J., Pattou, F., Alm, G., Lefebvre, J., Wattre, P., & Hober, D. (2000). Persistent infection of human pancreatic islets by coxsackievirus B is associated with alpha interferon synthesis in beta cells. *J Virol*, Vol. 74, pp 10153-10164, ISSN 1098-5514

Chehadeh, W., Weill, J., Vantyghem, M.C., Alm, G., Lefèbvre, J., Wattré, P., & Hober, D. (2000). Increased level of interferon-alpha in blood of patients with insulin-dependent diabetes mellitus: relationship with coxsackievirus B infection. *J Infect Dis*, Vol. 181, pp 1929-1939, ISSN 1344-6304

Choy, J.C., Granville, D.J., Hunt, D.W., & McManus, B.M. (2001). Endothelial cell apoptosis: biochemical characteristics and potential implications for atherosclerosis. *J Mol Cell Cardiol*, Vol. 33, pp 1673-1690, ISSN 0022-2828

Clements, G.B., Galbraith, D.N., & Taylor, K.W. (1995). Coxsackie B virus infection and onset of childhood diabetes. *Lancet*, Vol. 346, pp 221-223, ISSN 0140-6736

Cnop, M., Hughes, S.J., Igoillo-Esteve, M., Hoppa, M.B., Sayyed, F., van de Laar, L., Gunter, J.H., de Koning, E.J., Walls, G.V., Gray, D.W., Johnson, P.R., Hansen, B.C., Morris, J.F., Pipeleers-Marichal, M., Cnop, I., & Clark, A. (2009). The long lifespan and low turnover of human islet beta cells estimated by mathematical modelling of lipofuscin accumulation. *Diabetologia*, Vol. 53, pp 321-330, ISSN 0012-186X

Conaldi, P. G., Serra, C., Mossa, A., Falcone, V., Basolo, F., Camussi, G., Dolei, A., & Toniolo, A. (1997) Persistent infection of human vascular endothelial cells by Group B Coxsackieviruses. *J. Infect. Dis.*, Vol. 175, pp 693-696, ISSN 1344-6304

Corbett, J.A., Sweetland, M.A., Wang, J.L., Lancaster, J.R., & McDaniel. M.L. (1993). Nitric oxide mediates cytokine-induced inhibition of insulin secretion by human islets of Langerhans. *Proc Natl Acad Sci USA*, Vol. 90, pp 1731-1735, ISSN 0027-8424

Coyne, C.B., & Bergelson, J.M. (2006). Virus-induced Abl and Fyn kinase signals permit coxsackievirus entry through epithelial tight junctions. *Cell*, Vol. 124, pp 119-131, ISSN 0092-8674

D'Amore, P.A., & Ng, Y.S. (2002). Won't you be my neighbour? Local induction of arteriogenesis. *Cell*, Vol. 110, pp 289-292, ISSN 0092-8674

Datta, S.R., Brunet, A., & Greenberg, M.E. (1999). Cellular survival: a play in three Akts. *Genes Dev*, Vol. 13, pp 2905–2927, ISSN 1549-5477

Di Lorenzo, T.P., Peakman, M., & Roep, B.O. (2007). Translational mini-review series on type 1 diabetes: Systematic analysis of T cell epitopes in autoimmune diabetes. *Clin Exp Immunol*, Vol. 148, pp 1-16, ISSN 1365-2249

Dor, Y., Brown, J., Martinez, O.I., & Melton, D.A. (2004). Adult pancreatic beta-cells are formed by self-duplication rather than stem-cell differentiation. *Nature*, Vol. 429(6987), pp 41-46 ISSN 0028-0836

Dotta, F., Censini, S., van Halteren, A.G., Marselli, L., Masini, M., Dionisi, S., Mosca, F., Boggi, U., Muda, A.O., Del Prato, S., Elliott, J.F., Covacci, A., Rappuoli, R., Roep, B.O., & Marchetti, P. (2007). Coxsackie B4 virus infection of β cells and natural killer cell insulitis in recent-onset type 1 diabetic patients. *Proc Natl Acad Sci U S A*, Vol. 104, pp 5115–5120, ISSN 0027-8424

Elghazi, L., Balcazar, N., & Bernal-Mizrachi, E. (2006). Emerging role of protein kinase B/Akt signaling in pancreatic beta-cell mass and function. *Int J Biochem Cell Biol*, Vol. 38, pp 157–163, ISSN 1357-2725

Epperson, D.E., & Pober, J.S. (1994). Antigen-presenting function of human endothelial cells. Direct activation of resting CD8 T cells. *J Immunol*, Vol. 153, pp 5402-5412, ISSN 1550- 6606

Ercolini, A.M., & Miller, S.D. (2009). The role of infections in autoimmune disease. *Clin Exp Immunol*, Vol. 155, pp 1-15, ISSN 1365-2249

Favaro, E., Bottelli, A., Lozanoska-Ochser, B., Ferioli, E., Huang, G.C., Klein, N., Chiaravalli, A., Perin, P.C., Camussi, G., Peakman, M., Conaldi, P.G., & Zanone, M.M. (2005). Primary and immortalised human pancreatic islet endothelial cells: phenotypic and immunological characterisation. *Diabetologia*, Vol. 48, pp 2552-2562, ISSN ISSN 0012-186X

Favaro, E., Miceli, I., Bussolati, B., Schmitt-Ney, M., Cavallo Perin, P., Camussi, G., & Zanone, M.M. (2008). Hyperglycemia induces apoptosis of human pancreatic islet endothelial cells: effects of pravastatin on the Akt survival pathway. *Am J Pathol*, Vol. 173, pp 442-450, ISSN 0887-8005

Favaro, E. ,Miceli, I. , Settanni, F., Baragli, A., Granata, R., Camussi, G., Ghigo, E., Cavallo Perin, P., & Zanone, M.M. (2010). Obestatin and ghrelin bind to human pancreatic islet endothelial cells ad inhibit apoptosis in high glucose condition. *Diabetologia*, Vol. 53, [Suppl1]S1–S55, pp 14, ISSN 0012-186X

Fechner, H., Noutsias, M., Tschoepe, C., Hinze, K., Wang, X., Escher, F., Pauschinger, M., Dekkers, D., Vetter, R., Paul, M., Lamers, J., Schultheiss, H.P., & Poller, W.(2003). Induction of Coxsackievirus-adenovirus receptor expression during myocardial tissue formation and remodelling. *Circulation*, Vol. 107, pp 876-882, ISSN 0009-7322

Feldman, A. M. (2000). Medical progress: myocarditis. *N. Engl. J. Med.*, Vol. 343, pp 1388-1398, ISSN 1533-4406

Flickinger, B.D., & Olson, M.S. (1999). Localization of the platelet-activating factor receptor to rat pancreatic microvascular endothelial cells. *Am J Pathol*, Vol. 154, pp 1353-1358, ISSN 0887-8005

Folkman, J., Haudenschild, C., & Zetter, B.R. (1979). Long term culture of capillary endothelial cells. *Proc Natl Acad Sci USA*, Vol. 76, pp 5217, ISSN 0027-8424

Flodstrom, M., Maday, A., Balakrishna, D., Cleary, M. M., Yoshimura, A., & Sarvetnick., N. (2002). Target cell defense prevents the development of diabetes after viral infection. *Nat. Immunol*, Vol. 3, pp 373-382, ISSN 1529-2908

Flodström, M., Tsai, D., Fine, C., Maday, A., & Sarvetnick, N. (2003). Diabetogenic potential of human pathogens uncovered in experimentally permissive beta-cells. *Diabetes*, Vol. 52, pp 2025-2034, ISSN 1939-327X

Foulis, A.K., Farquharson, M.A., Meager, A. (1987). Immunoreactive alpha-interferon in insulin-secreting beta cells in type 1 diabetes mellitus. *Lancet*, Vol. 2, pp 1423-1427, ISSN 0140-6736

Foulis, A.K., McGill, M., Farquharson, M.A., & Hilton, D.A. (1997). A search for evidence of viral infection in pancreases of newly diagnosed patients with IDDM. *Diabetologia*, Vol. 40, pp 53-61, ISSN 0012-186X

Friedman, H.M., Macarak, E. J., MacGregor, R.R., Wolfe, J.A., & Kefalides, N.A. (1981) Virus infection of endothelial cells. *J. Infect. Dis.*, Vol. 143, pp 266-273, ISSN 1344-6304

Füchtenbusch, M., Irnstetter, A., Jäger, G., & Ziegler, A.G. (2001). No evidence for an association of Coxsackie virus infections during pregnancy and early childhood with development of islet autoantibodies in offspring of mothers or fathers with type 1 diabetes. *J Autoimmun*, Vol. 17, pp 333–340, ISSN 0896-8411

Fujimoto, T., & Singer, S.J. (1988). Immunochemical studies of endothelial cells in vivo: II. Chicken aortic and capillary endothelial cells exhibit different cell-surface distributions of the integrin complex. *J Histochem Cytochem*, Vol. 36, pp 1309–1317, ISSN 0022-1554

Fuse, K., Chan, G., Liu, Y., Gudgeon, P., Husain, M., Chen, M., Yeh, W.C., Akira, S., & Liu, P.P. (2005). Myeloid differentiation factor-88 plays a crucial role in the pathogenesis of Coxsackievirus B3-induced myocarditis and influences type I interferon production. *Circulation*, Vol. 112, pp 2276-2285, ISSN 0009-7322

Graves, P.M., Rotbart, H.A., Nix, W.A., Pallansch, M.A., Erlich, H.A., Norris, J.M., Hoffman, M., Eisenbarth, G.S., & Rewers, M. (2003). Prospective study of enteroviral infections and development of beta-cell autoimmunity: Diabetes Autoimmunity Study in the Young (DAISY). *Diabetes Res Clin Pract*, Vol. 59, pp 51–61, ISSN 0168-8227

Green, J., Casabonne, D., & Newton, R. (2004). Coxsackie B virus serology and Type 1 diabetes mellitus: a systematic review of published case-control studies. *Diabet Med*, Vol. 21, pp 507-514, ISSN 1464-5491

Greening, J.E., Tree, T.I., Kotowicz, K.T., van Halteren, A.G., Roep, B.O., Klein, N.J., & Peakman M. (2003). Processing and presentation of the islet autoantigen GAD by vascular endothelial cells promotes transmigration of autoreactive T-cells. *Diabetes*, Vol. 52, pp 717-725, ISSN 1939-327X

Hanafusa, T., Miyazaki, A., Miyagawa, J., Tamura, S., Inada, M., Yamada, K., Shinji, Y., Katsura, H., Yamagata, K., Itoh, N., & et al. (1990). Examination of islets in the pancreas biopsy specimens from newly diagnosed type 1 (insulin-dependent) diabetic patients. *Diabetologia*, Vol. 33, pp 105-111, ISSN 0012-186X

Hanninen, A., Jalkanen, S., Salmi, M., Toikkanen, S., Nikolakaros, G., & Simell, O. (1992). Macrophages, T cell receptor usage, and endothelial cell activation in the pancreas at the onset of insulin-dependent diabetes mellitus. *J Clin Invest*, Vol. 90, pp 1901-1910, ISSN 0021-9738

Hänninen, A., Salmi, M., Simell, O., & Jalkanen, S. (1993). Endothelial cell-binding properties of lymphocytes infiltrated into human diabetic pancreas. Implications for pathogenesis of IDDM. *Diabetes*, Vol. 42, pp 1656-1662, ISSN 1939-327X

Hartig, P.C., Madge, G.E., & Webb S.R. (1983). Diversity within a human isolate of coxsackie B4: relationship to viral-induced diabetes. *J Med Virol.*, Vol. 11, pp 23-30, ISSN 1096-9071

Hedrick, J. A., Saylor, V., Figueroa, D., Mizoue, L., Xu, Y., Menon, S., Abrams, J., Handel, T., & Zlotnik, A. (1997). Lymphotactin is produced by NK cells and attracts both NK cells and T cells in vivo. *J. Immunol.*, Vol. 158, pp 1533-1540, ISSN 1550- 6606

Heim, A., Canu, A., Kirschner, P., Simon, T., Mall, G., Hofschneider, P. H., & Kandolf, R. (1992). Synergistic interaction of interferon-beta and interferon-gamma in coxsackievirus B3-infected carrier cultures of human myocardial fibroblasts. *J. Infect. Dis.*, Vol. 166, pp 958-965, ISSN 1344-6304

Henningsson, R., Salehi, A., & Lundquist, I. (2002). Role of nitric oxide synthase isoforms in glucose-stimulated insulin release. *Am J Physiol Cell Physiol*, Vol. 283, pp 296-304, ISSN 1522-1563.

Henderson, J.R., & Moss, M.C. (1985). A morphometric study of the endocrine and exocrine capillaries of the pancreas. *Q J Exp Physiol*, Vol. 70, pp 347-356, ISSN 0144-8757

Hiltunen, M., Hyöty, H., Knip, M., Ilonen, J., Reijonen, H., Vähäsalo, P., Roivainen, M., Lonnrot, M., Leinikki, P., Hovi, T., & Akerblom H.K. (1997). Islet cell antibody seroconversion in children is temporally associated with enterovirus infections. *J Infect Dis*, Vol. 175, pp 554–560, ISSN 1344-6304

Hingorani, A.D., Cross, J.C., Kharbanda, R.K., Mullen, M.J., Bhagat, K., Taylor, M., Donald, A.E., Palacios, M., Griffin, G. E., Deanfield, J.E., MacAllister, R.J., & Vallance, P. (2000). Acute systemic inflammation impairs endothelium-dependent dilatation in humans. *Circulation*, Vol. 102, pp 994-999, ISSN 0009-7322

Homann, D., Jahreis, A., Wolfe, T., Hughes, A., Coon, B., van Stipdonk, M.J., Prilliman, K.R., Schoenberger, S.P., & von Herrath, M.G. (2002). CD40L blockade prevents autoimmune diabetes by induction of bitypic NK/DC regulatory cells. *Immunity* , Vol. 16, pp 403-415, ISSN 1074-7613

Honeyman, M.C., Coulson, B.S., Stone, N.L., Gellert, S.A., Goldwater, P.N., Steele, C.E., Couper, J.J., Tait, B.D., Colman, P.G., & Harrison, L.C. (2000). Association between rotavirus infection and pancreatic islet autoimmunity in children at risk of developing type 1 diabetes. *Diabetes*, Vol. 49, pp 1319-1324, ISSN 1939-327X

Horwitz, M. S., Bradley, L. M., Harbertson, J., Krahl, T., Lee, J., & Sarvetnick, N. (1998) Diabetes induced by Coxsackie virus: initiation by bystander damage and not molecular mimicry. *Nature Med.*, Vol. 4, pp 781-785, ISSN 1078-8956

Huang, X., Yuang, J., Goddard, A., Foulis, A., James, R. F., Lernmark, A., Pujol-Borrell, R., Rabinovitch, A., Somoza, N., & Stewart, T. A. (1995). Interferon expression in the pancreases of patients with type I diabetes. *Diabetes*, Vol. 44, pp 658-664, ISSN 1939-327X

Huber, S.A., Haisch, C., & Lodge, P. A. (1990) Functional diversity in vascular endothelial cells: role in Coxsackievirus tropism. *J. Virol.*, Vol. 64, pp 4516-4522, ISSN 1098-5514

Huber, S.A. (2006). Autoimmunity in coxsackievirus B3 induced myocarditis. *Autoimmunity*, Vol. 39, pp 55-61, ISSN 0891-6934

Huber, T.B., Hartleben, B., Kim, J., Schmidts, M., Schermer, B., Keil, A., Egger, L., Lecha, R.L., Borner, C., Pavenstädt, H., Shaw, A.S., Walz, G., & Benzing, T. (2003). Nephrin and CD2AP associate with phosphoinositide 3-OH kinase and stimulate AKT-dependent signaling. Mol Cell Biol., Vol. 23, pp 4917-28, ISSN 1098-5549

Hyöty, H., Leinikki, P., Reunanen, A., Ilonen, J., Surcel, H.M., Rilva, A., Käär, M.L., Huupponen, T., Hakulinen, A., Mäkelä, A.L., & et al. (1988). Mumps infections in the etiology of type 1 (insulin-dependent) diabetes. *Diabetes Res*, Vol. 9, pp 111-116, ISSN 0265-5985

Hyöty, H., & Taylor, K. W. (2002). The role of viruses in human diabetes. *Diabetologia*, Vol. 45, pp 1353-1361, ISSN 0012-186X

Itoh, N., Hanafusa, T., Miyazaki, A., Miyagawa, J., Yamagata, K., Yamamoto, K., Waguri, M., Imagawa, A., Tamura, S., Inada, M., & et al. (1993). Mononuclear cell infiltration and its relation to the expression of major histocompatibility complex antigens and adhesion molecules in pancreas biopsy specimens from newly diagnosed insulin-dependent diabetes mellitus patients. *J Clin Invest*, Vol. 92, pp 2313-2322, ISSN 0021-9738

Ito, M., Kodama, M., Masuko, M., Yamaura, M., Fuse, K., Uesugi, Y., Hirono, S., Okura, Y., Kato, K., Hotta, Y., Honda, T., Kuwano, R., & Aizawa, Y. (2000). Expression of coxsackievirus and adenovirus receptor in hearts of rats with experimental autoimmune myocarditis. *Circ Res*, Vol. 86, pp 275-280, ISSN 0009-7300

Johansson, M., Mattsson, G., Andersson, A., Jansson, L., & Carlsson, P.O. (2006). Islet endothelial cells and pancreatic beta-cell proliferation: studies in vitro and during pregnancy in adult rats. *Endocrinology*, Vol. 147, pp 2315-2324, ISSN 1945-7170

Jung, F., Haendeler, J., Goebel, C., Zeiher, A.M., & Dimmeler, S. (2000). Growth factor-induced phosphoinositide 3-OH kinase/Akt phosphorylation in smooth muscle cells: induction of cell proliferation and inhibition of cell death. *Cardiovasc Res*, Vol. 48, pp 148-157, ISSN 1755-3245

Kallewaard, N.L., Zhang, L., Chen, J.W., Guttenberg, M., Sanchez, M.D., & Bergelson, J.M. (2009). Tissue-specific deletion of the coxsackievirus and adenovirus receptor protects mice from virus-induced pancreatitis and myocarditis. *Cell Host Microbe*, Vol. 23;6, pp 91-98, ISSN 1931-3128

Karin, M., Liu, Z., & Zandi, E. (1997). AP-1 function and regulation. *Curr Opin Cell Biol*, Vol. 9, pp 240-246, ISSN 0955-0674

Karvonen, M., Tuomilehto, J., Libman, I., & LaPorte, R. (1993). A review of the recent epidemiological data on the worldwide incidence of type 1 (insulin-dependent) diabetes mellitus. World Health Organization DIAMOND Project Group. *Diabetologia*, Vol. 36, pp 883-892, ISSN 0012-186X

Kay, T.W., Campbell, I.L., Oxbrow, L., & Harrison, L.C. (1991). Overexpression of class I major histocompatibility complex accompanies insulitis in the non-obese diabetic mouse and is prevented by anti-interferon-gamma antibody. *Diabetologia*, Vol. 34, pp 779-785, ISSN 0012-186X

Kennedy, J., Kelner, G.S., Kleyensteuber, S., Schall, T.J., Weiss, M.C., Yssel, H., Schneider, P.V., Cocks, B.G., Bacon, K.B., & Zlotnik, A. (1995). Molecular cloning and functional characterization of human lymphotactin. *J. Immunol.*, Vol. 155, pp 203-209, ISSN 1550- 6606

King, A.M.Q. , Brown, F.,Christian, P., Hovi, T. ,Hyypiä, T., Knowles, N.J., & et al., (2002). *Family Picornaviridae.* In: M.H.V. Van Regenmortel, C.M. Fauquet, D.H.L. Bishop, C.H. Calisher and E.B. Carsten et al., Editors, Virus Taxonomy. Seventh Report of the International Committee for the Taxonomy of Viruses, Academic Press, New York, San Diego (2000), pp. 657–678.

Klingel, K., Hohenadl, C., Canu, A., Albrecht, M., Seemann, M., Mall, G., & Kandolf, R. (1992). Ongoing enterovirus-induced myocarditis is associated with persistent heart muscle infection: quantitative analysis of virus replication, tissue damage, and inflammation. *Proc. Natl. Acad. Sci. U. S. A.*, Vol. 89, pp 314-318, ISSN 0027-8424

Kolb, H., & Kolb-Bachofen, V. (1992). Nitric oxide: a pathogenetic factor in autoimmunity. *Immunol Today*, Vol. 13, pp 157-160, ISSN 0167-4919

Konstantinova, I., & Lammert, E. (2004). Microvascular development: learning from pancreatic islets. *Bioessays*, Vol. 26, pp 1069-1075, ISSN 1521-1878.

Kroncke, K.D., Kolb-Bachofen, V., Berschick, B., Burkart, V., & Kolb, H. (1991). Activated macrophages kill pancreatic syngeneic islet cells via arginine-dependent nitric oxide generation. *Biochem Biophys Res Commun*, Vol. 175, pp 752-758, ISSN 0006-291X

Kroncke, K.D., Rodriguez, M.L., Kolb, H., & Kolb-Bachofen, V. (1993). Cytotoxicity of activated rat macrophages against syngeneic islet cells is arginine-dependent, correlates with citrulline and nitrite concentrations and is identical to lysis by the nitric oxide donor nitroprusside. *Diabetologia*, Vol. 36, pp 17-24, ISSN 0012-186X

Kubota, Y., Kleinman, H., Martin, G.R., & Lawley, T.J. (1988). Role of laminin and basement in the differentiation of human endothelial cells into capillary-like structures. *J Cell Biol*, Vol. 107, pp 1589–1598, ISSN 1540-8140

Lammert, E., Cleaver, O., & Melton, D. (2001). Induction of pancreatic differentiation by signals from blood vessels. *Science*, Vol. 294, pp 564-567, ISSN 1095-9203

Lammert, E., Gu, G., McLaughlin, M., Brown D., Brekken, R., Murtaugh, L.C., Gerber, H.P., Ferrara, N., & Melton D.A. (2003). Role of VEGF-A in vascularization of pancreatic islets. *Curr Biol*, Vol. 13, pp 1070-1074, ISSN 0960-9822

Lee, K.H., Lawley, T.J., Xu, Y., & Swerlick, R.A. (1992). VCAM-1, ELAM-1, and ICAM-1 independent adhesion of melanoma cells to cultured human dermal microvascular endothelial cells. *J Invest Dermatol*, Vol. 98, pp 79, ISSN 0022-202X

Lidington, E.A., Moyes, D.L., McCormack, A.M., & Rose, M.L. (1999). A comparison of primary endothelial cells and endothelial cell lines for studies of immune interactions. *Transpl Immunol*, Vol. 7, pp 239–246, ISSN 0966-3274,

Like, A.A. (1970). The uptake of exogenous peroxidase by the beta cells of the islets of Langerhans. *Am J Pathol*, Vol. 59, pp 225-246, ISSN 0887-8005

Liu, S., Wang, H., Jin, Y., Podolsky, R., Reddy, M.V., Pedersen, J., Bode, B., Reed, J., Steed, D., Anderson, S., Yang, P., Muir, A., Steed, L., Hopkins, D., Huang, Y., Purohit, S., Wang, C.Y., Steck, A.K., Montemari, A., Eisenbarth, G., Rewers, M., & She, J.X. (2009). IFIH1 polymorphisms are significantly associated with type 1 diabetes and IFIH1 gene expression in peripheral blood mononuclear cells. *Hum Mol Genet*, Vol. 15;18, pp 358-365, ISSN 0964-6906

Lönnrot, M., Knip, M., Roivainen, M., Koskela, P., Åkerblom, H.K., & Hyöty, H. (1998). Onset of type I diabetes in infancy after enterovirus infections. *Diab Med*, Vol. 15, pp 431–434, ISSN 1464-5491.

Lönnrot, M., Salminen, K., Knip, M., Savola, K., Kulmala, P., Leinikki, P., Hyypiä, T., Åkerblom, H.K., & Hyöty, H. (2000). the Childhood Diabetes in Finland (DiMe) Study Group. Enterovirus RNA in serum is a risk factor for beta-cell autoimmunity and clinical type 1 diabetes: a prospective study. *J Med Virol*, Vol. 61, pp 214–220, ISSN 1096-9071

Lönnrot, M., Korpela, K., Knip, M., Ilonen, J., Simell, O., Korhonen, S., Savola, K., Muona, P., Simell, T., Koskela, P., & Hyöty, H. (2000). Enterovirus infection as a risk factor for beta-cell autoimmunity in a prospectively observed birth cohort: the Finnish Diabetes Prediction and Prevention Study. *Diabetes*, Vol. 49, pp 1314-1318, ISSN 1939-327X

Lozanoska-Ochser, B., & Peakman, M. (2005). CD86 on resting human islet endothelial cells co-stimulates CD4 T cell activation and facilitates T cell trans-endothelial migration in vitro. *Endocrine Journal*, Vol. 52 Suppl: 82, ISSN 0918-8959.

Luppi, P., Rudert, W. A., Zanone, M. M., Stassi, G., Trucco, G., Finegold, D., Boyle, G. J., del Nido, P., McGowan, F. X., & Trucco, M. (1998) Idiopathic dilated cardiomyopathy: a superantigen-driven autoimmune disease. *Circulation*, Vol. 98, pp 777-785, ISSN 0009-7322

Luppi, P., Zanone, M.M., Hyoty, H., Rudert, W.A., Haluszczak, C., Alexander, A.M., Bertera, S., Becker, D., & Trucco, M. (2000). Restricted TCR V beta gene expression and enterovirus infection in type I diabetes: a pilot study. *Diabetologia*, Vol. 43, pp 1484-1497, ISSN 0012-186X

Maedler, K., Sergeev, P., Ris, F., Oberholzer, J., Joller-Jemelka, H.I., Spinas, G.A., Kaiser, N., Halban, P.A. & Donath, M.Y. (2002). Glucose-induced beta cell production of IL-1beta contributes to glucotoxicity in human pancreatic islets. J Clin Invest , Vol. 110 pp 851-860, ISSN:0021-9738

Mach, F., Schönbeck, U., Sukhova, G.K., Bourcier, T., Bonnefoy, J.Y., Pober, J.S., & Libby, P. (1997). Functional CD40 ligand is expressed on human vascular endothelial cells, smooth muscle cells, and macrophages: implications for CD40-CD40 ligand signaling in atherosclerosis. *Proc Natl Acad Sci U S A* , Vol. 94, pp 1931-1936, ISSN 0027-8424

Marelli-Berg, F.M., Frasca, L., Weng, L., Lombardi, G., & Lechler, R.I. (1999). Antigen recognition influences transendothelial migration of CD4+ T cells. *J Immunol*, Vol. 162, pp 696-703, ISSN 1550- 6606

Marelli-Berg, F.M., James, M.J., Dangerfield, J., Dyson, J., Millrain, M., Scott, D., Simpson, E., Nourshargh, S., & Lechler, R.I. (2004). Cognate recognition of the endothelium induces HY-specific CD8+ T-lymphocyte transendothelial migration (diapedesis) in vivo. *Blood*, Vol. 103, pp 3111-3116, ISSN 1528-0020

Mattsson, G., Danielsson, A., Kriz, V., Carlsson, P.O., & Jansson, L. (2006). Endothelial cells in endogenous and transplanted pancreatic islets: differences in the expression of angiogenic peptides and receptors. *Pancreatology*, Vol. 6, pp 86-95, ISSN 1424-3911

Meier, J.J. (2008). Beta cell mass in diabetes: a realistic therapeutic target? *Diabetologia*, Vol. 51, pp 703-713, ISSN 0012-186X

Meier, J.J., Butler, A.E., Saisho, Y., Monchamp, T., Galasso, R., Bhushan, A., Rizza, R.A., Butler, & P.C. (2008). Beta-cell replication is the primary mechanism subserving the postnatal expansion of beta-cell mass in humans. *Diabetes*, Vol. 57, pp 1584-1594, ISSN 1939-327X

Middel, P., Thelen, P., Blaschke, S., Polzien, F., Reich, K., Blaschke, V., Wrede, A., Hummel, K.M., Gunawan, B., & Radzun, H.J. (2001). Expression of the T-cell chemoattractant chemokine lymphotactin in Crohn's disease. *Am. J. Pathol.*, Vol. 159, pp 1751-1761, ISSN 0887-8005

Mizuno, A., Noma, Y., Kuwajima, M., Murakami, T., Zhu, M., & Shima, K. (1999). Changes in islet capillary angioarchitecture coincide with impaired B-cell function but not with insulin resistance in male Otsuka-Long-Evans-Tokushima fatty rats: dimorphism of the diabetic phenotype at an advanced age. *Metabolism*, Vol. 48, pp 477-483, ISSN 1550-4131

Muir, P., Tizley, A.J., English, T. A.H., Nicholson, F., Signey, M., & Banatvala, J.E. (1989). Chronic relapsing pericarditis and dilated cardiomyopathy: serological evidence of persistent enterovirus infection. *Lancet*, Vol. 333, pp 804-807, ISSN 0140-6736.

Nejentsev, S., Walker, N., Riches, D., Egholm, M., & Todd, J.A. (2009). Rare variants of IFIH1, a gene implicated in antiviral responses, protect against type 1 diabetes. *Science*, Vol. 17; pp 387-389, ISSN 1095-9203

Nikolova, G., Jabs, N., Konstantinova, I., Domogatskaya, A., Tryggvason, K., Sorokin, L., Fässler, R., Gu, G., Gerber, H.P., Ferrara, N., Melton, D.A., & Lammert E (2006). The vascular basement membrane: a niche for insulin gene expression and Beta cell proliferation. *Dev Cell*, Vol. 10, pp 397-405, ISSN 1551-4005

Noutsias, M., Fechner, H., de Jonge, H., Wang, X., Dekkers, D., Houtsmuller, A.B., Pauschinger, M., Bergelson, J., Warraich, R., Yacoub, M., Hetzer, R., Lamers, J., Schultheiss, H.P., & Poller, W.(2001). Human coxsackie-adenovirus receptor is colocalized with integrins alpha(v) beta(3) and alpha(v) beta(5) on the cardiomyocyte sarcolemma and up-regulated in dilated cardiomyopathy: implications for cardiotropic viral infections. Circulation, Vol. 104, pp 275-280, ISSN 0009-7322

Noutsias, M., Seeberg, B., Schultheiss, H. P., & Kuhl, U. (1999). Expression of cell adhesion molecules in dilated cardiomyopathy: evidence for endothelial activation in inflammatory cardiomyopathy. *Circulation*, Vol. 99, pp 2124-2131, ISSN 0009-7322

Oikarinen, M., Tauriainen, S., Honkanen, T., Oikarinen, S., Vuori, K., Kaukinen, K., Rantala, I., Mäki, M., & Hyöty, H.(2008). Detection of enteroviruses in the intestine of type 1 diabetic patients. *Clin Exp Immunol*, Vol. 151, pp 71-75, ISSN 0009-9104

Ono, S.J., Issa-Chergui, B., Colle, E., Guttmann, R.D., Seemayer, T.A., & Fuks, A. (1988). IDDM in BB rats. Enhanced MHC class I heavy-chain gene expression in pancreatic islets. *Diabetes*, Vol. 37, pp 1411-1418, ISSN 1939-327X

Ostermann, G., Weber, K.S., Zernecke, A., Schroder, A., & Weber, C. (2002). JAM-1 is a ligand of the beta(2) integrin LFA-1 involved in transendothelial migration of leukocytes. *Nat Immunol*, Vol. 3, pp 151-8, ISSN 1529-2908

Otonkoski, T., Roivainen, M., Vaarala, O., & et al. (2000). Neonatal type I diabetes associated with maternal echovirus 6 infection: a case report. *Diabetologia*. 2000, Vol. 43, pp 1235–1238, ISSN 0012-186X

Petzelbauer, P., Bender, J.R., Wilson, J., & Pober, J.S. (1993). Heterogeneity of dermal microvascular endothelial cell antigen expression and cytokine responsiveness in situ and in cell culture. *J Immunol*, Vol. 151, pp 5062-5072, ISSN 1550- 6606

Pober, J.S., Kluger, M.S., & Schechner, J.S. (2001). Human endothelial cell presentation of antigen and the homing of memory/effector T cells to skin. *Ann N Y Acad Sci*, Vol. 941, pp 12-25, ISSN 0077-8923

Predescu, D., Predescu, S., McQuistan, T., & Palade, G.E. (1998). Transcytosis of alpha1-acidic glycoprotein in the continuous microvascular endothelium. *Proc Natl Acad Sci USA*, Vol. 95, pp 6175-6180, ISSN 0027-8424

Richardson, S.J., Willcox, A., Bone, A.J., Foulis, A.K., & Morgan, N.G. (2009). The prevalence of enteroviral capsid protein vp1 immunostaining in pancreatic islets in human type 1 diabetes. *Diabetologia*, Vol. 52, pp 1143–1151, ISSN 0012-186X

Roivainen, M., Rasilainen, S., Ylipaasto, P., Nissinen, R., Ustinov, J., Bouwens, L., Eizirik, D.L., Hovi, T., & Otonkoski, T.(2000). Mechanisms of coxsackievirus-induced damage to human pancreatic beta-cells. *J Clin Endocrinol Metab*, Vol. 85, pp 432-440, ISSN 1945-7197

Roivainen, M., Ylipaasto, P., Savolainen, C., Galama, J., Hovi, T., & Otonkoski, T. (2002). Functional impairment and killing of human beta cells by enteroviruses: the capacity is shared by a wide range of serotypes, but the extent is a characteristic of individual virus strains. *Diabetologia*, Vol. 45, pp 693-702, ISSN 0012-186X

Roivainen, M. (2006). Enteroviruses: new findings on the role of enteroviruses in type 1 diabetes. *Int J Biochem Cell Biol*, Vol. 38, pp 721-725, ISSN 1357-2725

Rose, N. R., Herskowitz, A., & Neumann, D. A. (1993) Autoimmunity in myocarditis: models and mechanisms. *Clin. Immunol. Immunopathol.*, Vol. 2, pp 95-99, ISSN 0090-1229

Ruotsalainen, V., Ljungberg, P., Wartiovaara, J. Lenkkeri, U., Kestilä, M., Jalanko, H., Holmberg, C., & Tryggvason, K. (1999). Nephrin is specifically located at the slit diaphragm of glomerular podocytes. *Proc Natl Acad Sci USA*, Vol. 96, pp 7962–7967, ISSN 0027-8424

Sadeharju, K., Hämäläinen, A.M., Knip, M., Lönnrot, M., Koskela, P., Virtanen, S.M., Ilonen, J., Åkerblom, H.K., & Hyöty, H. (2003). the Finnish TRIGR Study Group. Enterovirus infections as a risk factor for type I diabetes: virus analyses in a dietary intervention trial. *Clin Exp Immunol*, Vol. 132, pp 271–277, ISSN 0009-9104

Saijets, S., Ylipaasto, P., Vaarala, O., Hovi, T., & Roivainen, M. (2003) Enterovirus infection and activation of human umbilical vein endothelial cells. *J. Med. Virol.*, Vol. 70, pp 430-439, ISSN 1096-9071

Salminen, K., Sadeharju, K., Lönnrot, M., Vähäsalo, P., Kupila, A., Korhonen, S., Ilonen, J., Simell, O., Knip, M., & Hyöty, (2003). H. Enterovirus infections are associated with the induction of β-cell autoimmunity in a prospective birth cohort study. *J Med Virol*, Vol. 69, pp 91–98, ISSN 1096-9071

Savinov, A.Y., Wong, F.S., & Chervonsky, A.V. (2001). IFN-gamma affects homing of diabetogenic T cells. *J Immunol.*, Vol. 167, pp 6637-6643, ISSN 1550- 6606

Savinov, A.Y., Wong, F.S., Stonebraker, A.C., & Chervonsky, A.V. (2003). Presentation of antigen by endothelial cells and chemoattraction are required for homing of insulin-specific CD8+ T cells. *J Exp Med*, Vol. 197, pp 643-656, ISSN 1940-5901

Savinov, A.Y., Rozanov, D.V., & Strongin, A.Y. (2007). Specific inhibition of autoimmune T cell transmigration contributes to beta cell functionality and insulin synthesis in non-obese diabetic (NOD) mice. *J Biol Chem*, Vol. 282, pp 32106-32111, ISSN 1083-351X

Schmidt, H.H., Warner, T.D., Ishii, K., Sheng, H., & Murad, F. (1992). Insulin secretion from pancreatic B cells caused by L-arginine-derived nitrogen oxides. *Science*, Vol. 255, pp 721-723, ISSN 1095-9203

Seko, H., Matsuda, K., Kato, Y., Hashimoto, H., Yagita, K., Okumura, K., & Yasaki, Y. (1993). Expression of intercellular adhesion molecule 1 in murine hearts with acute myocarditis caused by coxsackievirus B3. *J. Clin. Invest.*, Vol. 91, pp 1327-1336, ISSN 0021-9738

Selinka, H. C., Wolde, A., Pasch, A., Klingel, K., Schnorr, J. J., Kupper, J. H., Lindberg, A. M., & Kandolf, R. (2004). Virus-receptor interactions of coxsackie B viruses and their putative influence on cardiotropism. *Med. Microbiol. Immunol*, Vol. 193, pp 127-131, ISSN 1432-1831

Shafren, D.R., Bates, R.C., Agrez, M.V., Herd, R.L., Burns, G.F., & Barry, R.D. (1995). Coxsackieviruses B1, B3, and B5 use decay accelerating factor as a receptor for cell attachment. *J Virol*, Vol. 69, pp 3873-3877, ISSN 1098-5514

Shafren, D. R. (1998). Viral cell entry induced by cross-linked decay-accelerating factor. J. Virol., Vol. 72, pp 9407-9412, ISSN 1098-5514

Shi, Y., Fukuoka, M., Li, G., Liu, Y., Chen, M., Konviser, M., Chen, X., Opavsky, M.A., & Liu, P.P. (2010). Regulatory T cells protect mice against coxsackievirus-induced myocarditis through the transforming growth factor beta-coxsackie-adenovirus receptor pathway. *Circulation*, Vol. 121, pp 2624-2634, ISSN 0009-7322

Somoza, N., Vargas, F., Roura-Mir, C., Vives-Pi, M., Fernández-Figueras, M.T., Ariza, A., Gomis, R., Bragado, R., Martí, M., Jaraquemada, D., & et al. (1994). Pancreas in recent onset insulin-dependent diabetes mellitus. Changes in HLA, adhesion molecules and autoantigens, restricted T cell receptor V beta usage, and cytokine profile. *J Immunol*, Vol. 153, pp 1360-1377, ISSN 1550- 6606

Southern, C., Schulster, D., & Green, I.C. (1990). Inhibition of insulin secretion by interleukin-1 beta and tumour necrosis factor-alpha via an L-arginine-dependent nitric oxide generating mechanism. *FEBS Lett*, Vol. 276, pp 42-44, ISSN

Stark, G.R., Kerr, I.M., Williams, B.R., Silverman, R.H., & Schreiber, R.D. (1988). How cells respond to interferons. *Annu Rev Biochem*, Vol. 67, pp 227-264, ISSN 0066-4154

Steiner, L., Kroncke, K., Fehsel, K., & Kolb-Bachofen, V. (1997). Endothelial cells as cytotoxic effector cells: cytokine-activated rat islet endothelial cells lyse syngeneic islet cells via nitric oxide. *Diabetologia*, Vol. 40, pp 150-155, ISSN 0012-186X

Stene, L.C., Oikarinen, S., Hyöty, H., Barriga, K.J., Norris, J.M., Klingensmith, G., Hutton, J.C., Erlich, H.A., Eisenbarth, G.S., & Rewers M. (2010). Enterovirus infection and progression from islet autoimmunity to type 1 diabetes: the Diabetes and

Autoimmunity Study in the Young (DAISY). *Diabetes*, Vol. 59, pp 3174-3180, ISSN 1939-327X

Stewart, T. A., Hultgren, B., Huang, X., Pitts-Meek, S., Hully, J., & MacLachlan, N. J. (1993). Induction of type I diabetes by interferon-alpha in transgenic mice. *Science*, Vol. 260, pp 1942-1946, ISSN 1095-9203

Stone, R. (1994). Post-polio syndrome: remembrance of virus past. *Science*, Vol. 264, pp 909, ISSN 1095-9203

Stork, P.J., & Schmitt, J.M. (2002). Crosstalk between cAMP and MAP kinase signaling in the regulation of cell proliferation. *Trends Cell Biol*, Vol. 12, pp 258-266, ISSN 0962-8924

Suschek, C., Fehsel, K., Kroncke, K.D., Sommer, A., & Kolb-Bachofen, V. (1994). Primary cultures of rat islet capillary endothelial cells. Constitutive and cytokine-inducible macrophagelike nitric oxide synthases are expressed and activities regulated by glucose concentration. *Am J Pathol*, Vol. 145, pp 685-695, ISSN 0887-8005

Swerlick, R.A., Garcia-Gonzalez, E., Kubota, Y., Xu, Y., & Lawley, T.J. (1991). Studies of the modulation of MHC antigen and cell adhesion molecule expression on human dermal microvascular endothelial cells. *J Invest Dermatol*, Vol. 97, pp 190–196, ISSN 0022-202X

Swerlick, R.A., Lee, K.H., Wick, T.M., & Lawley, T.J. (1992). Human dermal microvascular endothelial cells but not human umbilical vein endothelial cells express CD36 in vivo and in vitro. *J Immunol*, Vol. 148, pp 78–83, ISSN 1550- 6606

Swerlick, A.R., Lee, K.H., Li, L., Sepp, N.T., Wright Caughman, S., & Lawley T.J. (1992). Regulation of vascular cell adhesion molecule 1 on human dermal microendothelial cells. *J Immunol*, Vol. 149, pp 698-705, ISSN 1550- 6606

Takahashi, N., Kishimoto, T., Nemoto, T., Kadowaki, T., & Kasai, H. (2002). Fusion pore dynamics and insulin granule exocytosis in the pancreatic islet. *Science*, Vol. 297, pp 1349-1352, ISSN 1095-9203

Tam, P.E. (2006). Coxsackievirus myocarditis: interplay between virus and host in the pathogenesis of heart disease. *Viral Immunol*, Vol. 19, pp 133-146, ISSN 0882-8245

Tauriainen, S., Oikarinen, M., Keim, J., Oikarinen, S., & Hyöty, H. the nPOD Study Group. (2009). Detection of enterovirus in pancreatic tissues of cadaver organ donors: results from the Network for Pancreatic Organ Donors with Diabetes (nPOD) study. Abstract presented at the 10th International Congress of the Immunology of Diabetes Society, 17–20 May 2009, Malmö, Sweden

Tauriainen, S., Oikarinen, S., Oikarinen, M., & Hyöty, H. (2010). Enteroviruses in the pathogenesis of type 1 diabetes. Semin Immunopathol. 28 April 2010

Tough, D. F., & Sprent, J. (1996). Viruses and T cell turnover: evidence for bystander proliferation. *Immunol. Rev*, Vol. 150, pp 129-142, ISSN 1600-065X

Treutelaar, M.K., Skidmore, J.M., Dias-Leme, C.L., Hara, M., Zhang, L., Simeone, D., Martin, D.M., & Burant, C.F. (2003). Nestin-lineage cells contribute to the microvasculature but not endocrine cells of the islet. *Diabetes*, Vol. 52, pp 2503-2512, ISSN 1939-327X

Tryggvason, K., & Wartiovaara, J. (2001). Molecular basis of glomerular permselectivity. *Curr Opin Nephrol Hypertens*, Vol. 10, pp 543–549, ISSN 1062-4821

Varela-Calvino, R., Sgarbi, G., Wedderburn, L.R., Dayan, C.M., Tremble, J., & Peakman, M. (2001). T cell activation by coxsackievirus B4 antigens in type 1 diabetes mellitus: evidence for selective TCR Vbeta usage without superantigenic activity. *J Immunol*, Vol. 167, pp 3513-3520, ISSN 1550- 6606

Varela-Calvino, R., & Peakman, M. (2003). Enteroviruses and type 1 diabetes. *Diabetes Metab Res Rev*, Vol. 19, pp 431-441, ISSN 1520-7552

von Andrian U.H., & Mackay, C.R. (2000). T-cell function and migration. Two sides of the same coin. *N Engl J Med*, Vol. 343, pp 1020-1034, ISSN 1533-4406

von Herrath, M. (2009). Can we learn from viruses how to prevent type 1 diabetes? The role of viral infections in the pathogenesis of type 1 diabetes and the development of novel combination therapies. *Diabetes*, Vol. 58, pp 2–11, ISSN 1939-327X

Vreugdenhil, G.R., Wijnands, P.G., Netea, M.G., van der Meer, J.W., Melchers, W.J., & Galama, J.M. (2000). Enterovirus-induced production of pro-inflammatory and T-helper cytokines by human leukocytes. *Cytokine*, Vol. 12, pp 1793-1796, ISSN 1043-4666.

Wagner, A.H., Güldenzoph, B., Lienenlüke, B., & Hecker, M. (2004). CD154/CD40-mediated expression of CD154 in endothelial cells: consequences for endothelial cell-monocyte interaction. *Arterioscler Thromb Vasc Biol*, Vol. 24, pp 715-720, ISSN 1049-8834

Ward, K.P., & Galloway, W.H. (1979). Auchterlonie IA. Congenital cytomegalovirus infection and diabetes. *Lancet*, Vol. 1, pp 497, ISSN 0140-6736

Welsh, N., & Sandler, S. (1992). Interleukin-1 beta induces nitric oxide production and inhibits the activity of aconitase without decreasing glucose oxidation rates in isolated mouse pancreatic islets. *Biochem Biophys Res Commun*, Vol. 182, pp 333-340, ISSN 0006-291X

Williams, C.H., Oikarinen, S., Tauriainen, S., Salminen, K., Hyöty, H., & Stanway, G. (2006). Molecular analysis of an echovirus 3 strain isolated from an individual concurrently with appearance of islet cell and IA-2 autoantibodies. *J Clin Microbiol*, Vol. 44, pp 441-448, ISSN 1098-660X

Wucherpfennig, K. W. (2001) Mechanisms for the induction of autoimmunity by infectious agents. *J. Clin. Invest.*, Vol. 108, pp 1097-1104, ISSN 0021-9738.

Yang, Y., & Wilson, J.M. (1996). CD40 ligand-dependent T cell activation: requirement of B7-CD28 signaling through CD40. *Science*, Vol. 273, pp 1862-1864, ISSN 1095-9203

Ylipaasto, P., Klingel, K., Lindberg, A.M., Otonkoski, T., Kandolf, R., Hovi, T., & Roivainen, M. (2004). Enterovirus infection in human pancreatic islet cells, islet tropism in vivo and receptor involvement in cultured islet beta cells. *Diabetologia*, Vol. 47, pp 225–239, ISSN 0012-186X

Yoon, J.W., Onodera, T., & Notkins, A.L. (1978). Virus-induced diabetes mellitus. XV. Beta cell damage and insulin-dependent hyperglycemia in mice infected with coxsackie virus B4. *J Exp Med*, Vol. 148, pp 1068-1080, ISSN 1940-5901

Yoon, J.W., Austin, M., Onodera, T., & Notkins, A.L. (1979). Isolation of a virus from the pancreas of a child with diabetic ketoacidosis. *N Engl J Med*, Vol. 300, pp 1173-1179, ISSN 1553-2712

Yoshitomi, H., & Zaret, K.S. (2004). Endothelial cell interactions initiate dorsal pancreas development by selectively inducing the transcription factor Ptf1a. *Development*, Vol. 131, pp 807-817, ISSN 1011-6370.

Zanone, M. M., Favaro, E., Conaldi, P. G., Greening, J., Bottelli, A., Cavallo Perin, P., Klein, N. J., Peakman, M., & Camussi, G. (2003) Persistent infection of human microvascular endothelial cells by Coxsackie B viruses induces increased expression of adhesion molecules. *J. Immunol.*, Vol. 171, pp 438-446, ISSN 1550- 6606

Zanone, M.M., Favaro, E., Doublier, S., Lozanoska-Ochser, B., Deregibus, M.C., Greening, J., Huang, G.C., Klein, N., Cavallo Perin, P., Peakman, M., & Camussi, G. (2005). Expression of nephrin by human pancreatic islet endothelial cells. *Diabetologia*, Vol. 48, pp 1789-1797, ISSN 0012-186X

Zanone, M.M., Favaro, E., Ferioli, E., Huang, G.C., Klein, N.J., Perin, P.C., Peakman, M., Conaldi, P.G., & Camussi, G. (2007). Human pancreatic islet endothelial cells express Coxsackievirus and Adenovirus receptor and are activated by Coxsackie B virus infection. *Faseb J*, Vol. 21, pp 3308-3317, ISSN 1530-6860

Zanone, M.M., Favaro, E., & Camusi, G. From endothelial to beta cells: insights into pancreatic islet microendothelium. (2008). Curr Diabetes Rev. Vol 4 pp 1-9, ISSN: 1066-9442

Zautner, A.E., Körner, U., Henke, A., Badorff, C., & Schmidtke, M. (2003). Heparan sulfates and coxsackievirus-adenovirus receptor: each one mediates coxsackievirus B3 PD infection. *J Virol*, Vol. 77, pp 10071-10077, ISSN 1098-5514

Zheng, L., Dengler, T.J., Kluger, M.S., Madge, L.A., Schechner, J.S., Maher, S.E., Pober, J.S., & Bothwell, A.L. (2000). Cytoprotection of human umbilical vein endothelial cells against apoptosis and CTL-mediated lysis provided by caspase-resistant Bcl-2 without alterations in growth or activation responses. *J Immunol*, Vol. 164, pp 4665-4671, ISSN 1550- 6606

4

Type 1 Diabetes Mellitus and Co-Morbidities

Adriana Franzese, Enza Mozzillo, Rosa Nugnes,
Mariateresa Falco and Valentina Fattorusso
Department of Pediatrics, University Federico II of Naples
Italy

1. Introduction

Co-morbid conditions are relatively frequent in Type 1 Diabetes Mellitus (T1DM). They can severely affect clinical management of the disease, especially in pediatric age.
Furthermore, these conditions could present very interesting ethiopatogenetic mechanisms.

2. Associated autoimmune conditions

2.1 Genetic associations

Patients with type 1 diabetes (T1D) have an increased risk of other autoimmune conditions, such as autoimmune thyroid disease (AIT), celiac disease (CD), Addison's disease (AD) and vitiligo. These diseases are associated with organ-specific autoantibodies: AIT with thyroid peroxidase (TPO) and thyroglobulin autoantibodies (TG), CD with endomysial (EMA) and transglutaminase (TTG) autoantibodies, and AD with adrenal autoantibodies. Using these autoantibodies, organ-specific autoimmunity may be often detected before the development of clinical disease, in order to prevent significant morbidity related to unrecognized disease (Barker, 2006). The probable mechanism of these associations involves a shared genetic background (Myśliwiec et al., 2008; Smyth et al., 2008).
The majority of autoimmune endocrinopathies, including T1D, are inherited as complex genetic traits. Multiple genetic and environmental factors interact with each other to confer susceptibility to these disorders. Genetic risk factors associated with T1D, ATD, CD and AD include HLA genes and non-HLA genes.

2.1.1 HLA genes

The major histocompatibility complex (MHC) has been extensively studied in these diseases. HLA molecules are highly polymorphic and multiple different peptides can be presented to T cells by these molecules. In general it appears that the alleles associated with autoimmunity are not abnormal, but functional variants, that aid in determining specific targets of autoimmunity. The leading hypothesis is that these molecules contribute to determine risk through the peptides they bind and present to T-lymphocytes, either by influencing thymic selection, or peripheral antigen presentation. (Ide & Eisenbarth, 2003).
HLA DR4 and DR3 are strongly associated with T1D and approximately 30-50% of patients are DR3/DR4 heterozygotes. The DR3/DR4 genotype confers the highest diabetes risk with a synergistic mode of action, followed by DR4 and DR3 homozygosity, respectively. The

HLA-DQ (particularly DQ 2 and DQ8) locus has been found to be the most important determinant of diabetes susceptibility. Approximately 90% of individuals with T1D have either DQ2 or DQ8, compared to 40% of the general population (Ide & Eisenbarth, 2003). So, the highest-risk human leukocyte antigen (HLA) genotype for T1D is DR3-DQ2, DR4-DQ8. DR3-DQ2 shows a strong association with CD; homozygosity for DR3-DQ2 in a population with T1D carries a 33% risk for the presence of TTG autoantibodies (Bao et al., 1999). Moreover, in families with multiple members affected with T1D and AIT, DR3-DQ2 has been linked with AIT and T1D (Levin et al, 2004). AD has been associated with the presence of a rare subtype of DR3-DQ2, DR4-DQ8 in which the DR4 subtype is DRB1*0404. This subtype is found in less than 1% of the general population compared with 30% of the population with AD (Barker et al., 2005; Myhre et al., 2002; Yu et al., 1999). A schematic representation of the HLA region and its association with T1D is shown in the Figure 1.

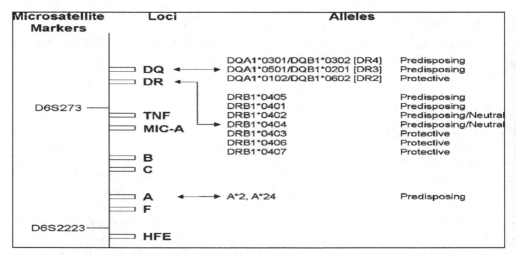

(from Pugliese A. and Eisenbarth G.S., Chapter 7, Type 1 Diabetes: Molecular, Cellular, and Clinical Immunology, www.barbaradaviscenter.org)

Fig. 1. The HLA Region and T1D susceptibility. Schematic representation of the HLA region showing microsatellite markers, loci, and alleles associated with T1D susceptibility. Distances between loci are grossly approximated.

2.1.2 Non-HLA genes

Non-HLA genes are also involved in the predisposition to T1D and other autoimmune diseases, such as MIC-A, PTPN22, CTLA-4 (Barker, 2006).

Polymorphisms of MIC-A (MHC I-related gene A) have been associated with T1D, CD and AD. This gene encodes for a protein that is expressed in the thymus and interacts with the receptor NKG2D, which is important for thymic maturation of T cells (Hue et al., 2003). It is hypothesized that the loss of this interaction is a way in which immunological tolerance may be lost. NKG2D also regulates the priming of human naïve CD8+ T cells, providing an alternative explanation for associations with autoimmune diseases (Maasho et al., 2005).

The PTPN22 gene is expressed in T cells and encodes lymphoid tyrosine phosphatase (LYP). LYP appears to be important in the signal cascade downstream from the T-cell receptor. A specific polymorphism, changing an arginine to tryptophan at position 620, has been associated with T1D (Bottini et al., 2004; Smyth et al., 2004) and also other autoimmune disorders, such as rheumatoid arthritis, systemic lupus erythematosus, Graves' disease and weakly with AD. The association with many autoimmune diseases suggests that this gene may be playing a role in susceptibility to autoimmunity in general.

Another non-HLA gene associated with T1D which has a generic role in susceptibility to autoimmunity is CTLA-4 (Cytotoxic T lymphocyte-associated antigen-4) (Vaidya & Pearce, 2004). CTLA-4 gene is an important susceptibility locus for autoimmune endocrinopathies and other autoimmune disorders, including T1D (Ueda et al., 2003). The CTLA-4 gene, which is located on chromosome 2, encodes a costimulatory molecule that is expressed on the surface of activated T cells. It plays a critical role in the T-cell response to antigen presentation, binding costimulatory molecules and inhibiting T-cell activation. (Vaidya & Pearce, 2004). The inhibitory effect of CTLA-4 on T-cell activation has led the investigations into its role in different human autoimmune disorders. Polymorphisms within the CTLA-4 gene have been linked to AIT (Vaidya et al., 1999). CTLA-4 has also been linked to AD and more strongly to subjects affected by AD in association with T1D and AIT compared with AD alone (Vaidya et al., 2000). CTLA-4 has been associated with a wide range of other autoimmune disorders, including primary biliary cirrhosis, multiple sclerosis, CD and rheumatoid arthritis. These observations have suggested that CTLA-4 is a general autoimmune locus, and that the susceptibility polymorphisms within the gene may lead to general defects in the immune regulation, while other tissue-specific (e.g. insulin gene polymorphisms) or antigen-specific (e.g. MHC) genetic factors and environmental factors determine the involvement of particular target organs (Vaidya & Pearce, 2004).

Gene	Associated diseases
MIC-A	T1D, CD, AD
PTPN22	AIT, AD
CTLA-4	T1D, AIT

Table 1. Non-HLA genes associated with T1D and other autoimmune diseases

2.2 Type 1 diabetes and celiac disease
2.2.1 Prevalence and age at starting
Traditional studies, both in children and adults, have shown that CD occurs in patients with T1D with a prevalence that varies from 1,5 to 10 % compared with 0.5 % of the general population (Cronin & Shanahan, 2007; Vaarala, 2000). The mean age at diagnosis of classical CD is commonly around 2-3 years, while the mean age at diagnosis of DM1 is 7-8 years. The age at onset of T1D is younger in patients with the double disease than in those with only T1D (Kaspers et al., 2004). The risk of CD is negatively and independently associated with age at onset of diabetes, with an higher risk being seen in children age < 4 years than in those age > 9 years (Cerutti et al., 2004). In patients with T1D, diabetes is usually diagnosed first, CD precedes diabetes onset only in 10-25% (Cerutti et al., 2004; Valerio et al., 2002), while generally CD diagnosis in T1D patients occurs, trough the screening performed at diabetes onset, in 70-80% of patients with a median age >8 years. Some authors hypothized that in genetically susceptible patients one disease could predispose to another. Particularly, it has been suggested that untreated (latent or silent) CD could be an immunological trigger and induce diabetes and/or thyroid disorders due to gluten as a driving antigen (Pocecco &

Ventura, 1995). In accordance with this, the prevalence of autoimmune disorders in CD is closely related to age at diagnosis or, in other words, to the duration of exposure to gluten (Ventura et al., 1999) and thyroid-related antibodies tend to disappear during twelve months of gluten-free diet, like CD-related antibodies (Ventura et al., 2000). However, at present, it is unknown whether treatment of CD reduces the likelihood of developing autoimmune disorders, or changes their natural history and actually others found no correlation between duration of gluten exposure in adult CD and risk of autoimmune disorders (Viljamaa et al., 2005).

2.2.2 Clinical features and follow up

The classic presentation of CD describes symptoms related to gastrointestinal malabsorption and includes malnutrition, failure to thrive, diarrhea, anorexia, constipation, vomiting, abdominal distension, and pain. This predominance of gastrointestinal symptoms is more common in children younger than three years of age. Non-gastrointestinal or atypical symptoms of CD include short stature, pubertal delay, fatigue, vitamin deficiencies, and iron deficiency anemia and are more commonly observed in older children. The classical presentation of CD can occur in T1D patients, but many patients with CD and T1D are either asymptomatic (silent CD) or present with only mild symptoms (Holmes, 2001a; Ventura et al., 2000). Diagnosis of CD is regularly performed because screening protocols are universally recommended and performed. In patients with overt CD, identifying and treating CD with gluten free diet (GFD) surely confer benefit in reducing complications such as malabsorption, infertility, osteoporosis, poor nutrition, impaired growth and reducing long-term malignancy risks and mortality rates (Collin et al., 2002; Freemark & Levitsky, 2003; Rubio-Tapia et al., 2009), while no evidence exists on long-term morbidity in silent CD. Similarly, children with T1D with evidence of symptomatic CD benefit from GFD (Hansen et al., 2006; Saadah et al., 2004); in symptom-free cases the demonstrated benefit is limited to weight gain and bone mineral density (BMD) changes.(Artz et al., 2008; Rami et al., 2005; Simmons et al., 2007). Recently a 2-year prospective follow up study has provided additional evidence that only in some of the children with T1D and few classical symptoms of CD, identified by screening as being TG+ present, the demonstrated benefit of GFD is limited to weight gain and BMD changes (Simmons et al., 2011); moreover, other authors have reported an improved glycemic control in GFD-compliant celiac patients (Sanchez-Albisua et al., 2005). On the contrary, silent untreated CD has no obvious effect on metabolic control in T1D patients, but could negatively influence weight gain (Rami et al., 2005). In any case, the adherence to GFD by children with T1D has been reported generally below 50% (Acerini et al., 1998; Crone et al., 2003; Hansen et al., 2006; Saadah et al., 2004, Westman et al., 1999). The different viewpoints highlight the need of a long follow up of patients affected by T1D and asymptomatic CD to clarify the role of a GFD. Actually some authors argument against the need to stress GFD in nonsymptomatic T1D patients (Franzese et al., 2007; Van Koppen et al., 2009). However, the wide spectrum of CD include also subjects with positive celiac-related antibodies without diagnostic small-bowel mucosal villous atrophy. This condition is defined as potential celiac disease (pot-CD) (Holmes, 2001b; Paparo et al., 2005; Troncone et al., 1996). Some authors described that the prevalence of pot-CD among patients with T1D recruited from the majority of childhood diabetes care centers in Italy is 12.2 %, with an higher prevalence of females. The prevalence of pot-CD in the CD control population is 8.4 % (Franzese et al., 2011). Case reports and small follow-up studies indicated that only few pot-CD patients may suffer from CD-related symptoms before the development of villous atrophy (Troncone et al., 1996). No definite consensus exists among experts about to treat pot-CD patients with GFD. No data are available on the natural history of these patients in the long term, nor on the risks they are exposed if left on normal gluten-containing diet, while a recent paper provided evidence that pot-CD children may benefit from GFD treatment (Kurppa et al., 2010).

Other studies have shown intestinal inflammation also in T1D patients without CD-related antibodies and structurally normal intestinal mucosa (Westerholm-Ormio et al., 2003). According to this, our group has observed a gluten-related inflammation either in rectal either in small bowel mucosa of children with T1D (Maglio et al,. 2009; Troncone et al., 2003). It can be speculated that gluten could be an optimal candidate to stimulate an abnormal innate immune reaction in intestinal mucosa due to its pro-inflammatory characteristics. It remains a crucial issue to estabilish to what the extented intestinal inflammation in T1D is gluten-dependent and whether it precedes the occurrence of the disease.

2.3 Type 1 diabetes and autoimmune thyroid disease
2.3.1 Prevalence and age at starting
Antithyroid antibodies have been shown to occur during the first years of diabetes in 11-16.9% of individuals with T1D (Kordonouri et al., 2002). Long-term follow up suggests that as much as 30 % of patients with T1D develop AIT (Umpierrez et al., 2003). The range of prevalence of AIT in patients with T1D is unusually wide (3.4-50%) (Burek et al., 1990; Radetti et al., 1995). Thyroid antibodies are observed more frequently in girls than in boys, often emerging along during pubertal maturation (Kordonouri et al., 2005).

2.3.2 Clinical features and follow-up
Hyperthyroidism is less common than hypothyroidism in association with T1D (Umpierrez et al., 2003), but still more common than in the general population. It may be due to Grave's disease or the hyperthyroid phase of Hashimoto's thyroiditis. The presence of abnormal thyroid function related to AIT in the population with T1D has the potential to affect growth, weight gain, diabetes control, menstrual regularity, and overall well-being. In particular clinical features of hypothyroidism may include the presence of a painless goitre, increased weight gain, retarded growth, tiredness, lethargy, cold intolerance and bradycardia while diabetic control may not be significantly affected. Clinical features of hyperthyroidism may include unexplained difficulty in maintaining glycaemic control, weight loss without loss of appetite, agitation, tachycardia, tremor, heat intolerance, thyroid enlargement or characteristic eye signs. The treatment of hypothyroidism is based on replacement with oral L-thyroxine (T4) sufficient to normalise TSH levels and usually this allows regression of the goitre if present. The treatment of hyperthyroidism is based on the use of carbimazole and beta-adrenergic blocking drugs, if necessary.

There are studies showing worse diabetes control in patients with a second autoimmunity, including AIT and CD (Franzese et al., 2000; Iafusco et al., 1998). The factors responsible for the worsened control have not been completely elucidated. Thyroid dysfunction could be responsible of variations in absorption of carbohydrates and increased insulin resistance. There are studies showing similar diabetes control in patients with and without a second autoimmunity, in these studies thyroid autoimmunity does not lead to worsening of diabetic metabolic control in children with T1D (Kordonouri et al., 2002; Rami et al., 2005; Sumnik et al., 2006). The thyroid status is not different between diabetic patients with and without CD: children with both T1D and CD do not have an increased risk of AIT development compared to diabetic patients without CD (Sumnik et al., 2006).

2.4 Type 1 diabetes, Addison disease and polyglandular syndromes
2.4.1 Prevalence and age at starting
Addison's disease (AD) affects approximately 1 in 10,000 of the general population. The autoimmune process resulting in AD can be identified by the detection of autoantibodies against the adrenal cortex (Anderson et al., 1957; Lovas & Husebye, 2002). Up 2 % of patients with T1D have antiadrenal autoantibodies (De Block et al.; 2001, Falorni et al., 1997; Peterson et al., 1997).

AD is occasionally associated with T1D in the Autoimmune Polyglandular Syndromes (APS I and II). APS I, also known as autoimmune polyendocrinopathy candidiasis ectodermal dysplasia (APECED), is a rare polyendocrine autoimmune disease caused by mutations of the autoimmune regulator gene (AIRE) on chromosome 21q22.3 (Aaltonen et al., 1994; Ahonen et al., 1990), which is characterized by the association of mucocutaneous candidiasis, adrenal insufficiency, and/or hypoparathyroidism. Follow-up of subjects with this disorder has revealed that many organ systems may be involved in the autoimmune process including the pancreatic β cell. Approximately 20% of subjects with APS-I develop T1D (Barker, 2006). APS II is more common in adults, but is also observed in children in association with autoimmune thyroiditis (Dittmar & Kahaly, 2003). Other less common disorders observed in APSII include Addison's disease, hypogonadism, vitiligo, alopecia, pernicious anemia and myasthenia gravis. Another rare disorder associated with T1D in early childhood is the Immunodysregulation Polyendocrinopathy X-linked Syndrome (IPEX), which is characterized also by severe enteropathy and autoimmune symptoms due to a clear genetic defect (FOX-P3) (Chatila et al., 2000). FOX-P3 is expressed in CD4+CD25+ regulatory T cells; mutations result in the inability to generate these regulatory T cells resulting in multiorgan autoimmunity (Barker, 2006).

2.4.2 Clinical features and follow-up
The condition of AD is suspected by the clinical picture of frequent hypoglycaemia, unexplained decrease in insulin requirements, increased skin pigmentation, lassitude, weight loss, hyponatraemia and hyperkalaemia. The diagnosis is based on the demonstration of a low cortisol, especially in response to ACTH test. Treatment with a glucocorticoid is urgent and life-threatening. In some cases the therapy has to be supplemented with a mineralocorticoid. In asymptomatic children with positive adrenal antibodies, detected on routine screening, a rising ACTH level suggests a failing adrenal cortex and the development of primary adrenal insufficiency (Kordonouri et al., 2009). There are no current recommendations for screening of adrenal autoimmunity.

2.5 Type 1 diabetes and vitiligo
Vitiligo is an acquired pigmentary disorder characterized by a loss of melanocytes resulting in white spots or leukoderma. The association of vitiligo with other autoimmune disorders, including thyroid disease, adrenal insufficiency, gonadal dysfunction, polyendocrine failure, diabetes mellitus, pernicious anemia, myasthenia gravis and alopecia areata, has been well documented (Bystryn, 1997; Handa & Dogra, 2003). This condition is present in about 6% of diabetic children (Hanas et al., 2009). Spontaneous re-pigmentation is rare and

not usually cosmetically acceptable. Treatment is difficult and multiple therapies have been tried with little success . (Ho et al., 2011)

2.6 Type 1 diabetes and collagenopathies
2.6.1 Rheumatoid arthritis
The tendency of autoimmune diseases to aggregate is well known as clusters of autoimmune diseases within families and individuals. Analysis of susceptible genetic loci for the distinct autoimmune disease shows considerable overlap that suggests the possibility of shared pathways in their pathogenesis. Reports on the clustering of T1D, AIT, CD and rheumatoid arthritis (RA) in the same patient are very scarce. The major genetic predisposition to RA is contributed by variants of the class II HLA gene, HLA DRB1. In exploring the overlap between T1D, CD and RA, there is strong evidence that variation within the TAGAP gene is associated with all three autoimmune diseases. Relatively little is known about the TAGAP gene, which encodes a protein transiently expressed in activated T cells, suggesting that it may have a role in immune regulation. So the TAGAP gene, previously associated with both T1D and CD, is also associated with RA susceptibility. Interestingly a number of loci appear to be specific to one of the three diseases currently studied suggesting that they may play a role in determining the particular autoimmune phenotype at presentation (Eyre et al., 2010). The majority of the published case reports are girls. The predominance of females among the affected individuals may reflect that certain genes play role in the pathogenesis as gender-specific factors or the penetrance of multiple risk genes are enhanced in females. In most reported patients, diabetes is diagnosed first, thyroid autoimmunity and juvenile rheumatoid arthritis develop after a period of several months to years. (Nagy et al., 2010; Pignata et al., 2000; Valerio et al., 2000).

2.6.2 Sclerodermia, systemic lupus erythematosus
The association of T1D with Systemic Lupus Erythematosus (SLE) and Sclerodermia is rare but reported in literature (Inuo et al., 2009, Zeglaoui et al., 2010). Some authors found a significant association between DQ2 allele and the presence of anti-SSA antibodies, while others described an association between CD and the presence of A1B8DR3 haplotype, which seems to be frequent in SLE and in Sclerodermia (Black et al., 1983; Mark, 2000; Sollid & Thorsby, 1993). In human, the CTLA-4 and PD-1 genes significantly contributed to the development of various autoimmune diseases in different genetic backgrounds (Inuo et al., 2009).). It has been suggest the involvement of CTLA-4 and PD-1 (inhibitor receptors of CD28) to the development of T1D, SLE or other autoimmune diseases.
Juvenile sclerodermia is present in 3% of sclerodermia cases, SLE in children is present in 9% of cases of SLE; one case of a 15 years girl with CD and SLE and Sclerodermia has been reported (Zeglaoui et al., 2010).

2.7 Screening for associated autoimmune disorders
Since Type 1 Diabetes is associated with the presence of additional autoimmune disease, such as AIT, CD and AD, which are associated with the production of organ-specific antibodies, it is possible to screen patients with T1D by means of these ones. However, only a subset of the subjects with organ-specific antibodies develops clinical disease. The frequency of screening and follow up of patients with positive antibodies remain controversial. The current American Diabetes Association (ADA) recommendations are to

screen for CD-associated antibodies at diagnosis of T1D and in presence of symptoms. The International Society of Pediatric Adolescent Diabetes (ISPAD) recommends to screen for CD at the time of diagnosis, annually for the first five years and every second year thereafter. More frequent assessment is indicated if the clinical situation suggests the possibility of CD or the child has a first-degree relative with CD. Respect to the screening for thyroid disease, current recommendations from the ADA are for screening TSH after stabilization at onset of diabetes, with symptoms of hypo- or hyperthyroidism, and every 1–2 yr thereafter. ISPAD recommends to screen by circulating TSH and antibodies at the diagnosis of T1D and, thereafter, every second year in asymptomatic individuals without goitre or in the absence of thyroid autoantibodies. More frequent assessment is indicated otherwise, subjects with positive TPO autoantibodies and normal thyroid function are screened on a more frequent basis (every 6 months to 1 yr). There are no current recommendations for screening of adrenal autoimmunity (Barker, 2006). Authors observed that the prevalence of adrenal antibodies in diabetic patients with thyroid antibodies compared with those without thyroid antibodies is increased (5,1 vs 0,6%) (Riley et al., 1981). It is possible conclude that routine screening for AD in children with T1D is not warranted unless there is a strong clinical suspicion or family history of AD (Marks et al., 2003)

Celiac disease	Transglutaminase antibodies	Yearly
Thyroiditis	TSH, FT4, thyroid antibodies	Yearly
Addison disease	Cortisolemia, adrenal antibodies	Screening if AD in family
Collagenopathies	Specific auto-antibodies	No screening

Table 2. Autoimmune diseases associated with T1D, recommended systems and frequency of the screening

3. Associated non-autoimmune conditions

3.1 Type 1 diabetes and growth

Type 1 diabetes and other chronic diseases are well known to adversely affect linear growth and pubertal development, this can include a wide spectrum of different conditions, from poor gain of weight to Mauriac Syndrome (MS); MS classically involves hepatomegaly, growth impairment, and Cushingoid features in poorly controlled diabetic patients. Although MS, the most important expression of growth alteration due to severe insulin deficiency in diabetic patients, is now rare, impaired growth in children with T1D is still reported. This is particularly true in patients with poor metabolic control (Chiarelli et al., 2004; Franzese et al., 2001). Some studies report that poorly controlled patients show a decrease in height standard deviation score over the next few years, while better controlled patients maintain their height advantage (Gunczler & Lanes, 1999; Holl et al., 1998).

Longitudinal bone growth is a complex phenomenon involving a multitude of regulatory mechanisms strongly influenced by growth hormone (GH) (Chiarelli et al., 2004) and by the interaction between insulin-like growth factors (IGF-I and IGF-II), that circulate bounded to specific insulin-like growth factor binding proteins (IGFBPs). IGFBP-3, the major circulating binding protein during post-natal life, is GH-dependent. Insulin is an important regulator of this complex. In fact, adequate insulin secretion and normal portal insulin concentrations are needed to support normal serum concentrations of IGFs and IGFBPs and indirectly to promote growth. Poor gain of height and weight, hepatomegaly, non alcoholic steatosis hepatis (NASH) and late pubertal development might be seen in children with persistently poorly controlled diabetes. Similar to healthy adolescents, the pubertal growth spurt represents the most critical phase for linear growth and final height in children with T1D. The pubertal phase is characteristically associated with reduction in insulin sensitivity, which is known to be more severe in patients with T1D, and might negatively influence growth and height gain (Chiarelli et al., 2004). Although the chronological age at onset of puberty and the duration of the pubertal growth spurt is not significantly different between subjects with T1D and healthy adolescents, several studies have shown a blunted pubertal growth spurt which seems to be associated with a reduced peak of height velocity SDS (Vanelli et al., 1992). Although loss of height from the onset of diabetes has been widely reported, an impaired final height has not been reported in children with T1D. In fact, while some studies, especially those performed in the pre-intensive insulin therapy era, showed an impaired final height in children with diabetes (Penfold et al., 1995), more recent studies show a normal or only slightly reduced final height (Salerno et al., 1997).

The Diabetes Control and Complications Trial (DCCT) and other studies have reported increased weight gain as a side effect of intensive insulin therapy with improved metabolic control (DCCT Research Group, 1993). As obesity is a modifiable cardiovascular risk factor, careful monitoring and management of weight gain should be emphasised in diabetes care. Girls seem to be more at risk of overweight and as well of eating disorders.

Monitoring of growth and development and the use of percentile charts is a crucial element in the care of children and adolescents with diabetes. Improvements in diabetes care and management and especially newer insulin schedules based on multiple daily injections or insulin pumps have led to a reduction in diabetic complications and seem to ameliorate growth in children with T1D. Start an intensive insulin regimen since the onset of diabetes might prevent the induction of abnormalities of the GH–IGF-I–IGFBP-3 axis potentially achieving near-normal portal insulin concentrations and thereby leading to normal IGF-I and IGFBP-3 levels and physiological growth in children and adolescents with T1D.

3.2 Type 1 diabetes and eating disorders

Eating disorders (EDs) are a significant health problem for many children and adolescents with T1D similar to that observed in other high risk groups, such as competitive athletes, models and ballet dancers. EDs and subclinical disordered eating behaviors (DEBs) have been described in adolescents with T1D with a higher prevalence than in a non-diabetic population. The start of insulin treatment and the need to comply with dietary recommendations both lead to weight gain, which in turn leads to body dissatisfaction and a drive for thinness. Since the dietary restraint usually requires ignoring internal cues of hunger and satiety, it has been suggested that it may be a triggering factor in the development of cycles of binge eating and purging. The concurrence of T1D and EDs can greatly increase morbidity and mortality. In diabetic subjects, EDs are associated with insulin omission for weight loss and impaired metabolic control. On the contrary, in a five year longitudinal study, the expected relationship between ED and poor metabolic control was not evident, although there was a trend for higher haemoglobin A1c in individuals with an EDs (Colton et al., 2007). This offers hope that early interventions might prevent the worsening metabolic control that is often associated with EDs. In addition subclinical DEBs among youth with T1D have been associated with increased risk of poor metabolic control and increased prevalence of microvascular complications such as retinopathy and nephropathy (Rydall et al., 1997). Some studies have examined the prevalence of EDs and DEBs in youth with T1D. Prevalence rates vary considerably from study to study possibly due to differences in sample, screening tools, and data collection methods. In a multi-site, cross sectional case-control study, the prevalence of ED meeting DSM-IV diagnostic criteria was about 10% and that of their sub-threshold variants about 14%: both were about twice as common in adolescent females with T1D than in their non-diabetic peers. (Jones et al., 2000). However there are also rare cases in childhood (Franzese et al., 2002a).

3.2.1 Management
Nutritional treatment is one of the main difficulties in managing diabetes in the young. Diabetes clinicians should be aware of the potential warning signs in an adolescent with diabetes as well as assessment and treatment options for eating disorders with concomitant T1D. Clinical approaches should focus on normalizing eating behaviour and enhancing self-esteem based on personal attributes unrelated to weight and eating, with a low threshold for referral for specialized EDs services (Colton et al., 2007). A multidisciplinary team, composed by clinicians, psychologist/psychiatric, dietitian/nutrition therapist, especially one with a background in EDs, is opportune to identify and treat unhealthy EDs and DEBs in T1D. Treatment for adolescents with T1D should include both diabetes management treatment and mental health treatment. The diabetes team and the mental health team have separate responsibilities but work collaboratively to address disordered eating in patients with T1D. Treatment begins with emphasis on nutritional rehabilitation, weight restoration, and adequate diabetes control. Psychotherapy should begin immediately for the patient and family (S.D. Kelly et al., 2005).

3.3 Necrobiosis lipoidica diabeticorum
Necrobiosis lipoidica diabeticorum (NBL) is an infrequent skin affection in pediatric age. The etiology is not clearly understood. The reported prevalence in children varies from 0.06% to 10% (De Silva et al., 1999). The female/male ratio is 3:1(Hammami et al., 2008). The average age of onset is 30–40 years. In the past, it has been described as a complication of diabetes and associated with microvascular complications (W.F. Kelly et al., 1993), but NBL has been observed also at the beginning of diabetes. NBL typically appears on the anterior lower legs. The lesions are usually bilateral and are characterized by well circumscribed yellow brown inflammatory plaques with raised borders and an atrophic center. Ulceration occurs in up to 35% of cases and is notoriously difficult to treat (Elmholdt et al., 2008). This complication negatively affects quality of life and implies a greater risk for secondary infection. Although NBL is usually observed in diabetic patients, there is some controversy regarding the degree of this association and it has been hypothesized that the strength of this association may have been overestimated in the past. Some authors have studied the effect of glucose control on NBL and found no correlation with glycosylated hemoglobin A1c levels (Dandona et al., 1981), while others found an association with a poor glucose control (Cohen et al., 1996).

3.3.1 Management
There is currently no standardized effective treatment of NBL. A wide variety of treatments have been used over the years in adults. These include: topical, systemic or intra-lesional

steroids, aspirin, cyclosporin, mycophenolate, becaplermin, excision and grafting, laser surgery, hyperbaric oxygen, topical granulocytemacrophage colony-stimulating factor and photochemotherapy with topical PUVA (Hanas et al., 2009). A recent study suggests the use of TNF inhibitors in selected patients for treatment of NBL (ulcerative forms) unresponsive to prior conventional therapies (Suárez-Amor et al., 2010). NBL in children can be hard to manage and may be associated with a long-term risk of malignant transformation to squamous cell carcinoma. Systemic therapies, such as corticosteroids and azathioprine are immunosuppressive and immunomodulatory and could facilitate malignant transformation (Beattie et al., 2006). Therefore, although NBL is not clearly related to poor metabolic control, we believe that the diabetic control may also be useful. Effective primary prevention strategies and new treatment options are needed to adequately control the disease and its progression.

3.4 Osteopenia
Children and adolescents with T1D can show several impairment of bone metabolism and structure, resulting in a higher risk of decreased bone mass and its related complications later in life. Consequently an assessment of quality of the bone through non-invasive methods (phalangeal ultrasonography) seems to be opportune in the care of diabetic patients, specially the ones with clusters of autoimmune diseases to define a possible involvement of the bone (Lombardi et al.,2010).
Bone impairment in multiple autoimmune diseases might be considered not only a complication due to endocrine or nutritional mechanisms, but also a consequence of an immunoregulatory imbalance.

3.4.1 Metabolic causes
Alterations of bone mineral density (BMD) are especially observed when diabetes is associated with CD and/or AIT. Bone loss, described in patients with T1D, AIT or CD is usually viewed as a complication of these diseases and is related to duration of diabetes and quality of metabolic control. The exact mechanisms accounting for bone loss in these diseases have been variably explained by metabolic derangements due to the impaired hormonal function in T1D or AIT (McCabe, 2007), or calcium malabsorption and secondary hyperparathyroidism in untreated CD patients (Selby et al., 1999). Alterations of homeostatic mechanisms might explain an imbalance of osteoclast activity leading to osteopenia (Lombardi et al.,2010; Wu et al., 2008).

3.4.2 Immune causes
Bone remodeling involves complex interactions between osteoclasts and other cells in their microenvironment (marrow stromal cells, osteoblasts, macrophages, T-lymphocytes and marrow cells) (Kollet et al., 2007; Teitelbaum, 2007). Besides their role in calcium mobilization from bone and initiation of bone remodeling, osteoclasts are now considered as the innate immune cells in the bone, since they are able to produce and respond to cytokines and chemokines. Some authors found altered levels of plasma Osteoprotegerin (OPG) in children with T1D. Osteoprotegerin is a circulating secretory glycoprotein and is a member of the tumor necrosis factor receptor (TNFR) family. It works as a decoy receptor for the cytokine receptor activator of NFkB ligand (RANKL). RANKL and OPG are a key agonist/antagonist cytokine system: RANKL increases the pool of active osteoclasts thus

increasing bone resorption, whereas OPG, which neutralizes RANKL, has the opposite effect. Alterations or abnormalities of the RANKL/OPG system have been implicated in different metabolic bone diseases characterized by increased osteoclast differentiation and activation, and by enhanced bone resorption (Galluzzi et al., 2005). Therefore, bone could be an additional target of immune dysregulation.

Cytotoxic T lymphocyte-associated antigen-4 (CTLA4), a well-known susceptibility gene for autoimmune disorders, might also represent a possible link between immune system and bone. In animal studies CTLA4 expressed on T regulatory (Treg) cells impairs osteoclast formation (Zaiss et al., 2007). Therefore the failure of Treg cell function in clustering of multiple autoimmune diseases could represent a mechanism to explain both the occurrence of poly-reactive autoimmune processes and the increase of bone resorption in the same individuals.

In patients affected by both T1D and CD, the risk of developing osteopenia is probably influenced by the compliance to gluten-free diet. Osteopenia occurs more frequently in patients with diabetes and CD with poor compliance to GFD. Interestingly, recent observations indicate also an imbalance of cytokines relevant to bone metabolism in untreated celiac patients' sera and the direct effect of these sera on in vitro bone cell activity. In particular the RANKL/osteoprotegerin (OPG) ratio was increased in patients not on gluten-free diet. Actually, the only presence of a second disease, either AIT or CD, do not seems to increase the frequency of osteopenia, provided a good compliance to GFD in CD patients, while the association of three autoimmune diseases significantly increases the occurrence of osteopenia (37.5%). In addition, poor compliance to GFD of CD patients could increase the occurrence of osteopenia more in patients with three autoimmune diseases (80%) than in those with two autoimmune diseases (18.8%) (Valerio et al., 2008).

3.5 Gastropathy

Gastrointestinal motility disorders are found in a consistent proportion of children with T1D and are associated with significant morbidity: they are usually associated with dyspeptic symptoms, such as nausea, vomiting, fullness and epigastric discomfort, and could be an important cause of morbidity in diabetic patients. Gastroparesis has been shown to be significantly correlated with a poor metabolic control in a population of T1D children with gastric electrical abnormalities. (Cucchiara et al., 1998). Furthermore it is conceivable that delayed gastric emptying may cause a mismatch between the onset of insulin action and the delivery of nutrients into the small intestine (Rayner et al., 2001). Diabetic children with unexplained poor glycemic control should be investigated for abnormalities in gastric motility (Shen & Soffer 2000). On the other hand, hyperglycaemia itself can affect the neuromuscular mechanisms regulating gastrointestinal motility and delay the gastric emptying process (Jebbink et al., 1994). Therefore, it is of great importance to try to reverse abnormalities of gastric motility and improve gastric emptying in patients with T1D and gastroparesis by the use of domperidone in children with T1D. (Franzese et al., 2002b).

3.6 Type 1 diabetes and limited joint mobility

Type 1 diabetes can be associated with other less common disabling conditions of locomotor system: Dupuytren's contracture, stiff hand, carpal tunnel syndrome, and limited joint mobility (LJM). Limited joint mobility is one of the earliest clinically apparent long-term complications of T1D in childhood and adolescence, characterized by a bilateral painless contracture of the finger joints and large joints, associated with tight waxy skin. Changes begin in the metacarpophalangeal and proximal interphalangeal joints of the fifth finger and extend radially with involvement of the distal interphalangeal joints as well. Involvement of larger joints includes particularly the wrist and elbow, but also ankles and cervical and thoracolumbar spine (Komatsu et al., 2004). The limitation is only mildly disabling even when severe. With rare exception, LJM appears after the age of 10 years. The prevalence of LJM in T1D, evaluated in several studies ranges from 9 to 58% in paediatric and adult patients (Lindsay et al., 2005).

The biochemical basis of LJM may be a consequence of changes in the connective tissue, probably due to alterations in the structural macromolecules of the extracellular matrix. The hyperglycaemia can alterate the glycation of protein with the formation of advanced glycation end products (AGEs), which resist to protein degradation and consequently increase thickness of basal membranes in the periarticular tissues (Shimbargger, 1987). Development of LJM is related to both age and diabetes duration (Cagliero et al., 2002), while others showed that it can be compromised also in a precocious age and with a short duration of diabetes (Komatsu et al., 2004). Of note, fluorescence of skin collagen, which reflects the accumulation of stable AGEs, increases linearly with age, but with abnormal rapidity in T1D and in correlation with the presence of retinopathy, nephropathy and neuropathy (Monnier et al., 1986).

Some authors have showed that there is a clear link between upper limb musculoskeletal abnormalities and poor metabolic control (Ramchurn et al., 2009). It has been observed a reduction in frequency of LJM between the mid-70s and mid-90s in children, most likely due to the improved glucose control during this era (Infante et al., 2001; Lindsay et al., 2005).

3.7 Type 1 diabetes and oedema

Insulin oedema is a well-recognized and extremely rare complication of insulin therapy. It was found to occur equally in both sexes in adults, but a clear female predominance was noted in younger ages. The condition is self-limiting, but a progression to overt cardiac failure and development of pleural effusion has been reported. (Chelliah & Burge, 2004).

The pathophysiology remains vague. Intensive fluid resuscitation in an insulin-deficient catabolic state may lead to extravasation of fluid to the subcutaneous tissue, resulting in peripheral oedema. This may be exacerbated by the increased capillary permeability associated with chronic hyperglycemia. Renal tubular sodium reabsorption is enhanced by insulin therapy via stimulating the Na+/K+-ATPase as well as the expression of Na+/H+ exchanger 3 in the proximal tubule. Transient inappropriate hyperaldosteronism has also been suggested to contribute to the fluid retention (Bas et al., 2010). Loss of albumin from the circulation due to increased transcapillary leakage probably contributed to the formation of oedema and the decreased serum albumin, but was not severe enough to account for the magnitude of oedema (Wheatly & Edwards 1985). Cases with normal serum albumin have also been reported.

Clinically, insulin oedema may present with a spectrum of severity until to frank anasarca. Pleural effusions have uncommonly been reported, although some of these patients were elderly and may have had pre-existing cardiac disease. Rarely, the oedema extended from peripheral tissues to serosal cavities with ascites and cardiac failure (Bas et al., 2010). Fluid and salt restriction should be implemented and this may be all that is necessary. Diuretic therapy may be indicated in more severe decompensated cases. Administration of an aldosterone antagonist such as spironolactone may be considered from a pathophysiological point of view in the presence of inappropriate hyperaldosteronism (Kalambokis et al., 2004). In most instances no specific therapy is needed and spontaneous recovery is noted.

Impaired growth	Poor metabolic control	Monitoring of growth and physical development using growth charts
Eating disorders	Dietary restriction	Ameliorating of nutritional assistance
Necrobiosis lipoidica diabeticorum	Parallel dermopathy	Routine clinical examination of the skin
Osteopenia	Probably even present, but worsened by poor metabolic control/comorbidity	Eventually controlled by Bone ultrasonography/ DEXA
Gastropathy	Poor metabolic control	Investigating of dyspeptic symptoms
Limited joint mobility	Parallel condition	Routine clinical examination of the joint mobility
Oedema	Unknown	Clinical examination

Table 3. Non autoimmune associated conditions to Type 1 diabetes, causes and detection

4. References

Aaltonen, J., Bjorses, P., Sandkuijl, L., Perheentupa, J. & Peltonen, L. (1994). An autosomal locus causing autoimmune disease: autoimmune polyglandular disease type I assigned to chromosome 21. *Nature Genetics*, Vol. 8, No. 1, (Sep 1994), pp. (83–87), 1061-4036

Acerini, C.L., Ahmed, M.L., Ross, K.M., Sullivan, P.B., Bird, G. & Dunger, D.B. (1998). Coeliac disease in children and adolescents with IDDM: clinical characteristics and response to gluten-free diet. *Diabetic Medicine*, Vol. 15, No. 1, (Jan 1998), pp. (38-44), 0742-3071

Ahonen, P., Myllarniemi, S., Sipila, I. & Perheentupa, J. (1990) Clinical variation of autoimmune polyendocrinopathy-candidiasis-ectodermal dystrophy (APECED) in a series of 68 patients. *New England Journal of Medicine*, Vol. 322, No. 26, (Jun 1990), pp. (1829–1836), 0028-4793

Anderson, J., Goudie, R.B., Gray, K.G. & Timbury, G.C. (1957). Auto-antibodies in Addison's Disease. *Lancet*, Vol. 269, No. 6979, (Jun 1957), pp. (1123–1124), 0140-6736

Artz, E., Warren-Ulanch, J., Becker, D., Greenspan, S. & Freemark, M. (2008). Seropositivity to celiac antigens in asymptomatic children with type 1 diabetes mellitus: association with weight, height, and bone mineralization. *Pediatric Diabetes*, Vol. 9, No. 4, (Jul 2008), pp. (277-284), 1399-543X

Bao, F., Yu, L., Babu, S., Wang, T., Hoffenberg, E.J., Rewers, M. & Eisenbarth, G.S. (1999). One third of HLA DQ2 homozygous patients with type 1 diabetes express celiac disease associated transglutaminase autoantibodies. *Journal of Autoimmunity*, Vol. 13, No. 1, (Aug 1999), pp. (143-148), 0896-8411

Barker, J.M., Ide, A., Hostetler, C., Yu, L., Miao, D., Fain, P.R., Eisenbarth, G.S. & Gottlieb, P.A. (2005). Endocrine and immunogenetic testing in individuals with type 1 diabetes and 21-hydroxylase autoantibodies: Addison's disease in a high-risk population. *Journal of Clinical Endocrinology and Metabolism*, Vol. 90, No. 1, (Jan 2005), pp. (128-134), 0021-972X

Barker, J.M. (2006). Clinical review: type 1 diabetes-associated autoimmunity: natural history, genetic associations and screening. *Journal of Clinical Endocrinology and Metabolism*; Vol. 91, No. 4, (Apr 2006) pp. (1210-1217), 0021-972X

Baş, V.N., Cetinkaya, S., Yılmaz Ağladıoğlu, S., Peltek Kendirici, H.N., Bilgili, H., Yıldırım, N. & Aycan, Z. (2010). Insulin oedema in newly diagnosed type 1 diabetes mellitus. *Journal of Clinical Research in Pediatric Endocrinology*, Vol. 2, No. 1, (Mar 2010), pp. (46-48), 1308-5727

Beattie, P.E., Dawe, R.S., Ibbotson, S.H. & Ferguson, J. (2006). UVA1 phototherapy for treatment of necrobiosis lipoidica. *Clinical and Experimental Dermatology*, Vol. 31, No. 2, (Mar 2006), pp. (235-238), 1365-2230

Black, C.M., Welsh, K.I., Walker, A.E., Bernstein, R.M., Catoggio, L.J., McGregor, A.R. & Jones, J.K. (1983). Genetic susceptibility to scleroderma-like syndrome induced by vinyl chloride. *Lancet*, Vol. 1, No. 8314-5, (Jan 1983), pp. (53–55), 0140-6736

Bottini, N., Musumeci, L., Alonso, A., Rahmouni, S., Nika, K., Rostamkhani, M., MacMurray, J., Meloni, G., Lucarelli, P., Pellechia, M., Eisenbarth, G., Comings, D. & Mustelin, T. (2004). A functional variant of lymphoid tyrosine phosphatase is associated with type 1 diabetes. *Nature Genetics*, Vol. 36, No. 4, (Apr 2004), pp. (337-338), 1061-4036

Burek, C.L., Rose, N.R., Guire, K.E. & Hoffman, W.H. (1990). Thyroid autoantibodies in black and in white children and adolescents with type 1 diabetes mellitus and their first degree relatives. *Autoimmunity*, Vol. 7, No. 2-3, pp. (157-167), 0891-6934

Bystryn, J.C. (1997). Immune mechanisms in vitiligo. *Clinical Dermatology*, Vol. 15, No. 6, (Nov-Dec 1997), pp. (853-861), 1507-5516

Cagliero, E., Apruzzese, W., Perlmutter, G.S. & Nathan, D.M. (2002). Musculoskeletal disorders of the hand and shoulder in patients with diabetes mellitus. *The American Journal of Medicine*, Vol.112, No. 6, (Apr 2002), pp. (487-490), 0002-9343

Cerutti, F., Bruno, G., Chiarelli, F., Lorini, R., Meschi, F. & Sacchetti, C. (2004). Diabetes study group of the Italian Society of Pediatric Endocrinology and Diabetology. Younger age at onset and sex predict celiac disease in children and adolescents with type 1 diabetes: an Italian multicenter study. *Diabetes Care*, Vol. 27, No. 6, (Jun 2004), pp. (1294-1298), 0149-5992

Chatila, T.A., Blaeser, F., Ho, N., Lederman, H.M., Voulgaropoulos, C., Helms, C., Bowcock, A.M. (2000). JM2, encoding a fork head-related protein, is mutated in Xlinked autoimmunity-allergic disregulation syndrome. *Journal of Clinical Investigation*, Vol.106, No. 12, (Dec 2000), pp. (R75–R81), 0021-9738

Chelliah, A. & Burge, M.R. (2004). Insulin edema in the twenty-first century: review of the existing literature. *Journal of Investigative Medicine*, Vol. 52, No. 2, (Mar 2004), pp. (104-108), 1081-5589

Chiarelli, F., Giannini, C. & Mohn, A. (2004). Growth, growth factors and diabetes. *European Journal of Endocrinology*, Vol. 151, Supplement 3, (Nov 2004), pp. (U109–U117), 0804-4643

Cohen, O., Yaniv, R., Karasik, A. & Trau, H. (1996). Necrobiosis lipoidica and diabetic control revisited. *Medical Hypotheses*, Vol. 46, No. 4, (Apr 1996), pp. (348-50), 0306-9877

Collin, P., Kaukinen, K., Valimaki, M. & Salmi, J. (2002). Endocrinological disorders and celiac disease. *Endocrine Reviews*, Vol. 23, No. 4, (Aug 2002), pp. (464-483), 0163-769X

Colton, P.A., Olmsted, M.P., Daneman, D., Rydall, A.C. & Rodin, G.M. (2007). Five-year prevalence and persistence of disturbed eating behavior and eating disorders in girls with type 1 diabetes. *Diabetes Care*, Vol. 30, No. 11, (Nov 2007), pp. (2861-2862), 0149-5992

Crone, J., Rami, B., Huber, W.D., Granditsch, G. & Schober, E. (2003). Prevalence of celiac disease and follow-up of EMA in children and adolescents with type 1 diabetes mellitus. *Journal of Pediatrics Gastroenterology and Nutrition*, Vol. 37, No. 1, (Jul 2003), pp. (67-71), 0277-2116

Cronin, C.C. & Shanahan, F. (2007). Insulin-dependent diabetes mellitus and coeliac disease. *Lancet*, Vol. 349, No. 9058, (Apr 1997), pp. (1096-1097), 0140-6736

Cucchiara, S., Franzese, A., Salvia, G., Alfonsi, L., Iula, V.D., Montisci, A. & Moreira, F.L. (1998). Gastric emptying delay and gastric electrical derangement in IDDM. *Diabetes Care*, Vol. 21, No. 3, (Mar 1998), pp. (438–443), 0149-5992

Dandona, P., Freedman, D., Barter, S., Majewski, B.B., Rhodes, E.L. & Watson, B. (1981). Glycosylated haemoglobin in patients with necrobiosis lipoidica and granuloma annulare. *Clinical and Experimental Dermatology*, Vol. 6, No. 3, (May 1981), pp. (299-302), 1365-2230

De Block, C.E., De Leeuw, I.H., Vertommen, J.J., Rooman, R.P., Du Caju, M.V., Van Campenhout, C.M., Weyler, J.J., Winnock, F., Van Autreve, J., Gorus, F.K. & The Belgian Diabetes Registry (2001). Beta-cell, thyroid, gastric, adrenal and celiac autoimmunity and HLA-DQ types in type 1 diabetes. *Clinical and Experimental Immunology*, Vol. 126, No. 2, (Nov 2001), pp. (236–241), 0009-9104

De Silva, B.D., Schofield, O.M. & Walker, J.D. The prevalence of necrobiosis lipoidica diabeticorum in children with type 1 diabetes. *The British Journal of Dermatology*, Vol. 141, No. 3, (Sep 1999), pp. (593-594), 0007-0963

Diabetes Control and Complication Trial (DCCT) Research Group. (1993). The effect of intensive treatment of diabetes on the development and progression of long-term complications in insulin-dependent diabetes mellitus. The Diabetes Control and Complications Trial Research Group. *The New England Journal of Medicine*, Vol. 329, No. 14, (Sep 1993), pp. (977–986), 0028-4793

Dittmar, M. & Kahaly, G.J. (2003) Polyglandular autoimmune syndromes: immunogenetics and long-term follow-up. *Journal of Clinical Endocrinology and Metabolism*, Vol. 88, No. 7, (Jul 2003), pp. (2983–2992), 0021-972X

Elmholdt, T.R., Sørensen, H.B. & Fogh, K. (2008). A severe case of ulcerating necrobiosis lipoidica. *Acta Dermato-Venereologica*, Vol. 88, No. 2, (Mar 2008), pp. (177–178), 0001-5555

Eyre, S., Hinks, A., Bowes, J., Flynn, E., Martin, P., Wilson, A.G., Morgan, A.W., Emery, P., Steer, S., Hocking, L.J., Reid, D.M., Harrison, P., Wordsworth, P., Yorkshire Early Arthritis Consortium, Biologics in RA Control Consortium, Thomson, W., Worthington, J. & Barton, A. (2010). Overlapping genetic susceptibility variants between three autoimmune disorders: rheumatoid arthritis, type 1 diabetes and coeliac disease. *Arthritis Research & Therapy*, Vol. 12, No. 5, (Sep 2010), p. (R175), 1478-6454

Falorni, A., Laureti, S., Nikoshkov, A., Picchio, M.L., Hallengren, B., Vandewalle, C.L., Gorus, F.K., Tortoioli, C., Luthman, H., Brunetti, P. & Santeusanio, F. (1997). 21-hydroxylase autoantibodies in adult patients with endocrine autoimmune diseases are highly specific for Addison's disease. Belgian Diabetes Registry. *Clinical and Experimental Immunology*, Vol. 107, No. 2, (Feb 1997), pp. (341–346), 0009-9104

Franzese, A., Buono, P., Mascolo, M., Leo, A.L. & Valerio, G. (2000). Thyroid autoimmunity starting during the course of type 1 diabetes denotes a subgroup of children with more severe diabetes. *Diabetes Care*, Vol. 23, No. 8, (Aug 2000), pp. 1(201-202), 0149-5992

Franzese, A., Iorio, R., Buono, P., Mascolo, M., Mozzillo, E. & Valerio, G. (2001). Mauriac Syndrome still exists. *Diabetes Research and Clinical Practice*, Vol. 54, No. 3, (Dec 2001), pp. (219–221), 0168-8227

Franzese, A., Valerio, G., Buono, P., Mozzillo, E., Gritti, A. & Lucariello, M.A. (2002). Comorbidity of type 1 diabetes and anorexia nervosa in a 6-year-old girl. *Diabetes Care*, Vol. 25, No. 4, (Apr 2002), pp. (800-801), 0149-5992

Franzese, A., Borrelli, O., Corrado, G., Rea, P., Di Nardo, G., Randinetti, A. L., Dito, L. & Cucchiara, S. (2002). Domperidone is more effective than cisapride in children with diabetic gastroparesis. *Alimentary Pharmacology & Therapeutics*, Vol. 16, No. 5, (May 2002), pp. (951-957), 1365-2036

Franzese, A., Lombardi, F., Valerio, G. & Spagnuolo, M.I. (2007). Update on Coeliac Disease and Type 1 Diabetes Mellitus in Childhood. *Journal of Pediatric Endocrinology and Metabolism*, Vol. 20, No. 12, (Dec 2007), pp. (1257-1264), 0334-018X

Franzese, A., Iafusco, D., Spadaro, R., Cavaliere, O., Prisco, F., Auricchio, R., Troncone, R., Valerio, G. & The Study-Group on Diabetes of Italian Society of Pediatric Endocrinology and Diabetology (2011). Potential celiac disease in type 1 diabetes: A multicenter study. *Diabetes Research in Clinical Practice*, Vol. 92, No. 1, (Apr 2011), pp. (53-56), 0168-8227

Freemark, M. & Levitsky, L.L. (2003). Screening for celiac disease in children with type 1 diabetes: two views of the controversy. *Diabetes Care*, Vol. 26, No. 6, (Jun 2003), pp. (1932-1939), 0149-5992

Galluzzi, F., Stagi, S., Salti, R., Toni, S., Piscitelli, E., Simonini, G., Falcini, F. & Chiarelli, F. (2005). Osteoprotegerin serum levels in children with type 1 diabetes: a potential modulating role in bone status. *European Journal of Endocrinology*, Vol. 153, No. 6, (Dec 2005), pp. (879–885), 0804-4643

Gunczler, P. & Lanes, R. (1999). Poor metabolic control decreases the growth velocity of diabetic children. *Diabetes Care*, Vol. 22, No. 6, (Jun 1999), p. (1012), 0149-5992

Hammami, H., Youssef, S., Jaber, K., Dhaoui, M.R. & Doss, N. (2008). Perforating necrobiosis lipoidica in a girl with type 1 diabetes mellitus: a new case reported. *Dermatology Online Journal*, Vol. 14, No. 7, (Jul 2008), p. (11), 1087-2108

Hanas, R., Donaghue, K.C., Klingensmith, G. & Swift, P.G. (2009). ISPAD clinical practice consensus guidelines 2009 compendium. Introduction. *Pediatric Diabetes*, Vol. 10, Supplement 12, (Sep 2009), pp. (1-2), 1399-543X

Handa, S. & Dogra, S. (2003). Epidemiology of childhood vitiligo: a study of 625 patients from north India. *Pediatric Dermatology*, Vol. 20, No. 3, (May-Jun 2003), pp. (207–210), 1525-1470

Hansen, D., Brock-Jacobsen, B., Lund, E., Bjorn, C., Hansen, L.P., Nielsen, C., Fenger, C., Lillevang, S.T. & Husby, S. (2006). Clinical benefit of a gluten-free diet in type 1 diabetic children with screening-detected celiac disease: a population-based screening study with 2 years' follow-up. *Diabetes Care*, Vol. 29, No. 11, (Nov 2006), pp. (2452-2456), 0149-5992

Ho, N., Pope, E., Weinstein, M., Greenberg, S., Webster, C. & Krafchik, B.R. (2011). A double-blind randomized placebo-controlled trial of topical tacrolimus 0.1% versus clobetasol propionate 0.05% in childhood vitiligo. *The British Journal of Dermatology*, Vol. 164, No. 4, (Apr 2011), 1365-2133

Holl, R.W., Grabert, M., Heinze, E., Sorgo, W. & Debatin, K.M. (1998). Age at onset and long-term metabolic control affect height in type-1 diabetes mellitus. *European Journal of Pediatrics*, Vol. 157, No. 12, (Dec 1998), pp. (972–977), 0340-6199

Holmes, G.K. (2001). Coeliac disease and Type 1 diabetes mellitus – the case for screening. *Diabetic Medicine*, Vol. 18, No. 3, (Mar 2001), pp. (169-177), 0742-3071

Holmes, G.K. (2001). Potential and latent coeliac disease. *European Journal of Gastroenterology and Hepatology*, Vol.13, No. 9, (Sep 2001), pp. (1057–1060), 0954-691X

Hue, S., Monteiro, R.C., Berrith-Aknin, S. & Caillat-Zucman, S. (2003). Potential role of NKG2D/MHC class I-related chain A interaction in intrathymic maturation of single-positive CD8 T cells. *Journal of Immunology*, Vol. 171, No. 4, (Aug 2003), pp. (1909-1917), 0022-1767

Iafusco, D., Rea, F. & Prisco, F. (1998). Hypoglycemia and reduction of the insulin requirement as a sign of celiac disease in children with IDDM. *Diabetes Care*, Vol. 21, No. 8, (Aug 1998), pp. (1379-1381), 0149-5992

Ide, A. & Eisenbarth, G.S. (2003). Genetic susceptibility in type 1 diabetes and its associated autoimmune disorders. *Reviews in Endocrine & Metabolic Disorders*, Vol. 4, No. 3, (Sep 2003), pp. (243-253), 1389-9155

Infante, J.R., Rosenbloom, A.L., Silverstein, J.H., Garzarella, L. & Pollock, B.H. (2001). Changes in frequency and severity of limited joint mobility in children with type 1 diabetes mellitus between 1976-78 and 1998. *Journal of Pediatrics*, Vol. 138, No. 1, (Jan 2001), pp. (33–37), 0022-3476

Inuo, M., Ihara, K., Matsuo, T., Kohno, H. & Hara, T. (2009). Association study between B- and T-lymphocyte attenuator gene and type 1 diabetes mellitus or systemic lupus erythematosus in the Japanese population. *International Journal of Immunogenetics*, Vol. 36, No. 1, (Feb 2009), pp. (65-68)

Jebbink, R.J., Samsom, M., Bruijs, P.P., Bravenboer, B., Akkermans, L.M., Vanberge-Henegouwen, G.P. & Smout, A.J. (1994). Hyperglycemia induces abnormalities of gastric myoelectrical activity in patients with type I diabetes mellitus. *Gastroenterology*, Vol. 107, No. 5, (Nov 1994), pp. (1390–1397), 0036-5521

Jones, J.M., Lawson, M.L., Daneman, D., Olmsted, M.P. & Rodin, G. (2000). Eating disorders in adolescent females with and without type 1 diabetes: cross sectional study. *The British Medical Journal*, Vol. 320, No. 7249, (Jun 2000), pp. (1563-1566), 0959-8138

Kalambokis, G., Tsatsoulis, A., Economou, G. & Tsianos, E.V. (2004). A case of insulin edema with inappropriate hyperaldosteronism. *Journal of Endocrinological Investigation*, Vol. 27, No. 10, (Nov 2004), pp. (957-960), 0391-4097

Kaspers, S., Kordonouri, O., Schober, E., Grabert, M., Hauffa, B.P., Holl, R.W. & German Working Group for Pediatric Diabetology (2004). Anthropometry, metabolic control, and thyroid autoimmunity in type 1 diabetes with celiac disease: A multicenter survey. *Journal of Pediatrics*, Vol. 145, No. 6, (Dec 2004), pp. (790-795), 0022-3476

Kelly, S.D., Howe, C.J., Hendler, J.P. & Lipman, T.H. (2005). Disordered Eating Behaviors in Youth With Type 1 Diabetes. *The Diabetes Educator*, Vol. 31, No. 4, (Jul-Aug 2005), pp. (572-583), 0145-7217

Kelly, W.F., Nicholas, J., Adams, J. & Mahmood, R. (1993). Necrobiosis lipoidica diabeticorum: association with background retinopathy, smoking, and proteinuria. A case controlled study. *Diabetic Medicine*, Vol. 10, No. 8, (Oct 1993), pp. (725-728), 0742-3071

Kollet, O., Dar, A. & Lapidot, T. (2007). The multiple roles of osteoclast in host defence: one remodeling and hematopoietic stem cell mobilization. *Annual Review of Immunology*, Vol. 25, (Apr 2007), pp. (51-69), 0732-0582

Komatsu, W.R., Gabbay, M.A. & Dib, S.A. (2004). Early subclinical limited axial and large joint flexibility in type 1 diabetes mellitus adolescents. *Journal of Diabetes and its Complications*, Vol. 18, No. 6, (Nov-Dec 2004), pp. (352-355), 1056-8727

Kordonouri, O., Klinghammer, A., Lang, E.B., Gruters-Kieslich, A., Grabert, M. & Holl, R.W. (2002). Thyroid autoimmunity in children and adolescents with type 1 diabetes: a multicenter survey. *Diabetes Care*, Vol. 25, No. 8, (Aug 2002), pp. (1346-1350), 0149-5992

Kordonouri, O., Hartmann, R., Deiss, D., Wilms, M. & Gruters-Kieslich, A. (2005). Natural course of autoimmune thyroiditis in type 1 diabetes: association with gender, age, diabetes duration, and puberty. *Archives of Disease in Childhood*, Vol. 90, No. 4, (Apr 2005), pp. (411-414), 0003-9888

Kordonouri, O., Maguire, A.M., Knip, M., Schober, E., Lorini, R., Holl, R.W. & Donaghue, K.C. (2009). Other complications and conditions associated with diabetes in children and adolescents. *Pediatric Diabetes*, Vol. 10 - Supplement 12; (Sep 2009), pp. (204-210), 1399-543X

Kurppa, K., Ashorn, M., Iltanen, S., Koskinen, L.L., Saavalainen, P., Koskinen, O., Mäki M. & Kaukinen, K. (2010). Celiac disease without villous atrophy in children: a prospective study. *Journal of Pediatrics*, Vol. 157, No. 3, (Sep 2010), pp. (373-380), 0022-3476

Levin, L., Ban, Y., Concepcion, E., Davies, T.F., Greenberg, D.A. & Tomer, Y. (2004). Analysis of HLA genes in families with autoimmune diabetes and thyroiditis. *Human Immunology*, Vol. 65, No. 6, (Jun 2004), pp. (640-647), 0198-8859

Lindsay, J.R., Kennedy, L., Atkinson, A.B., Bell, P.M., Carson, D.J., McCance, D.R. & Hunter, S.J. (2005). Reduced prevalence of limited joint mobility in type 1 diabetes in a U.K. clinic population over a 20-year period. *Diabetes Care*, Vol. 28, No. 3, (Mar 2005), pp. (658-661), 0149-5992

Lombardi, F., Franzese, A., Iafusco, D., Del Puente, A., Esposito, A., Prisco, F., Troncone, R. & Valerio, G. (2010). Bone involvement in clusters of autoimmune diseases: Just a complication? *Bone*, Vol. 46, No. 2, (Feb 2010), pp. (551-555), 8756-3282

Lovas, K. & Husebye, E.S. (2002). High prevalence and increasing incidence of Addison's disease in western Norway. *Clinical Endocrinology*, Vol. 56, No. 6, (Jun 2002), pp. (787-791), 0300-0664

Maasho, K., Opoku-Anane, J., Marusina, A.I., Coligan, J.E. & Borrego, F. (2005). NKG2D is a costimulatory receptor for human naïve CD8 + T cells. *Journal of Immunology*, Vol. 174, No. 8, (Apr 2005), pp. (4480-4484), 0022-1767

Maglio, M., Florian, F., Vecchiet, M., Auricchio, R., Paparo, F., Spadaro, R., Zanzi, D., Rapacciuolo, L., Franzese, A., Sblattero, D., Marzari, R. & Troncone, R. (2009). Majority of children with type 1 diabetes produce and deposit anti-tissue transglutaminase antibodies in the small intestine. *Diabetes*, Vol. 58, No. 7, (Jul 2009), pp. (1578-84), 0012-1797

Mark, M. (2000). Immunogénétique du lupus chez l'homme. *Médecine thérapeutique*, Vol.6, No. 7, (Aug-Sep 2000), pp. (522–528), 1264-6520

Marks, S.D., Girgis, R. & Couch, R.M. (2003). Screening for adrenal antibodies in children with type 1 diabetes and autoimmune thyroid disease. *Diabetes Care*, Vol. 26, No. 11, (Nov 2003), pp. (3187-3188), 0149-5992

McCabe, L. (2007). Understanding the pathology and mechanisms of Type 1 diabetic bone loss. *Journal of Cellular Biochemistry*, Vol. 102, No. 6, (Dec 2007), pp. (1343–1357), 1097-4644

Monnier, V.M., Vishwanath, V., Frank, K.E., Elmets, C.A., Dauchot, P. & Kohn, R.R. (1986). Relation between complications of type I diabetes mellitus and collagenlinked fluorescence. *New England Journal of Medicine*, Vol. 314, No. 7, (Feb 1986), pp. (403–408), 0028-4793

Myhre, A.G., Undlien, D.E., Lovas, K., Uhlving, S., Nedrebo, B.G., Kristian, J.F., Trovik, T., Sorheim, J.I. & Husebye, E.S. (2002). Autoimmune adrenocortical failure in Norway: autoantibodies and HLA class II associations related to clinical features. *Journal of Clinical Endocrinology and Metabolism*, Vol. 87, No. 2, (Feb 2002), pp. (618-623), 0021-972X

Myśliwiec, M., Myśliwska, J., Zorena, K., Balcerska, A., Malinowska, E. & Wiśniewski, P. (2008). Interleukin 6–174 (GNC) gene polymorphism is related to celiac disease and autoimmune thyroiditis coincidence in diabetes type 1 children. *Diabetes Research and Clinical Practice*; Vol. 82, No. 1, (Oct 2008), pp. (108-112), 0168-8227

Nagy, K.H., Lukacs, K., Sipos, P., Hermann, R., Madacsy, L. & Soltesz, G. (2010). Type 1 diabetes associated with Hashimoto's thyroiditis and juvenile rheumatoid arthritis: a case report with clinical and genetic investigations. *Pediatric Diabetes*, Vol. 11, No. 8, (Dec 2010), pp. (579-582), 1399-543X

Paparo, F., Petrone, E., Tosco, A., Maglio, M., Borrelli, M., Salvati, V.M., Miele, E., Greco, L., Auricchio, S. & Troncone, R. (2005). Clinical, HLA, and small bowel immunohistochemical features of children with positive serum antiendomysium antibodies and architecturally normal small intestinal mucosa. *The American Journal of Gastroenterology*, Vol. 100, No. 10, (Oct 2005), (pp. 2294–2298), 0002-9270

Penfold, J., Chase, H.P., Marshall, G., Walravens, C.F., Walravens, P.A. & Garg, S.K. (1995). Final adult height and its relationship to blood glucose control and microvascular complications in IDDM. *Diabetic Medicine*, Vol. 12, No. 2, (Feb 1995), pp. (129–133), 0742-3071

Peterson, P., Salmi, H., Hyoty, H., Miettinen, A., Ilonen, J., Reijonen, H., Knip, M., Akerblom, H.K. & Krohn, K. (1997). Steroid 21-hydroxylase autoantibodies in insulin-dependent diabetes mellitus. Childhood Diabetes in Finland (DiMe) Study Group. *Clinical Immunology and Immunopathology*, Vol. 82, No. 1, (Jan 1997), pp. (37–42), 0090-1229

Pignata, C., Alessio, M., Ramenghi, U., Bonissoni, S., Difranco, D., Brusco, A., Matrecano, E., Franzese, A., Dianzani, I. & Dianzani, U. (2000). Clustering of distinct autoimmune diseases associated with functional abnormalities of T cell survival in children.

Clinical and Experimental Immunology, Vol. 121, No. 1, (Jul 2000), pp. (53-58), 0009-9104

Pocecco, M. & Ventura, A. (1995). Coeliac disease and insulin-dependent diabetes mellitus: a causal association? Acta Paediatrica, Vol. 84, No. 12, (Dec 1995), pp. (1432-1433), 0803-5253

Radetti, G., Paganini, C., Gentili, L., Bernasconi, S., Betterle, C., Borkenstein, M., Cvijovic, K., Kadrnka-Lovrencic, M., Krzisnik, C., Battelino, T., et al. (1995). Frequency of Hashimoto's thyroiditis in children with type 1 diabetes mellitus. Acta Diabetologica, Vol. 32, No.2, (Jun 1995), pp. (121-124), 0940-5429

Ramchurn, N., Mashamba, C., Leitch, E., Arutchelvam, V., Narayanan, K., Weaver, J., Hamilton, J., Heycock, C., Saravanan, V. & Kelly, C. (2009). Upper limb musculoskeletal abnormalities and poor metabolic control in diabetes. European Journal of Internal Medicine, Vol. 20, No. 7, (Nov 2009), pp. (718-721), 0953-6205

Rami, B., Sumnik, Z., Schober, E., Waldhor, T., Battelino, T., Bratanic, N., Kurti, K., Lebl, J., Limbert, C., Madacsy, L., Odink, R.J., Paskova, M. & Soltesz, G. (2005). Screening detected celiac disease in children with type 1 diabetes mellitus: effect on the clinical course (a case control study). Journal of Pediatric Gastroenterology and Nutrition, Vol. 41, No. 3, (Sep 2005), pp. (317-321), 0277-2116

Rayner, C.K., Samsom, M., Jones, K.L. & Horowitz, M. (2001). Relationships of upper gastrointestinal motor and sensory function with glycemic control. Diabetes Care, Vol. 24, No. 2, (Feb 2001), pp. (371–381), 0149-5992

Riley, W.J., Maclaren, N.K., Lezotte, D.C., Spillar, R.P. & Rosenbloom, A.L. (1981). Thyroid autoimmunity in insulin-dependent diabetes mellitus: the case for routine screening. The Journal of Pediatrics, Vol. 99, No. 3, (Sep 1981), pp. (350-354), 0022-3476

Rubio-Tapia, A., Kyle, R.A., Kaplan, E.L., Johnson, D.R., Page, W., Erdtmann, F., Brantner, T.L., Kim, W.R., Phelps, T.K., Lahr, B.D., Zinsmeister, A.R., Melton, L.J. 3rd & Murray, J.A. (2009). Increased prevalence and mortality in undiagnosed celiac disease. Gastroenterology, Vol. 137, No. 1, (Jul 2009), pp. (88-93), 0036-5521

Rydall, A.C., Rodin, G.M., Olmsted, M.P., Devenyi, R.G. & Daneman, D. (1997). Disordered eating behavior and microvascular complications in young women with insulin-dependent diabetes mellitus. The New England Journal of Medicine, Vol. 336, No. 26, (Jun 1997), pp. (1849-1854), 0028-4793

Saadah, O.I., Zacharin, M., O'Callaghan, A., Oliver, M.R. & Catto-Smith, A.G. (2004). Effect of gluten-free diet and adherence on growth and diabetic control in diabetics with coeliac disease. Archives of Disease in Childhood, Vol. 89, No. 9, (Sep 2004), pp. (871-876), 0003-9888

Salerno, M., Argenziano, A., Di Maio, S., Gasparini, N., Formicola, S., De Filippo, G. & Tenore, A. (1997). Pubertal growth, sexual maturation, and final height in children with IDDM. Effects of age at onset and metabolic control. Diabetes Care, Vol. 20, No. 5, (May 1997), pp. (721–724), 0149-5992

Sanchez-Albisua, I., Wolf, J., Neu, A., Geiger, H., Wascher, I. & Stern, M. (2005) Coeliac disease in children with Type 1 diabetes mellitus: the effect of the gluten-free diet. Diabetic Medicine, Vol. 22, No. 8, (Aug 2005), pp. (1079-1082), 0742-3071

Selby, P.L., Davies, M., Adams, J.E. & Mawer, E.B. (1999). Bone loss in celiac disease is related to secondary hyperparathyroidism. Journal of Bone and Mineral Researh, Vol. 14, No. 4, (Apr 1999), pp. (652-657), 0884-0431

Shen, B. & Soffer, E.E. (2000). Diabetic gastropathy: a practical approach to a vexing problem. *Cleveland Clinical Journal of Medicine*, Vol. 67, No. 9, (Sep 2000), pp. (659–664), 0891-1150

Shimbargger, N.I. (1987). Limited joint mobility in adults with diabetes mellitus. *Physical Therapy*, Vol. 67, No. 2, (Feb 1987), pp. (2151–2158), 0031-9023

Simmons, J.H., Klingensmith, G.J., McFann, K., Rewers, M., Taylor, J., Emery, L.M., Taki, I., Vanyi, S., Liu, E. & Hoffenberg, E.J. (2007). Impact of celiac autoimmunity on children with type 1 diabetes. *Journal of Pediatrics*, Vol. 150, No. 5, (May 2007), pp. (461-466), 0022-3476

Simmons, J.H., Klingensmith, G.J., McFann, K., Rewers, M., Ide, L.M., Taki, I., Liu, E. & Hoffenberg, E.J. (2011). Celiac Autoimmunity in Children with Type 1 Diabetes: A Two-Year Follow-up. *Journal of Pediatrics*, Vol 158, No. 2, (Feb 2011), pp. (276-281), 0022-3476

Smyth, D., Cooper, J.D., Collins, J.E., Heward, J.M., Franklyn, J.A., Howson, J.M., Vella, A., Nutland, S., Rance, H.E., Maier, L., Barratt, B.J., Guja, C., Ionescu-Tirgoviste, C., Savage, D.A., Dunger, D.B., Widmer, B., Strachan, D.P., Ring, S.M., Walker, N. & Clayton, D.G. (2004). Replication of an association between the lymphoid tyrosine phospatase locus (LYP/PTPN22) with type 1 diabetes, and evidence for its role as a general autoimmunity locus. *Diabetes*, Vol. 53, No. 11, (Nov 2004), pp. (3020-3023), 0012-1797

Smyth, D.J., Plagnol, V., Walker, N.M., Cooper, J.D., Downes, K., Yang, J.H., Howson, J.M., Stevens, H., McManus, R., Wijmenga, C., Heap, G.A., Dubois, P.C., Clayton, D.G., Hunt, K.A., van Heel, D.A. & Todd, J.A. (2008). Shared and distinct genetic variant in Type 1 diabetes and celiac disease. *New England Journal of Medicine*; Vol. 359, No. 26, (Dec 2008) pp. (2837-2838), 0028-4793

Sollid, L.M. & Thorsby, E. (1993). HLA susceptibility genes in celiac disease: genetic mapping and role in pathogenesis. *Gastroenterology*, Vol. 105, No. 3, (Sep 1993), pp. (910–922), 0036-5521

Suárez-Amor, O., Pérez-Bustillo, A., Ruiz-González, I. & Rodríguez-Prieto, M.A. (2010). Necrobiosis Lipoidica Therapy with Biologicals: An Ulcerated Case Responding to Etanercept and a Review of the Literature. *Dermatology*, Vol. 221, No. 2, (Aug 2010), pp. (117–121), 1018-8665

Sumnik, Z., Cinek, O., Bratanic, N., Lebl, J., Rozsai, B., Limbert, C., Paskova, M. & Schober, E. (2006). Thyroid autoimmunity in children with coexisting type 1 diabetes mellitus and celiac disease: a multicenter study. *Journal of Pediatrics Endocrinology and Metabolism*, Vol. 19, No. 4, (Apr 2006), pp. (517-522), 0334-018X

Teitelbaum, S.L. (2007). Osteoclast: what do they do and how do they do? *The American Journal of Pathology*, Vol. 170, No. 2, (Feb 2007), pp. (427–435), 0002-9440

Troncone, R., Greco, L., Mayer, M., Paparo, F., Caputo, N., Micillo, M., Mugione, P. & Auricchio, S. (1996). Latent and potential celiac disease. *Acta Paediatrica*, Supplement 412, (May 1996), pp. (10–14), 0803-5253

Troncone, R., Franzese, A., Mazzarella, G., Paparo, F., Auricchio, R., Coto, I., Mayer, M. & Greco, L. (2003). Gluten sensitivity in a subset of children with insulin dependent diabetes mellitus. *The American Journal of Gastroenterology*, Vol. 98, No.3, (Mar 2003), pp. (590-595), 0002-9270

Ueda, H., Howson, J.M., Esposito, L., Heward, J., Snook, H., Chamberlain, G., Rainbow, D.B., Hunter, K.M., Smith, A.N., Di Genova, G., Herr, M.H., Dahlman, I., Payne, F., Smyth, D., Lowe, C., Twells, R.C., Howlett, S., Healy, B., Nutland, S., Rance, H.E.,

Smink, L.J., Lam, A.C., Cordell, H.J., Walker, N.M., Bordin, C., Hulme, J., Motzo, C., Cucca, F., Hess, J.F., Metzker, M.L., Rogers, J., Gregory, S., Allahabadia, A., Nithiyananthan, R., Tuomilehto-Wolf, E., Tuomilehto, J., Bingley, P., Gillespie, K.M., Undlien, D.E., Rønningen, K.S., Guja, C., Ionescu-Tîrgovişte, C., Savage, D.A., Maxwell, A.P., Carson, D.J., Patterson, C.C., Franklyn, J.A., Clayton, D.G., Peterson, L.B., Wicker, L.S., Todd, J.A. & Gough, S.C. (2003). Association of the T-cell regulatory gene CTLA-4 with susceptibility to autoimmune disease. *Nature*, Vol. 423; No. 6939, (May 2003), pp. (506-511), 0028-0836

Umpierrez, G.E., Latif, K.A., Murphy, M.B., Lambeth, H.C., Stentz, F., Bush, A. & Kitabchi, A.E. (2003). Thyroid Dysfunction in Patients With Type 1 Diabetes: A longitudinal study. *Diabetes Care*, Vol. 26, No. 4, (Apr 2003), pp. (1181-1185), 0149-5992

Vaarala, O. (2000). The role of the gut in beta-cell autoimmunity and type 1 diabetes: a hypothesis. *Pediatric Diabetes*, Vol. 1, No. 4, (Dec 2000), pp. (217-225), 1399-543X

Vaidya, B., Imrie, H., Perros, P., Young, E.T., Kelly, W.F., Carr, D, Large, D.M., Toft, A.D., McCarthy, M.I., Kendall-Taylor, P. & Pearce, S.H. (1999). The cytotoxic T lymphocyte antigen-4 is a major Graves' disease locus. *Human Molecular Genetics*, Vol. 8, No. 7, (Jul 1999), pp. (1195-1199), 0964-6906

Vaidya, B., Imrie, H., Geatch, D.R., Perros, P., Ball, S.G., Baylis, P.H., Carr, D., Hurel, S.J., James, R.A., Kelly, W.F., Kemp, E.H., Young, E.T., Weetman, A.P., Kendall-Taylor, P. & Pearce, S.H. (2000). Association analysis of the cytotoxic T lymphocyte antigen-4 (CTLA-4) and autoimmune regulator-1 (AIRE-1) genes in sporadic autoimmune Addison's disease. *Journal of Clinical Endocrinology and Metabolism*, Vol. 85, No. 2, (Feb 2000), pp. (688-691), 0021-972X

Vaidya, B. & Pearce, S. (2004). The emerging role of the CTLA-4 gene in autoimmune endocrinopathies. *European Journal of Endocrinology*, Vol. 150, No. 5, (May 2004), pp. (619-626), 0804-4643

Valerio, G., Franzese, A., Iovino, A.F., Tanga, M., Alessio, M. & Pignata, C. (2000). Simultaneous peripubertal onset of multireactive autoimmune diseases with an unusual long-lasting remission of type 1 diabetes mellitus. *Clinical Endocrinology (Oxf)*, Vol. 53, No. 5, (Nov 2000), pp. (649-653), 0300-0664

Valerio, G., Maiuri, L., Troncone, R., Buono, P., Lombardi, F., Palmieri, R. & Franzese, A. (2002). Severe clinical onset of diabetes and increased prevalence of other autoimmune diseases in children with coeliac disease diagnosed before diabetes mellitus. *Diabetologia*, Vol. 45, No. 12, (Dec 2002), pp. (1719-1722), 0012-186X

Valerio, G., Spadaro, R., Iafusco, D., Lombardi, F., Del Puente, A., Esposito, A., De Terlizzi, F., Prisco, F., Troncone, R. & Franzese, A. (2008). The influence of gluten free diet on quantitative ultrasound of proximal phalanxes in children and adolescents with Type 1 Diabetes mellitus and celiac disease. *Bone*, Vol. 43, No. 2, (Aug 2008), pp. (322-326), 8756-3282

van Koppen, E.J., Schweizer, J.J., Csizmadia, C.G., Krom, Y., Hylkema, H.B., van Geel, A.M., Koopman, H.M., Verloove-Vanhorick, S.P., Mearin, M.L. (2009). Long-term health and quality-of-life consequences of mass screening for childhood celiac disease: a 10-year follow-up study. *Pediatrics*, Vol. 123, No. 4, (Apr 2009), pp. (582-588), 0031-4005

Vanelli, M., De Fanti, A., Adinolfi, B. & Ghizzoni, L. (1992). Clinical data regarding the growth of diabetic children. *Hormone Research*, Vol. 37, Supplement 3, (1992), pp. (65-69), 0301-0163

Ventura, A., Magazzù, G. & Greco, L. (1999). Duration of exposure to gluten and risk for autoimmune disorders in patients with celiac disease. SIGEP Study Group for Autoimmune Disorders in Celiac Disease. *Gastroenterology*, Vol. 117, No. 2, (Aug 1999), pp. (297-303), 0016-5085

Ventura, A., Neri, E., Ughi, C., Leopaldi, A., Citta, A. & Not, T. (2000). Gluten-dependent diabetes-related and thyroid-related autoantibodies in patients with celiac disease. *Journal of Pediatrics*, Vol. 137, No. 2, (Aug 2000), pp. (263-265), 0022-3476

Viljamaa, M., Kaukinen, K., Huhtala, H., Kyronpalo, S., Rasmussen, M. & Collin, P. (2005). Coeliac disease, autoimmune diseases and gluten exposure. *Scandinavian Journal of Gastroenterology*, Vol. 40, No. 4, (Apr 2005), pp. (437-443), 0036-5521

Westerholm-Ormio, M., Vaarala, O., Pihkala, P., Ilonen, J. & Savilahti, E. (2003). Immunologic Activity in the Small Intestinal Mucosa of Pediatric Patients With Type 1 Diabetes. *Diabetes*, Vol. 52, No. 9, (Sep 2003), pp. (2287-2295), 0012-1797

Westman, E., Ambler, G.R., Royle, M., Peat, J. & Chan, A. (1999). Children with celiac disease and insulin dependent diabetes mellitus–growth, diabetes control and dietary intake. *Journal of Pediatric Endocrinology and Metabolism*, Vol. 12, No. 3, (May-Jun 1999), pp. (433-442), 0334-018X

Wheatly, T. & Edwards, O.M. (1985). Insulin oedema and its clinical significance: metabolic studies in three cases. *Diabetic Medicine*, Vol. 2, No. 5, (Sep 1985), pp. (400-404), 0742-3071

Wu, Y., Humphrey, M.B. & Nakamura, M.C. (2008). Osteoclasts—the innate cells of the bone. *Autoimmunity*, Vol. 41, No. 3, (Apr 2008), pp. (183–194), 0891-6934

Yu, L., Brewer, K.W., Gates, S., Wu, A., Wang, T., Babu, S., Gottlieb, P., Freed, B.M., Noble, J., Erlich, H., Rewers, M. & Eisenbarth, G. (1999). DRB1*04 and DQ alleles: expression of 21 hydroxylase autoantibodies and risk of progression to Addison's disease. *Journal of Clinical Endocrinology and Metabolism*, Vol. 84, No. 1, (Jan 1999), pp. (328-335), 0021-972X

Zaiss, M.M., Axmann, R., Zwerina, J., Polzer, K., Gückel, E., Skapenko, A., Schulze-Koops, H., Horwood, N., Cope, A. & Schett, G. (2007). Treg cells suppress osteoclast formation. A new link between the immune system and bone. *Arthritis and Rheumatism*, Vol. 56, No. 12, (Dec 2007), pp. (4104–4112), 0004-3591

Zeglaoui, H., Landolsi, H., Mankai, A., Ghedira, I. & Bouajina, E. (2010). Type 1 diabetes mellitus, celiac disease, systemic lupus erythematosus and systemic scleroderma in a 15-year-old girl. *Rheumatology International*, Vol. 30, No. 6, (Apr 2010), pp. (793-795), 0172-8172

5

Hypoglycemia as a Pathological Result in Medical Praxis

G. Bjelakovic[1], I. Stojanovic[1], T. Jevtovic-Stoimenov[1], Lj. Saranac[2],
B. Bjelakovic[2], D. Pavlovic[1], G. Kocic[1] and B.G. Bjelakovic[3]

[1]*Institute of Biochemistry, Faculty of Medicine, University of Niš*
[2]*Department of Pediatrics, Clinical Center Nis, Faculty of Medicine, University of Niš*
[3]*Clinic of Internal Medicine, Department of Hepato-Gastroenterology,*
Faculty of Medicine, University of Niš
Serbia

1. Introduction

Maintenance of blood glucose homeostasis is fundamentally important for health. The maintain of stable levels of glucose in the blood is one of the most finely regulated of all homeostatic mechanisms and one in which the liver, the extrahepatic tissues, and several hormones play a part. Even mild disruptions of glucose homeostasis can have adverse consequences.

The physiological post absorptive serum glucose concentration in healthy humans range is 4, 4-5,8 mmol/L (80 to 105 mg/dL). The stability of the plasma glucose level is a reflection of the balance between the rates of whole body glucose production and glucose utilization.

Generally, hypoglycemia is defined as a serum glucose level below 3. 8 mmol/L (70 mg/dL).As a relatively rare disorder, hypoglycemia most often affects those humans at the extremes of age, such as infants and the elderly, but may happen at any age.

As a medical problem, hypoglycemia is diagnosed by the presence of three key features (known as Whipple's triad). Whipple's triad is:

1. symptoms consistent with hypoglycemia,
2. a low plasma glucose concentration, and
3. relief of symptoms after the plasma glucose level is raised.

The etiology of hypoglycemia is numerous:

1. Inborn error of metabolism (more common in the pediatric patient than in adults). Disturbance in carbohydrates metabolism: Malabsorption of glucose/galactose, alactasia, asucrasia, galactosemia, fructose intolerance. Glycogen storage disease, Type I ,or von Gierke Disease, glycogen storage disease, Type III, a deficiency of glycogen disbranching enzyme activity (limit dextrinosis), Type VI glycogen storage disease, a deficiency of liver phosphorylase)

2. **Hormonal disturbance** .The hormone insulin plays a central role in the regulation of the blood glucose concentration. It is produced by the β cells of islets of Langerhance in the pancreas. Insulin exerts hypoglycemic effect. Glucagon is the hormone produced by the α

cells of Langerhance islets in the pancreas. Its secretion is stimulated by hypoglycemia. The hormone glucagon, epinephrine, norepinephrine, growth hormone, and cortisol exert the opposite effects to insulin and they belong in the counter-regulatory hormones

3. The disorders of some organs (Liver and Kidney Disorders especially). Any abnormality in the functioning of the liver can disturb the process of blood-sugar regulation, resulting in hypoglycemia. On the other hand, kidney disorder can be one of the major causes of low blood sugar.
4. Infection-related hypoglycemia (in older adults)
5. The adverse medication reactions
6. Hypoglycemia as the complication of treatment of diabetes mellitus.

The central nervous system requires glucose as its primary fuel. The brain uses more than 30% of blood glucose. The brain does not produce the glucose required for its functioning and it is completely dependent on the rest of the body for its supply. So, fluctuations in blood sugar levels can prove to be harmful for the brain; a continual supply of glucose is necessary as a source of energy for the nervous system and some other organs like erythrocytes, testes and kidney medulla .Gluconeogenesis, the biosynthesis of new glucose, (i.e. not glucose from glycogen) from other metabolites (lactic acid, amino acids and glycerol) is necessary for use as a fuel, since glucose is the sole energy source for these organs.

The symptoms caused by low blood sugar come from two sources and may resemble other medical conditions. The first symptoms are caused by the release of epinephrine from the nervous system. These include sweating, pale skin color, shakiness, trembling, rapid heart rate, a feeling of anxiety, nervousness, weakness, hunger, nausea and vomiting. Lowering of the brain's glucose causes: headache, difficulty in thinking, changes in vision, lethargy, restlessness, inability to concentrate or pay attention, mental confusion, sleepiness, stupor, and personality changes.

To treat low blood sugar immediately the patients should eat or drink something that has sugar in it, such as orange juice, milk, or a hard candy. It is need to find out the causes of hypoglycemia.

Laboratory diagnosis of hypoglycemia is very important in medical praxis especially in pediatric, internal medicine (hepatology, renal failure, and cardiology) neuropsychiatry disorders and so on.

Glucose is the name of the simple sugar found in plant and animal tissues. It is made within plants as a product of photosynthesis. Although glucose can be produced within the human body, most of it is supplied to people by dietary carbohydrate intake principally as starch. Once consumed and digested, glucose will either be used immediately or stored as glycogen for future use, (Caraway & Watts,1986; Mayer,1975).

Glucose is the major energy source for human body and is derived primarily from dietary carbohydrates (grains, starchy vegetables, and legumes), from body stores of carbohydrates (glycogen) and from the synthesis of glucose from protein and glycerol moiety of triglycerides (gluconeogenesis) (King, 2011).

The glucose level in blood is kept within narrow range through a variety of influences. While there is some variation in blood glucose as circumstance changes (feeding, prolonged fasting), levels above or below the normal range usually indicate disease.

High blood glucose due to diabetes mellitus is the most commonly encountered disorder of carbohydrate metabolism. Low blood glucose is an uncommon cause of serious diseases. There are numerous rare conditions that cause hypoglycemia in neonatal period and early childhood. In adults, low blood glucose in the fasting state is almost always due to a serious underlying condition (Caraway & Watts,1986; King, 2011; Mayer, 1975; Service,1992).

2. Digestion and absorption of carbohydrates

Carbohydrates are important components of the diet. The carbohydrates that we ingest range from simple monosaccharides (glucose, fructose and galactose) to disaccharides (lactose, sucrose) and complex polysaccharides, starch and glycogen. Most carbohydrates are digested by salivary and pancreatic amylases, and are further broken down into monosaccharides by enzymes in the brush border membrane (BBM) of enterocytes. Maltase, lactase and sucrase-isomaltase are disaccharidases involved in the hydrolysis of nutritionally important disaccharides, maltose, lactose, saccharose. Once monosaccharides are presented to the BBM, mature enterocytes, expressing nutrient transporters, transport the sugars into the enterocytes, (Drozdowski & Thomson, 2006).

The resultant glucose and other simple carbohydrates, galactose (from lactose) and fructose (from succrose) are transported across the intestinal wall to the hepatic portal vein and then to liver parenchymal cells. Both fructose and galactose are readily converted to glucose by hepatocytes Absorption of glucose and galactose occurs by an active carrier-mediated transfer process. Fructose is absorbed by facilitated diffusion (Harper,1975; King, 2011; www.deo.ucsf.edu/type1/understanding-diabetes).

Fructose and galactose are phosphorylated by specific enzymes, fructokinase and galactokinase, presented only in the liver, and converted to glucose. Glucose is transported from the liver via the bloodstream to be used by all the body cells as the most important source of energy. Glucose, as unique sugar in systemic blood circulation, leaves the blood, enters cells through specific transport proteins and has one principal fate: it is phosphorylated by ATP to form glucose-6-phosphate by hexokinase in all human body cells or by the action of glucokinase in hepatocytes. This step is notable because glucose-6-phosphate cannot diffuse through the membrane out of the cells (Haris, 1997; Harper,1979; King,2011; Tietz,1986; Voet & Voet, 2004a).

3. Glycemia - Physiological regulation

Maintenance of blood glucose homeostasis is fundamentally important for health. The plasma glucose level is tightly controlled throughout life in the normal individual, in spite of intermittent food ingestion and periods of fasting, as the net balance between the rates of glucose production and utilization. The stability of the plasma glucose level is a reflection of the balance between the rates of whole body glucose production and glucose utilization.

The amount of plasma glucose level in healthy humans is usually maintained within a range of 4.4 to 5.8 mmol/L , 80 to 110 mg/dL), (Caraway & Watts,1986; King, 2011; Mayes,1975; Service, 1992; Voet & Voet, 2004a).

4. Intermediary metabolism of carbohydrates

4.1 Glycogen synthesis

Glycogen is the storage form of glucose and serves as a tissue reserve for the body's glucose needs. Glycogen synthesis occurs in virtually all animal tissues, but it is especially prominent in the liver and skeletal muscles. In the liver, glycogen serves as a reservoir of glucose, readily converted into blood glucose for distribution to other tissues, whereas in muscles glycogen is broken down via glycolysis to provide energy for muscle contraction. In human body, glycogen is synthesized and stored when glucose levels are high and is broken down during starvation or periods of high glucose demand.

Glycogen is a highly branched polymeric structure containing glucose as the basic monomer (Mayes, 1975; Voet & Voet, 2004b). It is composed of polymers of α-1-4 linked glucose, interrupted by α 1-6 linked branch point every 4-10 residues (Fig 1).

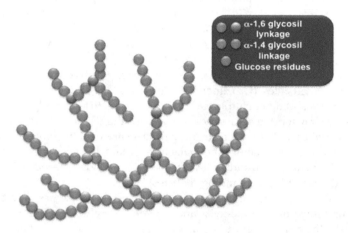

Fig. 1. Glycogen structure

Uridine diphosphate glucose (UDP-glucose) is the immediate precursor for glycogen synthesis. Glycogen synthase will only add glucose units from UDP-glucose onto a preexisting glycogen chain that has at least four glucose residues. Linkage of the first few glucose units to form the minimal "primer" needed for glycogen synthase recognition is catalyzed by a protein called glycogenin, which attaches to the first glucose and catalyzes linkage of the first eight glucoses by alpha(1,4) bonds. The enzyme, glycogenin, initiates glycogenynthesis (oregonstate.edu/.../summer09/lecture/glycogennotes.html; Voet & Voet, 2004b).

The enzyme glycogen synthase then catalyzes elongation of glycogen chains initiated by glycogenin to a chane of 9 – 11 glucose molecule. Glycogen synthase catalyzes transfer of the glucose moiety of UDP-glucose to the hydroxyl at C_4 of the terminal residue of a glycogen chain to form an α(1-4)-glycosidic linkage (Fig 2) (Mayes,1975; King, 2011; Voet & Voet, 2004b; www.uic.edu/.../glycogen%20metab/Glycogen%20biochemistry.htm).

A branching enzyme forms the branching points in glycogen. The branches arise from α-(1-6) linkages which occur every 8 to 12 residues. Glycogen branches are formed by amylo-(1,4-1,6)-transglycosylase, also known as branching enzyme. The branching enzyme transfers a segment from the end of a glycogen chain to the C6 hydroxyl of a glucose residue of glycogen to yield a branch with an α-(1-6) linkage. In the presence of glycogenin, glycogen synthase, branching enzyme and UDP glucose (active glucose) form glycogen as a highly branched polymeric structure, containing glucose as the basic monomer (Figure 2).

Glycogen is synthesized and stored mainly in the liver and the muscles as well as in the cytoplasm of all human body cells as granules named "residual bodies", (Voet & Voet, 2004b).

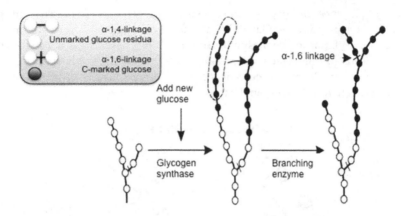

Fig. 2. Glycogenesis

4.2 Glycogen breakdown (glycogenolysis)

In the proceses of glycogen catabolism or glycogenolysis, glycogen, stored in the liver and muscles, is converted first to glucose-1-phosphate and then into glucose-6-phosphate. (Mayes,1975; Voet &;Voet, 2004b). Three enzymes participate in glycogenolysis: glycogen phosphorylase, oligo-1,4-1,4–glucan transferase or trisaccharide transferase, and α(1-6) glucosidase or γ- amylase. Glycogen phosphorylase catalyzes phosphorolytic cleavage of the α-1,4 glycosidic linkages of glycogen (using inorganic phosphate), releasing glucose-1-phosphate as reaction product and limit dextrin. After extensive phosphorylase action on glycogen, the molecule contains four glucose residues in α-1,4-glucosidic bond attached by a(1,6)-link to the glycogen molecule.

These structures can be further degraded by the action of a debranching enzyme, which carries out two distinct reactions. The first of these, known as oligo-a1,4-a-1,4) glucan transferase activity or trisaccharide transferase, removes a trisaccharide unit from limit branch and transfers this group to the end of another nearby glycogen chain, with resynthesis of the α-1,4 bond. This leaves a single glucose residue in a-(1,6) linkage to the main chain. The α-1,6-glucosidase or γ-amylase activity of the debranching enzyme then catalyzes hydrolysis of the α(1,6) linkage, leaving a polysaccharide chain with one branch fewer and yielding free glucose. This is a minor fraction of free glucose released from glycogen (Fig 3), since that the major product of glycogen breakdown by phosphorylase activity is glucose-1-phosphate. Phosphoglucomutase catalyzes the reaction: glucose-1-phosphate $\rightarrow$ glucose-6-phosphate.

Glucose-6-phosphate is the first step of the glycolysis pathway if glycogen is the carbohydrate source of further energy needed. If energy is not immediately needed, the glucose-6-phosphate is converted to glucose, by the action of the enzyme glucose-6-phosphatase (mainly in liver), for distribution to various cells by blood, such as brain, erythrocytes, adipocytes, etc.

The reactions involved in tissue glycogen synthesis and degradation are carefully controlled and regulated by hormones. The primary hormone responsible for conversion of glucose to glycogen is insulin. Opposite effects to glycogen metabolism have its antagonists: glucagon, adrenaline, cortisol, growth hormone which facilitate glycogenolysis in liver and muscles.

The principal enzymes of glycogen metabolism are glycogen synthase and glycogen phosphorylase, reciprocally regulated by allosteric effectors and covalent modification (through phosphorylation or dephosphorylation). Glycogen synthase is active when high blood glucose leads to intracellular glucose-6-P increase. Glycogen phosphorylase is active in the presence of high level of cyclic adenosine monophosphate (cAMP) which suggests that the cells need chemical energy in the form of ATP.

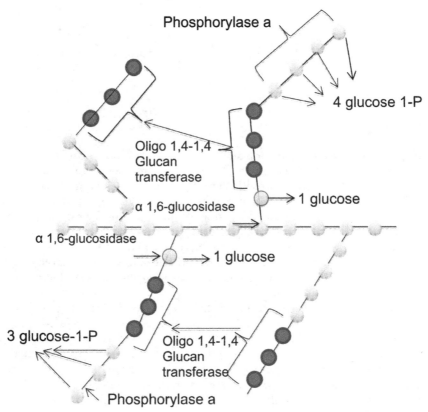

Fig. 3. Glycogenolysis

Glucagon, synthesized by pancreatic α-cells, and epinephrine (adrenaline), synthesized by adrenal medulla, regulate glycogen metabolism by covalent modification (phosphorylation and dephosphorylation) through cAMP cascades. Both hormones are produced in response to low blood glucose level. Glucagon activates cAMP formation in liver, while adrenaline activates its formation in muscle. Phosphorylation of the enzyme, via cAMP cascade, induced by adrenaline, results in further activation of glycogen phosphorylase. These regulatory processes ensure release of phosphorylated glucose from glycogen, for entry into glycolysis to provide ATP needed for muscle contraction.
Insulin, produced in response to high blood glucose, antagonizes effects of the cAMP cascade induced by glucagon and adrenaline. It is the only hormone inducing cAMP decrease (Mayes, 1975; Voet & Voet, 2004b).

4.3 Glycolysis

ATP depletion in cells, or low blood glucose level, lead to the activation of glycogenolysis and the enhancement of glucose degradation through glycolysis. Glycolysis is a central metabolic pathway of glucose metabolism, starting with glucose-6-phosphate, produced by glycogenolysis or gluconeogenesis. Glucose-6-phosphate could also be synthesized directly from blood-derived glucose by the action of hexokinase in all human body cells or by the action of glucokinase in hepatocytes.

Glycolysis is the anaerobic catabolism of glucose. It occurs in cytosol of virtually all cells. The glycolytic pathway converts a molecule of glucose into 2 molecules of pyruvic acid and captures 2 molecules of ATP. If glycolysis proceeds in aerobic conditions 2 molecules of pyruvic acid enter mitochondria, transforms into acetyl-CoA which is oxidized by the citric acid cycle. One cycle provides 12 mol ATP per one molecule of pyruvate. Aerobic conditions provide a mechanism for converting NADH back to NAD$^+$ which is essential for glycolysis to operate (Fig 4).

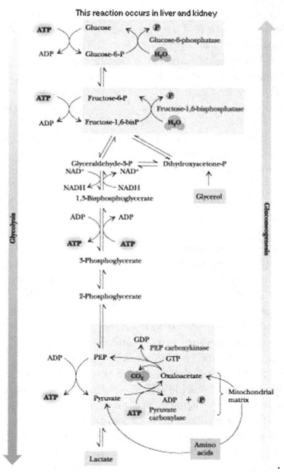

Fig. 4. Glycolysis and Gluconeogenesis

Under anaerobic conditions 2 molecules of pyruvate, under the action of lactate dehydrogenaze, and by using $NADH_2$, convert to 2 molecules of lactate. The reaction is freely reversible (Haris, 1997; Mayes, 1975; Voet & Voet, 2004b;   users.rcn.com/.../I/ IntermediaryMetabolism.html).

4.4 Gluconeogenesis

If glucose is not obtained in the diet, during fasting , the body must produce new glucose from noncarbohydrate precursors by the proces of gluconeogenesis. The term gluconeogenesis means the generation (*genesis*) of new (*neo*) glucose.

The production of glucose from other metabolites is necessary to maintain the glucose level in the blood as a fuel source by the brain, erythrocytes, kidney medulla and testes, since glucose is the sole energy source for these organs. During starvation, however, the brain can derive energy from ketone bodies which are converted to acetyl-CoA. The adipose tissue needs glucose which is also necessary for the synthesis of triacylglycerls and glycerophospholipids. The main precursors for gluconeogenesis are lactate and alanine from muscle, glycerol from adipose tissue, and glucogenic amino acids from the proteolysis in peripheral tissues and proteins from the diet. The most of the amino acids, as well as their α-keto acids, are TCA cycle intermediates. In addition, the gluconeogenetic processes are used to clear the intermediary products of metabolism of other tissues from the blood, e.g. lactate, produced by muscles and erythrocytes, and glycerol, which is continuously produced by adipose tissue.The principal organs responsible for gluconeogenesis are the liver and kidneys, which account for about 90% and 10% of the body's gluconeogenic activity, respectively. Interestingly, the mammalian organs that consume the most glucose, namely, brain and muscle, carry out very little glucose synthesis (Gerich et al, 2001; King, 2011; Mayes,1975; Voet & Voet, 2004b; Woerle & Stumvoll, 2001).

Gluconeogenesis is similar but not the exact reverse of glycolysis; some of the steps are the identical in reverse direction and three of them are new ones (Fig 4). In glycolysis energy barriers obstruct a simple reversal of glycolysis: reactions catalyzed by pyruvate kinase, phospho-fructokinase and hexokinase. These barriers are circumvented by new, special enzymes of gluconeogenesis: pyruvate carboxylase, phosphoenolpyruvate carboxykinase, fructoso-1,6-diphosphatase and glucose-6-phosphatase. The conversion of lactate to glucose begins with the oxidation of lactate, by the action of lactate dehydrogenase, to pyruvate. In the presence of ATP, pyruvate carboxylase and CO_2 convert pyruvat to oxaloacetate. The enzyme, phosphoenolpyruvate carboxykinase (PEPCK) transfers oxaloacetate to phosphoenolpyruvate in the presence of GTP and by elimination of CO_2. Thus, with the help of these two enzymes, and lactate dehydrogenase, lactate can be converted to oxaloacetate. The pyruvate and oxaloacetate are the intermediary products of catabolic pathway of many glycolytic amino acids. The next steps of reversal glycolysis continue just to formation of fructose-1,6-diphosphate, the substrate for fructose-1, 6-diphosphatase. Fructose-6-phosphate, formed by elimination of inorganic phosphate, converts to glucose-6-phosphate (G6P). The energy required for the hepatic synthesis of glucose from lactate is derived from the oxidation of fatty acids. In the liver and kidney, G6P can be dephosphorylated to glucose by the enzyme glucose 6-phosphatase. This is the final step in the gluconeogenesis pathway.

4.4.1 Cory cycle

Lactate, formed by the oxidation of glucose in skeletal muscles and by erythrocytes through the proceses of anaerobic glycolysis, is transported to the liver and kidney, where it re-forms glucose, which again become available via the circulation for oxidation in the tissues. This process is known as the Cory cycle or lactic acid cycle (Fig 5).

4.4.2 Glucose-alanine cycle

It has been noted that of the amino acids transported from muscles to the liver during starvation or under the action of cortisol, alanine predominate. Glucose-alanine cycle represents a cycling glucose from the liver to the muscles and alanine from muscles to liver, effecting a net transfer of amino nitrogen from muscle to liver and free energy from liver to muscle. At the level of muscles, pyruvate, formed by glycolysis, transforms to alanine by the action of alanine transaminase (ALT) or glutamate pyruvat transaminase (GPT). The reaction is freely reversible; at the level of hepatocytes alanine transfers to pyruvate by the action of the same anzyme (Fig 5).

Glycerol, necessary for the synthesis of triacylglicerols and glycerophosholipids is derived, initially, from the blood glucose since free glycerol cannot be utilised readily for the synthesis of these lipids in tissues. Instead of free glycerol, adipose tissue uses α-glycero phosphate or "active glycerol" produced during degradation of glucose by glycolysis.

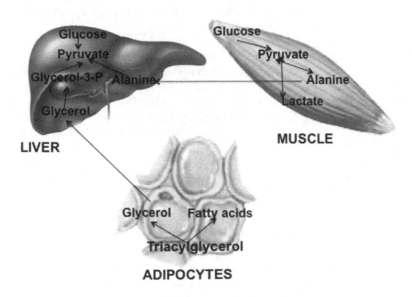

Fig. 5. Cory cycle , glucose-alanine cycle and glycerol-glucose cycle

4.4.3 Glycerol - Glucose cycle

Glycerol, a product of the continual lipolysis, diffuses out of the tissue into the blood. It is converted back to glucose by gluconeogenic mechanisms in the liver and kidney. Thus, a continous cycle exists in which glucose is transported from the liver to adipose tissue and, hence, glycerol is returned to be synthesized into glucose by the liver. Glycerokinase, which requires ATP, catalyzes the conversion of glycerol to α-glycero phosphate. Glycerokinase is present in liver and kidney. The enzyme α -glycero phosphate dehydrogenase oxidizes α-glycero phosphate to the dihydroxyacetone phosphate, the component of glycolysis, which enters the glycolytic pathway as a substrate for triose phosphate isomerase (Fig 4). Thus, liver is able to convert glycerol to blood glucose by making use of above enzymes - some of the enzyme of glycolysis and specific enzymes of gluconeogenic pathway, fructose-1,6-diphosphatase and glucose-6-phosphatase(Harris & Crabb, 1997; King, 2011; Mayes,1975).

Glucose produced by gluconeogenesis in the liver and kidney is released into the blood and is subsequently absorbed by all human body cells especially brain, heart, muscle, and red blood cells to meet their metabolic needs. In turn, pyruvate, lactate and glycerol produced in these tissues are returned to liver and kidney to be used as gluconeogenic substrates.

5. The physiological regulation of carbohydrate metabolism

5.1 Glucose homeostasis

The maintaining of stable levels of blood glucose is one of the most finely regulated of all homeostatic mechanisms and one in which the liver, extrahepatic tissues and several hormones play a part. Even mild disruptions of glucose homeostasis can have adverse consequences. The physiological post absorptive serum glucose concentration in healthy humans range is 4. 4-5.8 mmol/L (80 to 110 mg/dL).

Glycemia is controlled by several physiological processes. It tends to fluctuate to higher levels after meals, due to intestinal absorption of carbohydrates of low molecular weight present in the diet or broken down polysaccharides, such as starch or glycogen. On the other hand, glucose tends to decrease to lower levels induced by cell metabolism, particularly after stress, temperature regulation and physical exercise. Glucose can also be supplied via breakdown of cellular reserves of glycogen. Another input to glycemia levels is gluconeogenesis, whereby glycogen stored in the liver and skeletal muscles are depleted.

The stability of the glycemia is a reflection of the balance between the rates of whole body glucose production and glucose utilization. The glucose homeostasis is tightly regulated by the levels of hormones and substrates in blood and by the physiologic functions of body tissues and organs (Carraway & Watts, 1986; Haris, 1997; King,2011).

5.2 Hormonal regulation of glycemia

The hormones involved in glycemia regulation include insulin (which lowers the blood sugar level) and other hormons which raise blood sugar, namely antagonists of insulin such as glucagon, epinephrine, cortisol, growth hormone, thyreoid hormones (T3 and T4) and many others. The proper functions of these hormones is precise control of glucose concentration in the blood. Insulin and glucagon are two major hormones involved in regulation of blood glucose level. They are both secreted in response to blood sugar levels, but in opposite fashion. At the same time, enhanced insulin secretion induced increased glucagon secretion.

Insulin has a hypoglycemic effect. Secretion of insulin is a response to increased glucose level in the blood. In addition to the direct effects of hyperglycemia in enhancing the uptake of glucose into both the liver and peripheral tissues, the hormon insulin plays a central role in the regulation of the blood glucose concentration. Similarly, as blood glucose falls, the amount of insulin secreted by the pancreatic islets goes down.

Glucagon, as a direct antagonist of insulin, has a hyperglycemic effect. Secretion of glucagon is a response to decreased glucose level in the blood (Chattoraj & Watts,1986; Ginsberg, 1990 a, 1990b; Mayes,1975; King, 2011).

5.2.1 Insulin

Insulin is a small protein consisting of an alpha chain of 21 amino acids linked by two disulfide (S−S) bridges to a beta chain of 30 amino acids. The precursor of insulin is a proinsulin, which contains C peptide (conective peptide). The conversion of proinsulin to insulin requires biologic proteolysis (Ginsberg,1990; Bowen, 2010; Harper, 1975; Chattoraj & Watts,1986).

The stimulus for insulin secretion is a high blood glucose. Insulin is produced by β cells of Langerhans islets in pancreas and is secreted into the blood as a direct response to hyperglycemuia. Beta cells have channels in their plasma membrane that serve as glucose detectors. When blood glucose levels rise (after a meal), insulin is secreted from the pancreas into the pancreatic vein, which empties into the portal vein system, so that insulin traverses the liver before it enters the systemic blood supply. Insulin acts to rapidly lower blood glucose concentration in several ways. It stimulates the active transport of glucose across plasma membranes through glucose transporter (GLUT 4) of muscle and adipose tissue. The liver, brain and red blood cells do not require insulin for glucose uptake. Insulin is an anabolic hormone. It promotes anabolic processes in these cells, such as increasing the rate of glycogenesis, lipidogenesis and proteins synthesis. The cellular uptake of glucose from the blood have the net effect of lowering the high blood glucose levels into the normal range. Insulin stimulates cells in most tissues of the body to preferentially use glucose as their metabolic fuel. It increases cellular glucose utilization by inducing the synthesis of several important glycolytic enzymes, namely, hexokinase, glucokinase, phosphofructokinase, and pyruvate kinase. In addition, insulin inhibit gluconeogenesis in liver. All of these physiological effects of insulin serve to lower blood glucose levels. In each case, insulin triggers these effects by binding to the insulin receptor - a transmembrane protein embedded in the plasma membrane of the responding cells. When the the glucose concentration in the blood falls, pancreas stops releasing insulin (Ginsberg, 1990 a, 1990b; Bowen, 2007; King, 2011).

5.2.2 Amylin

Pancreatic beta cells secrete amylin, a peptide of 37 amino acids. All of its actions (inhibition of glucagon secretion, slowing down the stomach emptying, sending a satiety signal to the brain) tend to supplement those of insulin, reducing the level of glucose in the blood (King, 2011; Silvestre et al, 2001; Young, 2005; users.rcn.com/.../I/IntermediaryMetabolism.html).

5.2.3 Glucagon

Glucagon is another 29 amino acid peptide hormone produced by pancreas. It is a hyperglycemic hormone (Bowen, 2007). Glucagon is produced by alpha (α) cells of

Langerhans islets as proglucagon and proteolytically processed to yield glucagon within alpha cells of the pancreatic islets. Proglucagon is also expressed within the intestinal tract, where it is processed not into glucagon, but to a family of glucagon-like peptides (GLP) (Ginsberg,1990b; Bowen, 2007). Glucagon is secreted in response to hypoglycemia. It is active in liver and adipose tissue, but not in other tissues. This peptide hormone travels through the blood to specific receptors on hepatocytes and adipocytes. When the concentration of glucose in blood decreases, α cells of the pancreas begin to release glucagon. Glucagon stimulates hepatocytes to glycogenolysis and gluconeogenesis, resulting in hyperglycemia. It increases the amount of cAMP and stimulates lipolysis, contributing to reduction of the cellular glucose utilization, the increasing of lipolysis in adipose tissue, providing glycerol and free fatty acids which enter β oxidation cycle, producing the chemical energy (ATP) to most cells. Glycerol leaves the adipose tissue, and through the blood enters the hepatocytes where it may serve as the substrate in the process of gluconeogenesis (Fig 5).

5.2.4 Epinephrine (adrenaline)

Epinephrine is a hormone of adrenal medulla, which consists of masses of neurons that are the part of the sympathetic branch of the autonomic nervous system. Instead of releasing their neurotransmitters at a synapse, these neurons release them into the blood. Thus, although part of the nervous system, the adrenal medulla functions as an endocrine gland. It releases catecholamines: adrenaline (epinephrine) and noradrenalin (also called norepinephrine).

Synthesis of both catecholamines begins with the amino acid tyrosine, which is taken up by chromaffin cells. Called the "fight or flight" hormone, adrenaline prepares the organism for mobilization of large amounts of energy and dealing with stress. Together with cortisol and growth hormone   they are named "stress hormones". Following release into blood, these hormones bind adrenergic receptors on target cells, where they induce essentially the same effects as direct sympathetic nervous stimulation. Adrenaline acts on liver and muscles. Mechanisms of the actions of adrenaline are the same as the mechanisms of glucagon. Through augmentation of cAMP in the cells, adrenaline initiates the enzyme cascade which leads to the activation of glycogen phosphorylase, leading to rapid breakdown of glycogen, inhibition of glycogen synthesis, stimulation of glycolysis and production of energy. In fat cell, it stimulates lipolysis, providing fatty acids as energy source in many tissues. Stimulation of lipolysis contributes to the reduction of the cellular glucose utilization and aids in conservation of dwindling reserves of blood glucose. The stimulation of hepatocytes to glycogenolysis and gluconeogenesis results in regulation of glycemia (Ginsberg,1990a; Chattoraj, & Watts, 1986; www.ncbi.nlm.nih.gov/books/NBK22429/).

5.2.5 Glucocorticoids

The glucocorticoids (cortisol as the principal one) get their name from their effect of raising the level of blood glucose. Glucocorticoids are a class of steroid hormones, synthesized and secreted from zone fasciculate of adrenal cortex, that exert distinct effects on liver, skeletal muscles, and adipose tissue (Bjelakovic et al,2008,2009). The effects of cortisol are best described as catabolic, because it promotes protein breakdown and decreases protein synthesis in skeletal muscles. However, in the liver, it stimulates gluconeogenesis, inducing increased gene expression of several enzymes of the gluconeogenic pathway. Cortisol-induced gluconeogenesis results, primarily, in increased conversion of glycogenic amino acids (from protein breakdown in peripheral tissues) and glycerol (from fat) into glucose (Ginsberg, 1992c; Chattoraj & Watts, 1986; Gil, 1992; Litwak & Schmidt, 1997a; users.rcn.com/.../I/IntermediaryMetabolism.html.)

5.2.6 Growth hormone (GH)

Human growth hormone (GH; also called somatotropin), the protein of 191 amino acids, secreted by somatotrophs of the anterior part of pytuatary gland, regulates overall body and cell growth, carbohydrate, protein and lipid metabolism, and water-electrolyte balance. The GH-secreting cells are stimulated by growth hormone releasing hormone (GHRH) from hypothalamus and inhibited by somatostatin. The release of GH might be regulated not only by hypothalamic GHRH, but also by ghrelin derived from the stomach (Kojima et al., 2005). GH promotes body growth by binding to receptors on the surface of liver cells and stimulates them to release insulin-like growth factor-1 (IGF-1, also known as somatomedin). GH exerts the hyperglycemic effect, stimulating glycogenolysis and lypolysis in peripheral tissues. In liver, GH also stimulates glycogenolysis and glyconeogenesis (Barry, 1992c; Frohman,1992; Litwak.& Schmidt, 1997b).

5.2.7 Thyroid hormones

Thyroid hormones are derivatives of the amino acid tyrosine bound covalently to iodine. The two principal thyroid hormones are: triiodothyronin (T3) and thyroxin (T4). Thyroid hormones receptors are intracellular DNA-binding proteins that function as hormone-responsive transcription factors. The effect of the hormone-receptor complex binding to DNA is to modulate gene expression, either by stimulating or inhibiting transcription of specific genes. It is likely that all cells in the body are targets for thyroid hormones. Thyroid hormones affect oxidative metabolism, especially the metabolism of carbohydrates. Thyroid hormones enhance glucose absorption and the utilization of carbohydrates. They stimulate both the synthesis and disposal of glucose Hypothyroidism or thyroid hormone deficiency leads to decrease in basal metabolic rate and hypoglycemia (Bowen, 2010; Harper, 1975; Zmire et al, 1999).

6. Physiological functions of liver, kidneys and brain in carbohydrate metabolism

Beside hormones, some organs have the important roles in glycemia regulation. Among them, the most important are liver, kidneys and brain.

6.1 The role of liver in carbohydrate metabolism

The metabolic activities of the liver are essential for providing fuel to the brain, muscle, and other peripheral organs. The liver removes two-thirds of the glucose from the blood and all of the remaining monosaccharides (Lehninger,1977; Cherrington,1999). The absorbed glucose is converted into glucose 6-phosphate by hexokinase and the liver-specific glucokinase, whose K_m (Michaelis constant) for glucose is sufficiently higher than the normal circulating concentration of glucose (5mM). The liver plays a unique role in controlling carbohydrate metabolism by maintaining glucose concentrations in a normal range. It possesses the key enzymes for glucose intake (hexokinase and glucokinase) and for releasing of glucose from hepatocytes (glucose-6-phosphatase). The liver has a great capability for synthesis and storing of glycogen (glycogenesis), and, in opposite direction, for glycogen breakdown (glycogenolysis). Also, the liver is the place for gluconeogenesis. (King.2011, Nordlie et al, 1999; Radziuk & Pye, 2001).

Glucose-6-phosphatase liberates free glucose molecules from hepatocytes into blood, catalyzing the following reaction: glucose-6-phosphate + H_2O → glucose + Pi.The substrate for this enzyme is glucose-6-phosphate, the product of glycogenolysis or the end product of gluconeogenesis (Berg, 2002; Radziuk & Pye, 2001; Raddatz & Ramadori, 2007; Yamashita et al, 2001; Berg, 2002) .

6.2 The role of kidney in carbohydrate metabolism

Kidney may play a significant role in carbohydrate metabolism under both physiological and pathological conditions due to renal gluconeogenesis (King, 2011; Gerich et al., 2001). Although the liver is the major site of glucose homeostasis, the kidney plays a vital role in the overall process of regulating the level of blood glucose. Glucose is continually filtered by the glomeruli but is ordinarily returned completely to the blood by the enzymatic reabsorptive system of the renal tubules. The reabsorption of glucose is a process which is similar to that responsible for the absorption of this sugar from the intestine. The capacity of tubular system to reabsorb glucose is limited by the capacity of enzymatically systems of the tubule cells to a rate of about 350 mg/ minute, representing as tubular maximum for glucose (Tmg). Due to that capacity of the kidney, the definitive urine doesn't contain glucose. When the blood levels of glucose are elevated, the glomerular filtrate may contain more glucose then can be reabsorbed; the excess passes into urine to produce glycosuria. In normal individuals, glucosuria occures when the venous blood sugar excesss 9.5-10 mmol/L (170-180 mg/100 ml). This level of the venous blood sugar is termed the renal threshold for glucose (Mayes,1975; Woerle & Stumvoll, 2001).

6.3 The role of brain in carbohydrate metabolism

Glucose is the major energy source for maintenance of brain metabolism and function, except during prolonged starvation. However, the brain has limited glucose reserves and needs a continuous supply of glucose. Endogenous glucose provides more than 90% of energy needed for brain function (Cryer, 1997; Gerich et al, 2001; Halmos & Suba,2011; King, 2011). Since the brain cannot synthesize glucose or store more than a few minutes' supply as glycogen, it is critically dependent on a continuous supply of glucose from the circulation. Fatty acids do not serve as fuel for the brain, because they are bound to albumins in plasma and so do not traverse the blood-brain barrier. In prolonged starvation, ketone bodies, generated by the liver, partly replace glucose as fuel for the brain, (Cahill, 2006).

Glucose is transported into brain cells by the glucose transporter GLUT3. This transporter has a low KM for glucose (1.6 mM). Thus, the brain is usually provided with a constant supply of glucose. At normal (or elevated) arterial glucose concentrations, the rate of blood-to-brain glucose transport exceeds the rate of brain glucose metabolism. However, as arterial glucose levels fall below the physiological range, blood-to-brain glucose transport becomes limiting to brain glucose metabolism, and ultimately survival.

Nowadays it is hypothesised that the brain, in particular the hypothalamus, has a great role in carbohydrate metabolism and glucose homeostasis. The brain is an insulin-sensitive organ. Brain-insulin action is required for intact glucose homeostasis. Receptors for insulin are concentrated in hypothalamic area. Hypothalamus is the site of afferent and efferent stimuli between special nuclei and β- cells and α cells of pancreas, and it regulates induction/inhibition of glucose output from the liver. Insulin gets across the blood-brain barrier, links to special hypothalamic receptors, regulating peripheral glucose (the hypothalamus-pancreas) (Halmos & Suba, 2011). In addition, the hypothalamus can affect metabolic functions by neuroendocrine connections: the hypothalamus-pancreas axis (the control of insulin and glucagone release), the hypothalamus-adrenal axis (the control of the release of adrenaline and noradrenaline) and the hypothalamus-pituitary axis (release of glucocorticoids and thyroid hormones through adrenocorticotrophic hormone (ACTH) and thyroid-stimulating hormone (TSH) control, respectively, which modulate glucose metabolism.

Recently, evidence is accumulating demonstrating that gastrointestinal hormones (peptides) are involved in regulating glucose metabolism through humoral gut–brain axis. Some of them are: ghrelin, neuropeptide Y (NPY), cholecystokinin - CCK, gastric inhibitory polypeptide - GIP, glucagon-like peptide (GLP) etc. (Kojima & Kangawa, 2005; King, 2011; Korner & Leibel, 2003; Neary et al, 2004 ; Young, 2005).

7. Neuro-endocrine defence to hypoglycemia

Generally, hypoglycemia is defined as a serum glucose level below (3.8 mmol/L or, 70 mg/dL). Hypoglycemia is a rare disorder, considered as pathophysiological state rather than a disease. Just as pain and fever require identification of the underlying condition, hypoglycemia warrants diagnosis of the primary disorder causing the low plasma glucose concentration.

The symptoms of hypoglycemia are not specific. For this reason it is necessary to demonstrate a low plasma glucose concentration concomitant with symptoms and subsequent relief of symptoms by correction of the hypoglycemia, i.e., Whipple's tirade. This triade can be considered to be the basis for a patient's symptoms, regardless of the cause of hypoglycemia (Service,1992). Whipple's triad considers: 1) symptoms consistent with hypoglycemia, 2) a low plasma glucose concentration, and 3) relief of symptoms after the plasma glucose level is raised. Hypoglycemia most often affects those at the extremes of age, such as infants and the elderly, but may happen at any age. Given the survival value of maintenance of the plasma glucose concentration, it is not surprising that very effective physiological mechanisms prevent or rapidly correct hypoglycemia have evolved.

Hypoglycemic symptoms are related to the brain and the sympathetic nervous system. The central nervous system requires glucose as the preferred energy substrate. Though the brain accounts for only about 10% of body weight, it uses more than 30% of blood glucose. Hypoglycemic symptoms are mediated through both central and peripheral nervous systems. Once plasma glucose concentration fall belows 3.8 mmol/L or 70 mg/dL, a sequence of events begins to maintain glucose delivery to the brain and prevent hypoglycemia.

The first of all events is the stimulation of the autonomic nervous system and, after that, release of neuroendocrine hormones (counter-regulatory or anti-insulin hormones). Peripheral autonomic symptoms (adrenergic), including sweating, irritability, tremulousness, anxiety, tachycardia, and hunger, serve as an early warning system and preceed the central neuroglycopenic symptoms due to cerebral glucose deprivation (e.g., confusion, paralysis, seizures, and coma) (Zammitt & Frier, 2005).

A hierarchical hormonal response exists in response to decreasing blood glucose levels. As blood glucose drops, pancreatic β-cell reduce insulin secretion. If blood glucose drops further, the pancreatic α-cell secrete glucagon and the adrenal medulla release adrenaline. Both, glucagon and adrenaline, act rapidly to increase glucose availability and therefore are the two major counter-regulatory hormones. Cortisol and growth hormone are also released, but they are unable to prevent prolonged hypoglycemia withouth the preliminary actions of glucagone and adrenaline. In sensing hypoglycemia, the nutritionally deprived brain also stimulates the sympathetic nervous system, leading to neurogenic symptoms.Decreased levels of glucose lead to deficient cerebral glucose availability i.e., neuroglycopenia, that can manifest as confusion, headache, difficulty with concentration. If the symptoms are overlooked, there can be irreversible brain damage. Eventually, the patient may go into coma and death. The adrenergic symptoms often precede the neuroglycopenic symptoms and, thus, provide an early warning system for the patient, (Cryer,1997; Heijboer et., 2006).

8. Hypoglycemia as a result of inherited or acquired disorder of carbohydrates metabolism

8.1 Hypoglicemia and inborn errors of carbohydrate metabolism

Hypoglycemia is not a disease by itself, but its presence is an indication of a problematic health condition. As a relatively frequent common event in the pediatric newborn period (childhood), hypoglicemia may be a consequence of some inborn errors of carbohydrate metabolism (Service,1992; Sinclair,1979; Caraway & Watts, 1986).

8.1.1 Defects in digestion & absorption of carbohydrates

8.1.1.1 Inherited lactase deficiency (alactasia)

Enzyme lactase is necessary to digest lactose to glucose and galactose in the small intestine. Lactase deficiency is a rare congenital disorder in which infants are born without lactase. If lactase is deficient,undigested lactose enters the large intestine, where it is fermented by colonic bacteria, producing lactic acid and gases (hydrogen, methane, carbon dioxide).The gas produced creates the uncomfortable feeling of gut distention and the annoying problem of flatulence. The lactic acid produced by the microorganisms is osmotically active and draws water into the intestine, as does any undigested lactose, resulting in diarrhea. As children are weaned and milk becomes less prominent in their diets, lactase activity normally declines to about 5 to 10% of the level at birth (Gary,1978; Sinclair,1979; Tietz et al,1986). The simplest treatment is to avoid the consumption of products containing much lactose. Alternatively, the enzyme lactase can be ingested with milk products.

8.1.1.2 Lactose intolerance

Lactose intolerance is an inability to digest significant amounts of lactose due to an absence of the enzyme lactase in adult intestines. The symptoms of this disorder, which include diarrhea and general discomfort, can be relieved by eliminating milk from the diet (Maxton et al, 1990; Tietz et al,1986).

8.1.1.3 Sucrase deficiency

Enzyme sucrase decomposes disaccharide sacharose to glucose and fructose molecules. There is a number of reports of an inherited deficiency of the disaccharidases, sucrase and isomalatase, occurring within the mucosa of the small intestine. Symptoms occur in early childhood following ingestion of sucrose. The symptoms are the same as those described in lactase deficiency except that they are evoked by the ingestion of table sugar (Gary,1978 ; Sinclair,1979; Tietz et al,1986)

8.1.1.4 Glucose galactose malabsorption

Glucose Galactose Malabsorption (GGM) is a genetic disorder caused by a defect in glucose and galactose transport across the intestinal brush border membrane. Normally, lactose in milk is broken down into glucose and galactose by lactase, an ectoenzyme on the brush border, and the hexoses, having nearly identical chemical structure, are transported into the cell by the Na$^+$-glucose cotransporter SGLT1 (Fig 6). The mutations causing the defect in sugar transport have been identified (Gary, 1978; Wright, 1998; Wright et al, 2002; Wright et al, 2004; Wright, 2003).

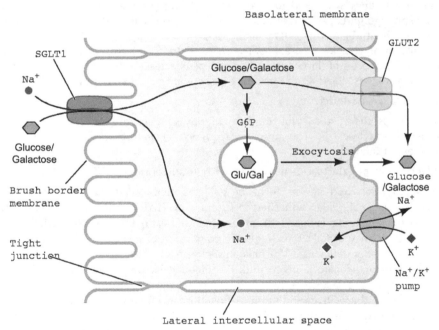

Fig. 6. Sugar transport across intestinal apithelium (Wright et al., 2004, modified)

Glucose-galactose malabsorption is an autosomal recessive disorder in which affected individuals inherit two defective copies of the SGLT1 gene, located on chromosome 22. This disease presents in newborn infants as a life-threatening diarrhea. The diarrhea ceases within 1 h of removing oral intake of lactose, glucose and galactose, but promptly returns with the introduction of one or more of the offending sugars into the diet. We conclude that mutations in the SGLT1 gene are the cause of glucose-galactose malabsorption, and sugar transport is impaired mainly because the mutant proteins are either truncated or are not targeted properly to the cell membrane. The glucose and galactose, if left untransported, draw water out of the body into the intestinal lumen, resulting in diarrhea.

Although no cure exists for GGM, patients can control their symptoms (diarrhea) by removing lactose, sucrose and glucose from their diets. Infants showing a prenatal diagnosis of GGM will thrive on a fructose-based replacement formula and will later continue their "normal" physical development on a fructose-based solid diet. Older children and adults with severe GGM can also manage their symptoms on a fructose-based diet and may show improved glucose tolerance and even clinical remission as they age (Wright et al., 2001; Wright,1998; Gary, 1978).

8.1.2 Galactosemia

Galactose is found in the disaccharide lactose, the principal milk sugar, made from galactose and glucose. It will be recalled that galactose is required in the body, not only in the formation of milk lactose during lactogenesis in lactating mammary glands, but also as a constituent of the glucosphyngolipids (cerebrosides, globosides, gangliosides) and for the synthesis of mucopolysaccharides (MPS) or glucosaminoglycanes (GAG). Glucosaminoglycanes are linked to core proteins forming proteoglycanes. Proteoglycanes and glucosphyngolipids perform numerous vital functions within the body, some of which still remain to be studied (King, 2011; Segal, 1989).

The disruption of galactose metabolism is referred to as galactosemia. Galactosemia can result from deficiencies of three different enzymes: galactose-1-phosphate uridyl transferase (GALT), galactokinase (GALK) and uridine diphosphate galactose 4-epimerase (GALE).

8.1.2.1 Galactokinase deficiency

Galactokinase is the first enzyme in the pathway of galactose metabolism, converting galactose to galactose-1-P. The only consequence of galactokinase deficiency is the development of cataract.

8.1.2.2 Deficiency of galactose-1-phosphate uridyl transferase (GALT)

The most common and severe form of galactosemia, called classic galactosemia or Galactosemia Type 1, is an inherited deficiency of GALT, the enzyme that converts galactose-1-phosphate (galactose-1-P) to uridine diphosphate galactose (UDPgalactose). Absence or deficiency of GALT prevents the conversion of galactose into glucose in liver. People with absent or deficient GALT have intolerance to galactose.

When an infant or neonate is given milk the blood galactose level is markedly elevated (galactosemia), and galactose is found in urine (galactosuria). These can cause severe damage to eyes, kidneys, liver and brain. Afflicted infants fail to thrive. They vomit or have diarrhea after consuming milk and enlargement of liver and jaundice are common, sometimes progressing to cirrhosis. Cataracts will form, and lethargy and retarded mental development are also common. A cataract, the clouding of the normally clear lens of the eye, is a consequence of the accumulation of galactose in the lens of the eye; in the presence of high galactose amount and of aldose reductase, galactose is reduced to galactitol. The absence of the transferase in red blood cells is a definitive diagnostic criterion (Mayatepek et al, 2010).

These problems can be prevented by removing galactose and lactose from the diet. In classic galactosemia conversion of UDP-galactose to UDP-glucose is blocked. The epimerase reaction is, however, present in adequate amounts, so that the galactosemic individual can still form UDP-galactose from glucose. This explains the normal growth and development of affected children in spite of the galactose-free diets which are used to control the symptoms of the disease (Harper, 1975).

In adults, the toxicity of dietary galactose appears to be less severe, due, in part, to the metabolism by alternative metabolic pathway of galactose-1-P by UDP-glucose pyrophosphorylase, which apparently can accept galactose-1-P in place of glucose-1-P. The levels of this enzyme may increase in the liver of galactosemic individuals, in order to accommodate the metabolism of galactose, later, after 10 years.

8.1.2.3 Uridine diphosphate galactose 4-epimerase deficiency

Uridine diphosphate galactose-4-epimerase (UDP-galactose-4-epimerase, GALE) converts UDP-galactose to UDP-glucose. Reaction is freely reversible (Fig 7). In this manner, glucose, as a unique monosaccharide in systemic blood circulation in healthy subects , can be converted to galactose in many different tissues of human body if UDP-galactose-4-epimerase is present. Galactosemia due to epimerase deficiency is the rarest and most poorly understood form. In most patients with GALE (or epimerase) deficiency, the defect presenting with clinical features is similar to classic galactosemia. The treatment for children with generalised GALE deficiency, as with GALT deficiency is the restriction of dietary galactose.

Since galactose is an essential component of galactoproteins and galactolipids, theoretically, in generalised GALE deficiency, no endogenous production of galactose is possible, with a resulting deficiency in galactolipids and galacto-proteoglycanes production.

The most common treatment is to remove galactose (and lactose) from the diet. The enigma of galactosemia is that, although elimination of galactose from the diet prevents liver disease and cataract development, the majority of patients still suffer from central nervous system malfunction, most commonly a delayed acquisition of language skills. Females will also display ovarian failure (Sarkar et al, 2010; Segal, 1989; Walter et al, 1999).

8.1.3 The inherited abnormalities in fructose metabolism

Fructose is monosacharide found in honey and in numerous vegetables and fruits. Disacharide sucrose consists of one molecule fructose attached to a molecule of glucose. It should be mentioned that fructose constitutes the main sugar of seminal fluid. Three inherited abnormalities in fructose metabolism have been identified: essential fructosuria, hereditary fructose intolerance and hereditary fructose-1,6-bisphosphatase deficiency (Baerlocher et al,1978; Gitzelmann et al., 1989; Froesch, 1978).

After absorption by the proces of facilitated diffusion, fructose enters hepatocytes , by the portal blood. A specific kinase, fructokinase, in liver and kidney catalyzes the phosphorylation of fructose to fructose 1-phosphate. Fructose 1-phosphate is cleaved to D-glyceraldehyde and dihydroxyacetone phosphate by aldolase B, an enzyme found in the liver. D-glyceraldehyde enters glycolysis via phosphorylation to glyceraldehyde 3-phosphate catalyzed by triokinase. The two triose phosphates, dihydroxyacetone phosphate and glyceraldehyde 3-phosphate, may either be degraded by glycolysis or may be substrates for aldolase A , the enzyme which forms fructose1,6-diphosphate and hence gluconeogenesis, which is the fate of much of the fructose metabolized in the liver.

$$Fructose + ATP \; \textit{fructokinase} \rightarrow Fructose - 1 - P + ADP$$

$$Fructose - 1 - P \; \textit{aldolaseB} \rightarrow dihydroxyacetone - P + glyceraldehyde$$

8.1.3.1 Essential fructosuria

Essential fructosuria is a benign metabolic disorder caused by the lack of fructokinase, which is normally present in liver and kidney cortex. The disorder is asymptomatic and it may go undiagnosed.

8.1.3.2 Hereditary fructose intolerance (aldolase B deficiency)

Hereditary fructose intolerance is a potentially lethal disorder resulting from a lack of aldolase B which decomposes fructose-1-phosphate to dihydroxyaceton-phosphate plus glycerine aldehyde. The disorder is characterized by severe hypoglycemia and vomiting following fructose or sacharose intake. Prolonged intake of fructose by infants with this defect leads to vomiting, poor feeding, jaundice, hepatomegaly, hemorrhage and eventually death. The hypoglycemia that results, following fructose uptake, is caused by fructose-1-phosphate inhibition of glycogenolysis, by interfering with the phosphorylase reaction and inhibition of gluconeogenesis at the deficient aldolase step. Patients remain symptom free on a diet devoid of fructose and sucrose(Baerlocher et al, 1978; Gitzelman at al, 1989; Odièvre et al, 1978).

8.1.3.3 Hereditary fructose-1,6-bisphosphatase deficiency

This disordered is characterized by hypoglycemia, ketosis and lactic acidosis and oftern lethal course in newborn infants. Due to enzyme defect gluconeogenesis is severely impaired. Gluconeogenis precursors, such as amino acids, lactate and ketones, accumulate as soon as liver glycogen stores are depleted (Asberg et al, 2010; Baerlocher et al, 2010; Froesch, 1978; Mortensen, 2006; Song, 2010; Zaidi, 2009).

8.1.4 The glycogen storage diseases (GSDs)

Glycogen is the storage form of glucose and is present in virtually all living cells, although the liver is primary organ for storage and subsequent release of glucose into the circulation. Glycogen biosynthesis from glucose (glycogenesis), along with the release of glucose from glycogen by the process of glycogenolysis, is highly regulated process that aids in the maintaing of normal blood glucose concentration during fasting.

During the last century, patients who have deficient activity in virtually every enzyme important in the normal synthesis, degradation or regulation of glycogen have been identified. Most of them are inherited in an autosomal recessive manner. Several inborn errors of glycogen metabolism have been described, and they result from mutations in genes that code for proteins involved in various steps of glycogen synthesis, degradation, or regulation. Glycogen storage diseases are characterized by an abnormal tissue concentration (>70 mg per gram of liver or 15 mg per gram of muscle tissue of normal or abnormal structure of glycogen). Hypoglycemia is the main biochemical consequence of GSD type I and some of the other GSDs. The basis of dietary therapy is nutritional manipulation to prevent hypoglycemia and improve metabolic dysfunction (Heller et al, 2008; Mayatepek et al, 2010).

All glycogenosis may divide in two groups: hepatic and muscular forms of glycogenosis. The various hepatic enzyme deficiencies are expressed primarily as hypoglycemia and hepatomegaly. In glycogenosis type I, III and VI there is limitation in the output of glucose from hepatic tissue, and hypoglycemia is an prominent laboratory sing. (Goldberg & Slonim, 1993; Heller et al, 2008; Howell, 1978; Wolfsdorf.& Weinstein, 2003).

8.1.4.1 Glycogen storage disease type I

Glycogen storage disease type I (glucose-6-phosphatase deficiency; von Gierke disease; Hepato-renal glycogenoses). GSD type I (or von Gierke disease) is an autosomal recessive disorder that is caused by deficient G6Pase activity. Glucose-6-phosphatase (G6Pase), an enzyme found mainly in the liver and kidneys, plays a critical role in blood glucose homoeostasis, providing glucose during starvation. One of the important functions of the liver and, to a lesser extent, of the kidney cortex is to provide glucose during conditions of starvation. Glucose is formed from gluconeogenic precursors in both tissues, and in the liver also from glycogen. Both glycogenolysis and gluconeogenesis result in the formation of glucose 6-phosphate, which has to be hydrolysed by G6Pase before being liberated as glucose into the circulation.

Glucose-6-phosphatase is the enzyme that catalyzes the last step of glycogenolysis and gluconeogenesis in liver and kidneys, i.e. the hydrolysis of glucose 6-phosphate to free glucose and inorganic phosphate. Its genetic deficiency is characterized by the association of hepatomegaly and nephromegaly due to the accumulation of large amounts of glycogen in these organs, with hypoglycaemia and lactic acidosis.

GSD type Ia is the most frequent form of glycogenosis, accounting for about 80% of the cases. It is caused by a lack of G6Pase activity, which is easily demonstrated by measuring the activity of this enzyme in a liver biopsy specimen. The deficiency of G6Pase activity is caused by mutations in the gene encoding this enzyme.

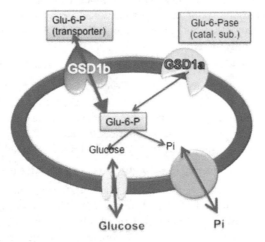

Fig. 7. The glucose-6-phosphatase system

On the basis of the imunological studies, by using the antibodies against to several of five components of glucose-6-phosphatase, GSD type I has been subcategorised into types a, b, and c, with type a as the most common, but all types have similar clinical manifestation as hypoglycemia and hepatomegaly due to the deposition of glycogen with normal structure. Fasting-induced hypoglycemia may be extreme, and with combination with lactic acidosis. Although severely affected patients may suffer brain damage in early infancy, this is not usually the case, and the most patients have normal intelligence. During starvation, however, the brain can derive energy from ketone bodies which are converted to acetyl-

CoA. It is likely that the nervous system is able to metabolise such substance as ketones and lactic acid.

Glucose-6-phosphatase consists of a hydrolase, whose catalytic site faces the lumen of the organelle and of translocases required for the transport of glucose 6-phosphate, Pi and glucose (Figure 7). Glucose 6-phosphate is transported into the lumen of the endoplasmic reticulum by a specific transporter before being hydrolysed by glucose-6-phosphatase, a transmembrane protein with its catalytic site oriented towards the lumen of the endoplasmic reticulum. Glycogen storage disease type Ia (GSD Ia) is due to a defect in glucose-6-phosphatase catalytic site and glycogen storage disease type Ib, to a defect in the glucose 6-phosphate transporter (Schaftingen and Gerin, 2002).

8.1.4.2 Debranching enzyme deficiency (type III glycogen storage disease; limit dextrinosis; Cori's disease)

Type III glycogen storage disease (amylo-1, 6-glucosidase (debrancher) deficiency) most often affects only liver, but may affect muscles as well. In this form of glycogen storage disease, a glycogen accumulates which has a structure resembling the limit dextrin produced by degradation of of glycogen by phosphorylase a , which is free of debrancher (amylo-1, 6-glucosidase) activity. Early in life, hepatomegaly and growth retardation may be striking. In contrast to patients with Type I glycogenosis, moderate enlargement of the spleen is sometime seen. Glycogen of abnormal structure frequently accumulates in muscle and heart, as well as in the liver. In the older patients it may cause a chronic progressive myopathy and cardiomegaly. With muscle involvement, the serum creatine phosphokinase (CPK) activity is elevated, and patients are usually classified as having type III b diseases. There is no renal enlargement in this disease. Generally, the clinical course of this disease is milder than that of Type I glycogenoses.

8.1.4.3 Type VI glycogenosis (hepatic phosphorylase deficiency; Hers' disease)

Large group of patients with hepatic forms of the glycogen storage diseases have increased hepatic glycogen (with normal structure) and a reduction to about 25 percent normal of hepatic phosphorylase activity. Patients with increased liver glycogen and profound reduction in liver phosphorylase activity (and normal activating system) continued to be observed. Hypoglycemia is present (Wolfsdorf & Weinstein, 2003; Heller et al, 2008).

8.1.4.4 Glycogen synthase deficiency (type 0 glycogen storage disease; GSD0)

Type 0 glycogen storage disease (GSD0) is caused by deficiency of the hepatic isoform of glycogen synthase (Weinstein et al, 2006). Although GSD0 has been classified as a glycogen storage disease, this is a misnomer. In contrast to all other types of glycogenoses, which are characterized by increased glycogen storage, deficiency of glycogen synthase causes a marked decrease in liver glycogen content. GSD0 is the only GSD not associated with hepatomegaly and hypoglycemia typically is milder than in the other types of GSD (Wolfsdorf & Weinstein, 2003; Weinstein, 2006).

Patients with GSD0 have fasting ketotic hypoglycemia. Most children are cognitively and developmentally normal. Until recently, the definitive diagnosis of GSD0 depended on the demonstration of decreased hepatic glycogen on a liver biopsy. The need for an invasive procedure may be one reason that this condition has been infrequently diagnosed. Mutation analysis of the GYS2 gene (12p12.2) is a non-invasive method for making this diagnosis in patients suspected to have this disorder.

8.1.5 Disorders of gluconeogenesis

A key role of gluconeogenesis is in the maintenance of blood sugar. Deficiency of any enzyme participating in gluconeogenesis can lead to hypoglycemia with lactic acidosis. Inborn deficiencies are known of each of the four enzymes of the glycolytic-gluconeogenic pathway that ensure a unidirectional flux from pyruvate to glucose: pyruvate carboxylase, phosphoenolpyruvate carboxykinase, fructose-1,6-bisphosphatase, and glucose-6-phosphatase (van den Berghe, 1996).

8.1.5.1 Pyruvate carboxylase deficiency (PCD)

Pyruvate carboxylase, a member of the biotin-dependent enzyme family, catalyses the ATP-dependent carboxylation of pyruvate to oxaloacetate. Pyruvate carboxylase is an important enzyme in gluconeogenesis. Deficiency of pyruvate carboxylase can lead to hypoglycemia with lactic acidosis. Pyruvate carboxylase deficiency is a rare disorder that can cause developmental delay and failure to thrive starting in the neonatal or early infantile period. PCD results in malfunction of the citric acid cycle and gluconeogenesis, thereby depriving the body of energy. Based on the severity of the clinical presentation and the biochemical disturbances, two clinical forms have been described. The milder form A presents in infancy with delayed neurological development, chronic lactic acidemia and a normal lactate to pyruvate ratio. Longer survival, but with severe clinical sequelae, is common in the mild form A. The complex form B presents neonatally or in early infancy with severe metabolic acidosis, lactic acidosis, ketosis, and hepatomegaly (Jitrapakdee &. Wallace, 1999; Ahmad et al., 1999).

8.1.5.2 Phosphoenolpyruvate carboxykinase deficiency

Phosphoenolpyruvate carboxykinase is an important enzyme in gluconeogenesis. It is found in both cytosol and mitochondria of the liver cells. Deficiency of the enzyme, a rare inherited disorder, can cause severe, persistent neonatal hypoglycaemia and liver impairment (Hommes et al, 1976; Vidnes & Sovik, 1976).

8.1.5.3 Fructose-1,6-diphosphatase (FDPase) deficiency

Fructose-1,6-diphosphatase (F1,6DPase) catalyzes the conversion of fructose-1,6-diphosphate (F1,6DP) to fructose-6-phosphate. The F1,6BPase reaction is a major point of control of gluconeogenesis. Fructose-1,6-diphosphatase (FDPase) deficiency is an autosomal recessive disorder caused by a mutation of the FDP1 gene and results in impaired gluconeogenesis (Froesch, 1978; Gitzelmann et al, 1989; Hellerud, 2010).

Patients with FDPase deficiency typically present in the newborn period with symptoms or signs related to hypoglycemia and metabolic acidosis following ingestion of fructose. Patients lacking FDPase accumulate intrahepatocellular fructose-1,6-bisphosphate (FDP) which inhibits gluconeogenesis and, if intracellular phosphate stores are depleted, inhibits glycogenolysis. The inability to convert lactic acid or glycerol into glucose leads to hypoglycemia and lactic acidosis (Asberg et al, 2010; Hellerud, 2010; Song, 2011; Zaidi, 2009; Mortensen, 2006). The accumulation of fructose 1,6-diphosphate (FDP) inhibits phosphorylase a in liver, the first enzyme of glycogenoslysis.

8.1.5.4 Glycero kinase deficiency

Glycerol kinase (GK) catalyzes the phosphorylation of glycerol to glycerol 3-phosphate (G3P) which is important in the formation of triacylglycerol (TAG) and fat storage. GK is at the interface of fat and carbohydrate metabolism. GK deficiency (GKD) is an X-linked inborn error of metabolism that is characterized biochemically by hyperglycerolemia and glyceroluria and is due to mutations within or deletions of the GK gene on Xp21 (Rahib et al, 2007). Isolated GKD can occur in patients with or without symptoms, mainly due to disturbed energy homeostasis associated with hyperketotic hypoglycemia (Sjarif et al, 2004). The greater importance of glycerol as a gluconeogenetic substrate in children than in adults may explain the episodes in young patients with GKD, often elicited by catabolic stress (Hellerud et al, 2004).

8.1.6 Leucine-sensitive hypoglycemia

This type of hypoglycemia was reported in 1956 by Cochrane who described children who became hypoglycemic on a casein-rich diet and whose symptoms worsened on feeding on high protein and low carbohydrate diet. The one-third of all infants with unexplained hypoglycemia may be sensitive to leucin. Presentation is most often in the first year of life. A common symptom is the development of convulsion after milk-feeding, (MacMullen et al., 2001) .

Leucine produces hypoglycemia by causing the release of insulin from the pancreas islet cells. The hypoglycemia found in maple syrup urine diseases is probably caused by high circulating levels of leucin. Two-thirds of the infants who have had leucine-sensitive hypoglycemia have subsequently mental retardation and neurological disorders (Roe &, Kogut, 1982; Sinclair, 1979).

8.1.7 Hyperinsulinism/hyperammonemia (HI/HA) syndrome

Hyperinsulinism is the most common cause of hypoglycemia in early infancy. Congenital hyperinsulinism, is usually caused by genetic defects in beta-cell regulation, including a syndrome of hyperinsulinism plus hyperammonemia (Kelly et al., 2001; Kogut, 1982; Stanley, 1997).

The hyperinsulinism/hyperammonemia (HI/HA) syndrome is a form of congenital hyperinsulinism in which affected children have recurrent symptomatic hypoglycemia together with asymptomatic, persistent elevations of plasma ammonium levels. The disorder is caused by dominant mutations of the mitochondrial enzyme, glutamate dehydrogenase (GDH), that impair sensitivity to the allosteric inhibitor, GTP. These data confirm the importance of allosteric regulation of GDH, as a control site for amino acid-stimulated insulin secretion and indicate that the GTP-binding site is essential for the regulation of GDH activity by both GTP and ATP (MacMullen et al, 2001; Kogut,1982).

9. Hypoglycemia as results of acquired disorders of carbohydrates metabolism

9.1 Liver and kidney disorders

Although hypoglycemia is usually linked with diabetes, there are various types of conditions, which are generally rare, that can cause it even in those who do not have diabetes. Any disorder or abnormality in the functioning of the liver can disturb the process of blood-sugar regulation, resulting in hypoglycemia. On the other hand, disorders in kidney can cause problems in excretion of certain medications. Hence, kidney disorders can be one of the major causes of low blood sugar.

9.1.1 Hypoglycemia in liver disorders

Symptomatic hypoglycemia is uncommon in liver diseases because glucose homeostasis can be maintained with as little as 20 per cent of healthy parenchymal cells, but biochemical hypoglycemia has been reported in a wide variety of aquired hepatic diseases. The hypoglycemia of Reye's syndrome and sepsis, as well as alcohol hypoglycemia, are considered to be the consequence of hepatic disturbance. Acute viral hepatitis results in serious impairment in hepatic glycogen synthesis and gluconeogenesis and frequently gives rise to fasting hypoglycemia (Felig et al., 1970). Glycogen stores rapidly disappear as liver disease (including cirrhosis due to alcoholism) progresses, causing recurrent hypoglycemia (Service, 1992).

Reye syndrome is a fatal disease, most commonly occuring following some virus infections (influenza A, influenza B, herpes, varicella zoster and several other common viral infections). Epidemiologic evidence suggests that aspirin plays a potentiating role in the pathogenesis of this syndrome. The hepatic dysfunction appears to be the primary error and the direct result of a mitochondrial disturbance that causes secondary metabolic derangement, (hyperamoniemia, hypoprotrombinemia without hyperbilirubinemia), including hypoglycemia.

Hypoglycaemia in patients with hepatocellular carcinoma usually occurs during the terminal stage of the illness, but there are patients with hepatocellular carcinoma who develop hypoglycaemia early in the course of their illness. Hypoglycemia occurs predominantly as a paraneoplastic manifestation of hepatocellular carcinoma, (Sorlini et al., 2010; Thipaporn et al., 2005; Young, 2007).

Ethanol is a potent hypoglycemic agent, causing decreased endogenous glucose production and glycogenolysis. The volume of alcohol intake is correlated with the degree of resulting hypoglycemia (Raghavan et al., 2007; Smeeks, 2008). Ethanol-induced hypoglycemia arises from inhibition of gluconeogenesis as a result of the increase in the NADH-NAD ratio, which suppresses the conversion of lactate to pyruvate, glycerophosphate to dihydroxyacetone phosphate, and glutamate to α-ketoglutarate and several tricarboxylic cycle reactions. Ethanol reduces rates of hepatic glucose production, supresses plasma insulin concentration, increases plasma lactate concentration, beta hydroxybutirate, glycerol and free fatty acids, and increases lactate-pyruvate and beta-hydroxybutirate-acetoacetate ratios. Hypoglycemia usually develops within 6 to 36 hours of the ingestion, of even moderate amounts of ethanol by persons chronically malnouriched or by healthy persons who have missed one of the meals. Healthy children are especially susceptible to ethanol hypoglycemia. Blood ethanol levels may not be elevated when the patient is hypoglycemic. Healthy children are especially susceptible to ethanol hypoglycemia. Blood ethanol levels may not be elevated when the patient is hypoglycemic(Arky, 1989; Badawy, 1977; Service, 1992).

9.1.2 Hypoglycemia in kidney disorders

Kidneys play a significant role in carbohydrate metabolism under both physiological and pathological conditions due to renal gluconeogenesis. Hypoglycemia in patients with renal failure may be due to inadequate gluconeogenic substrate availability. It seems that disturbances in renal gluconeogenesis together with lower degradation of insulin played the key role in creating hypoglycaemia in patients with renal diseases. Hypoglycemia should be suspected in any patient with renal failure who exhibits any change in mental or neurologic status (Arem, 1989; Rutsky,1978). Also, kidney disease is a frequent cause of adverse medication reactions due to the problems in excretion of certain medications and, therefore, causing hypoglycemia in older adults (Gerich, 2001).

9.2 Hormonal disturbances and hypoglycemia

Adrenocortical insufficiency or **Adrenocortical hypofunction** is defined as the deficient production of glucocorticoids or mineralocorticoids, or both. Hypoglycemia is common in adrenocortical insufficiency. Primary adrenocortical insufficiency (Addison's disease) is due to destruction of the adrenal cortex, whereas in secondary adrenocortical insufficiency impaired cortisol production is due to deficient ACTH production. Spontaneous hypoglycemia has been reported to be a frequent finding in isolated ACTH deficiency. The cause for primary adrenocortical insufficiency is autoimmune destruction or tuberculosis of the adrenal cortex.

Hypoglycemia in hypopituitarism is common in children under 6 years of age but less so beyond that age. Asymptomatic hypoglycemia has been observed in isolated growth hormone deficiency after prolonged fasting (Tyrrell, 1992).

Insulinoma. Insulin-producing tumors of pancreas can cause severe hypoglycemia; among these are islet cell adenoma and carcinoma (insulinoma). Insulinoma is uncommon in persons less than 20 years of age and is rare in those less than 5 years of age. Of the patients with insulinoma, approxymately 87 per cent have single benign tumors. These tumors are most common in women (60%), with median age of diagnosis 50 years (Service, 1992).

9.3 Reactive hypoglycemia

The post-prandial hypoglycemia occurs immediately following meals, with no known causes (idiopathic reactive hypoglycemia, RH) (Krinsley & Grover, 2007).

Alimentary hypoglycemia, another form of RH related to prior upper GI surgery (Guettier, 2006), results from rapid glucose absorption into the intestine and increased insulin secretion after every meal. The food stimulated hypoglycemia usually cause symptomes mediated by the autonomic nervous system - sweating, shakiness, anxiety, palpitations, and weakness, and rarely those of impairment of central nervous system function. The food deprived hypoglycemia, on the other hand, usually result in impariment of central nervous system functions - reduced intellectual capacity, confusion, irritability, abnormal behavior, convulsions and coma (Service,1992).

Infections. Hypoglycemia often occurs during or following acute infections in older adults. Infection-related hypoglycemia increases the risk of death and morbidity among persons over age 70 Secretion of glucagon, epinephrine, and growth hormone during hypoglycemia diminishes significantly after age 65, reducing autonomic warning symptoms in older adults.

Sepsis as a cause of hypoglycemia should be readily apparent. The mechanism for hypoglycemia with sepsis is not well defined. Depleted glycogen stores, impaired gluconeogenesis, and increased peripheral utilization of glucose may all be contributing factors. Laboratory testing can confirm the suspicion of hepatic dysfunction (Rattarasarn, 1997).

9.3.1 Hypoglycemia due to drug medications

Insulin treatment of Diabetes mellitus. Hypoglycaemia is a serious, frequent and recurrent complication of treatment of diabetes mellitus with insulin, which may become a direct danger to the patient's life. Hypoglycaemia represents the limiting factor to obtain good glycemic control. Dysregulation of counteracting mechanisms and autonomic nervous system neuropathy contribute to a strong increase in the incidence of hypoglycaemia in type 1 diabetic patients, but also in long lasting type 2 diabetic patients (Cryer, 2001, 2008).

Predictors of hypoglycemia in patients with type 2 diabetes include treatment with insulin and duration of insulin treatment, a history of previous hypoglycemia. Primary risk factors for hypoglycemia in decreasing importance have been reported as age over 64, current insulin treatment, sulfonylurea treatment, polypharmacy, renal impairment and previous hypoglycemic episodes (Miller et al., 2001).

Antibiotics. Pentamidine used in treating opportunistic infections associated with immunosuppression (e.g. Pneumocystis pneumonia) and protozoan parasites, causes severe hypoglycemia by increasing insulin secretion. Isoniazid causes hypoglycemia through cytotoxic hepatic damage (Service, 1992).

Sulfonamides and Fluorquinolones have been known to cause significant, life-threatening hypoglycemia by increasing insulin secretion.

Cardiac medications. Beta-blockers inhibit glycogenolysis and are most likely to be associated with hypoglycemia in older adults. Isolated reports indicate that angiotensin-converting enzyme inhibitors can cause hypoglycemia by increasing insulin sensitivity.

Salicylates. It has been determined more recently that salicylates, such as aspirin, decrease serum glucose by reversing or inhibiting the process of insulin resistance related to generalized inflammatory responses.

Psychotropic medications. It should be avoided haloperidol in older adults with a history of hypoglycemia, or sulfonylurea or insulin use, due to the risk of severe hypoglycemic interactions. Tricyclic antidepressants, chlorpromazine, MAO inhibitors, and lithium also have been reported to cause severe hypoglycemia.

Quinolines. Quinines, used as an anti-malarial and anti-arrhythmic agents, have strong hypoglycemic properties, increasing insulin secretion as the sulfonylureas do (Service, 1992).

10. Conclusion

Hypoglycemia is defined as a serum glucose level below (3.8 mmol/L or, 70 mg/dL). The plasma glucose level is tightly controlled throughout life in the normal individual. The stability of the plasma glucose level is a reflection of the balance between the rates of whole body glucose production and glucose utilization. The physiological post absorptive serum glucose concentration in healthy humans range is 4.4-5.8 mmol/L (80 to 110 mg/dL). Variation in blood glucose levels above or below the normal range usually indicate to serious diseases. Even mild disruptions of glucose homeostasis can have adverse consequences.

Hypoglycemia most often affects those at the extremes of age, such as infants and the elderly, but may happen at any age, in neonatal period and early childhood As a relatively frequent common event in the pediatric newborn period (childhood), hypoglicemia may be a consequence of some inborn errors of carbohydrate metabolism. In adults, hypoglycemia is a result of acquired disorders, primarily due to disturbance of physiological function of some organs (liver, kidney, CNS) or manifests disorders of some endocrine glands, involved in carbohydrate metabolism .

The symptoms of hypoglycemia are not specific and are related to disturbance of the brain and the sympathetic nervous system. The stimulation of the autonomic nervous system produces sweating, pale skin, irritability, anxiety, weakness, hunger, nausea, serving as an early warning system and preceding the neuroglycopenic symptoms due to cerebral glucose deprivation, e.g. headache, confusion, inability to concentrate or pay attention, mental confusion, difficulty in thinking, changes in vision, lethargy, sleepiness, stupor.

Biochemical hypoglycemia has been reported in a wide variety of acquired hepatic and renal diseases. Also, kidney disease is a frequent cause of adverse medication reactions due to the problems in excretion of certain medications and, therefore, causing hypoglycemia in older adults due to drug medications. Hypoglycaemia is a serious, frequent and recurrent complication of diabetes mellitus treatment with insulin, which may become a direct danger to the patient's life.

Laboratory diagnosis of hypoglycemia is very important in medical praxis, especially in pediatric praxis, suggesting some inborn errors of carbohydrate metabolism, or, in adults, suggesting hepatic disorders, renal failure, and cardiac disorders, neuropsychiatric disorders, etc.

11. References

Ahmad, A., Kahler, S.G., Kishnani, P.S., Artigas-Lopez, M., Pappu, A.S., Steiner, R., Millington, D.S., & Van Hovel, J.L.K. (1999). Treatment of Pyruvate Carboxylase Deficiency With High Doses of Citrate and Aspartate. *Am J Med Genet*, Vol.87, pp.331–338, ISSN 0148-7299.

Alan, D., Rinkler, R., & Henderson, A. (1986). Gastric, pancreatic, and intestinal function, Chapter 14, In: *Textbook of Clinical Chemistry*, Tietz, N.W. (ed.), pp.1434-1493, WB Saunders Company, ISBN 0-7216-8886-1, Philadelphia, London, Toronto.

Ardigo, S., & Philippe J. (2008) Hypoglycemia and diabetes. *Rev Med Suisse*, Vol.4, No.160, pp.1376-1378, ISSN 1660-9379.

Arem, R. (1989). Hypoglycemia associated with renal failure. *Endocrinol Metab Clin North Am*, Vol.18, No.1, (Mar 1989), pp.103-121, ISSN 0889-8529.

Arky, R.A. (1989). Hypoglycemia associated with liver disease and ethanol. *Endocrinol Metab Clin North Am*, Vol.18, No.1, pp. 75-90, ISSN 0889-8529.

Asberg, C., Hjalmarson, O., Alm, J., Martinsson, T., Waldenström, J., & Hellerud C. Fructose 1,6-bisphosphatase deficiency: enzyme and mutation analysis performed on calcitriol-stimulated monocytes with a note on long-term prognosis. *J Inherit Metab Dis*, 2010 Feb 12. [Epub ahead of print], ISSN 0141-8955.

Badawy, A.A.B. (1977). A Review of the Effects of Alcohol on Carbohydrate Metabolism. *Br J Alcohol and Alcoholism*, Vol.12, pp.30-42.

Baerlocher, K., Gitzelmann, R., Steinmann, B. & Gitzelmann-Cumarasamy, N. (1978). Hereditary fructose intolerance in early childhood: a major diagnostic challenge. Survey of 20 symptomatic cases. *Helv Paediatr Acta*, Vol.33, No.6, (Dec 1978), pp.465-487, ISSN:0018-022X.

Bjelakovic G, Stojanovic I, Jevtovic-Stoimenov T, Bjelakovic B. (2008). Glucocorticoids, thymus function and sex hormone in human body Growing. In: *Adverse effects of steroids*. Inoue, Y., Watanabe, K. (eds.), pp.187-210, Nova Science Publishers Inc, ISBN 978-1-60456-880-6, New York.

Bjelaković, G., Stojanovic, I., Jevtovic-Stoimenov, T., Pavlović, D., Kocić, G., Kamenov, B., Saranac, L., Nikolić, J., Bjelaković, B., Sokolović, D., & Basić, J. (2009). Thymus as a target tissue of glucocorticoid action: what are the consequences of glucocorticoid thymectomy ? *J Basic Clin Physiol Pharmacol*, Vol.20, No.2, pp.99-125, ISSN 0792-6855.

Bowen R. (2006) *Pathophysiology of endocrine system*. November 11, 2007, Available at: http://www.vivo.colostate.edu/hbooks/pathphys/endocrine/index.html.

Cahill G.F.Jr. (2006). Fuel metabolism in starvation. *Annu Rev Nutr*, Vol.26, pp.1-22, ISSN 0199-9885.

Caraway TW & Watts NB. (1986). Carbohydrates..Chapter 6, In: *Textbook of Clinical Chemistry*, Tietz, N.W. (ed.), pp.775-826, W.B.Saunders Company, ISBN 0-7216-8886-1, Philadelphia, London, Toronto.

Chattoraj, S.C., & Watts, N.B. (1986). Endocrinology, In: *Textbook of Clinical Chemistry*, Tietz, N.W. (ed.), pp.997-1171, WB Saunders Company, ISBN 0-7216-8886-1, Philadelphia, London, Toronto.

Cherrington, A.D. (1999). Banting Lecture 1997 Control of Glucose Uptake and Release by the Liver In Vivo. *Diabetes*, Vol.48, (May 1999), pp.1198-1214, ISSN 0012-1797.

Cryer, P.E.(1997). Hierarchy of physiological responses to hypoglycemia: relevance to clinical hypoglycemia in type I (insulin dependent) diabetes mellitus. *Horm Metab Res*, Vol.29, No.3, (Mar 1997), pp.92-96, ISSN 0018-5043.

Cryer, P.E. (2008). Hypoglycemia: still the limiting factor in the glycemic management of diabetes. *Endocr Pract*, Vol.14, No.6, (Sep 2008), pp.750-756, ISSN 1530-891X.

Cryer, P.E., Davis, S.N. & Shamoon H. (2003). Hypoglycemia in diabetes. *Diabetes Care*, Vol.26, No.6, (Jun 2003), pp.1902-1912, ISSN 0149-5992.

Drozdowski, L.A. & Thomson, A.B.R. Intestinal sugar transport. *World J Gastroenterol*, Vol.12, No.11, (March 2006), pp. 1657-1670. ISSN 1007-9327

Felig, P., Brown,W.V., Levine, R.A., & Klatskin, G. (1970). Glucose Homeostasis in Viral Hepatitis. *N Engl J Med*, Vol.283, pp.1436-1440, ISSN 0028-4793.

Frohman, L.A. (1992). The anterior pituitary, In: *Cecil Textbook of Medicine*. Wyngaarden, B.J., Smith, H.L., & Bennett W.B. (ed), pp.1224-1238, Saunders Company, ISBN 0-721608886-1, Phyladelphia, London, Toronto, Montreal, Sydney, Tokyo.

Froesch, E.R. (1978). Essential fructosuria, hereditary fructose intolerance and fructose-1,6-diphosphate deficiency, Chapter 6, In: *The metabolic Basis of inherited diseases*, Fourth Edition, John J. Stanbury, James B. Wyngarden, Donald S. Fredrickson (eds), pp.121-138, McGraw-Hill Book Company, ISBN 0-07-060725-7, New York.

Gary, G.M. (1978). Intestinal disaccharidase deficiencies and glucose-galactose malabsorption, Chapter 64, In: *The metabolic Basis of inherited diseases*, Fourth Edition, John J. Stanbury, James B. Wyngarden, Donald S. Fredrickson (eds), pp.1526-1536, McGraw-Hill Book Company, ISBN 0-07-060725-7, New York.

Gerich, J.E., Meyer, C., Woerle, H.J., & Stumvoll, M.(2001). Renal Gluconeogenesis. Its importance in human glucose homeostasis. *Diabetes Care* , Vol.24, No.2, pp. 382-391, ISSN 0149-5992.

Gill, N.G. (1992). Endocrine end Reproductive diseases, Part XVI, In: *Cecil Textbook of Medicine*. Wyngaarden, B.J., Smith, H.L., & Bennett W.B. (ed), pp.1194-1290, Saunders Company, ISBN 0-721608886-1, Phyladelphia, London, Toronto, Montreal, Sydney, Tokyo.

Ginsberg, H.B. (1990a). Molecular endocrinology: mechanism of hormonal action, Chapter 17, In: *Biochemistry. A Case oriented Approch*, Fifth Edition, Montgomery R., Conway W.T., Spector A.A. (eds), pp.721-748, The C.V. Mosby Company, ISBN 0-8016-3549-7, USA, Canada.

Ginsberg, H.B. (1990b). Molecular endocrinology: hormones active at the cell surface. Chapter 18, In: *Biochemistry. A Case oriented Approaach*, Fifth Edition, Montgomery R., Conway W.T., Spector A.A. (eds), pp.749-795, The C.V. Mosby Company, ISBN 0-8016-3549-7, USA, Canada.

Ginsberg H.B. (1990c). Molecular endocrinology:hormones active inside the cell. Chapter 19, In: Montgomery In: *Biochemistry. A Case oriented Approach*, Fifth Edition,

Montgomery R., Conway W.T., Spector A.A. (eds), pp.797-836, The C.V. Mosby Company, ISBN 0-8016-3549-7, USA, Canada.

Gitzelmann, R., Steinmann, B., & VanDenBerg, G. (1989), Disorders of Fructose metabolism, Chapter 11, In: *The Metabolic Basis of Inherited diseases I*, 6th Edition, Scriver, C.R., Beaudet, A.L., Sly, W.S., Valle, D. (eds), pp.399-424, McGraw-Hill Information Services Company, ISBN 0-07-060726-1, New York.

Goldberg, T., & Slonim, A.E. (1993). Nutrition therapy for hepatic glycogen storage diseases. *J Am Diet Assoc.* Vol.93, No.12, pp.1423-1430.

Greene, H.L. (1992). The glycogen storage disease, In: *Cecil Textbook of Medicine*. Wyngaarden, B.J., Smith, H.L., & Bennett W.B. (ed), pp.1078-1081, W.B.Saunders Company, ISBN 0-721608886-1, Phyladelphia, London, Toronto, Montreal, Sydney, Tokyo.

Hakimi, P., Johnson, M.T., Yang, J., Lepage, D.F., Conlon, R.A., Kalhan, S.C., Reshef, L., Tilghman, S.M., & Hanson, R.W. (2005). Phosphoenolpyruvate carboxykinase and the critical role of cataplerosis in the control of hepatic metabolism. *Nutr Metab (Lond)*. Vol.21, No.2, (Nov 2005), pp.33, ISSN 1743-7075.

Halmos, T., & Suba, I. (2011). The role of the brain in the regulation of metabolism and energy expenditure: the central role of insulin, the insulin resistance of the brain. *Orv Hetil*. Vol.152, No.3, (Jan 2011), pp.83-91, ISSN 0030-6002.

Harris, R.A., & Crabb, D.W. (1997). Metabolic interrelationships, In: *Textbook of biochemistry with clinical correlations*. Devlin, T.M. (ed), pp.525-672, Wiley-Liss, ISBN 0-471-15451-2, New York.

Haris, R.A.. (1997). Carbohydrate metabolism I: Major metabolic pathways and their control, Chapter 7. In: *Textbook of biochemistry with clinical correlations*. Devlin, T.M. (ed), pp 267-327, Wiley-Liss, ISBN 0-471-15451-2, New York.

Harper, A.H. (1975). Digestion & Absorption from the gastrointestinal tract, Chapter 12, In: *Rewiew of Physiological Chemistry*, 15th edition, pp.243-278, Lange Medical Publications, ISNB:0-87041-033-4, Los Altos, California.

Heijboer, CH., Van den Hoek, P.A.M., Havekes, L.M., Romijn, J.A., & Corssmit, E.P.M. (2006). Gut–Brain Axis: Regulation of Glucose Metabolism. *J Neuroendocrinol*. Vol.18, No.12, pp.883–894, ISSN 0953-8194.

Heller, S., Worona, L., & Consuelo, A. (2008). Nutritional therapy for glycogen storage diseases. *J Pediatr Gastroenterol Nutr*. Vol.47, Suppl 1, (Aug 2008), pp.S15-21, ISSN 0277-2116.

Hellerud, C. (2010). Fructose 1,6-bisphosphatase deficiency: enzyme and mutation analysis performed on calcitriol-stimulated monocytes with a note on long-term prognosis. *J Inherit Metab Dis*. DOI: 10.1007/s10545-009-9034-5, ISSN 0277-2116.

Hellerud, C., Wramner, N., Erikson, A., Johansson, A. Samuelson, G., & Lindstedt, S. (2004). Glycerol kinase deficiency: follow-up during 20 years, genetics, biochemistry and prognosis. *Acta Paediatr*. Vol 93, No.7, pp. 911-921, ISSN 0001-656X.

Hers, H.G., Van Hoof, F., & de Barsa, T. (1989). Glycogen storage diseases, Chapter 12, In: *The Metabolic Basis of Inherited diseases I*, 6th Edition, Scriver, C.R., Beaudet, A.L., Sly, W.S., Valle, D. (eds), pp. 425-452, McGraw-Hill Information Services Company, ISBN 0-07-060726-1, New York.

Hommes, F.A., Bendien, K., Elema, J.D., Bremer, H.J., & Lombeck, I. (1976). Two cases of phosphoenolpyruvate carboxykinase deficiency. *Acta Paediatr Scand*. Vol.65, No.2, pp.233-240, ISSN 0001-656X.

Howell, R.R. (1978). The glycogen storage diseases, Chapter 7, In: *The metabolic Basis of inherited diseases*, Fourth Edition, John J. Stanbury, James B. Wyngarden, Donald S.

Fredrickson (eds), pp.137-159, McGraw-Hill Book Company, ISBN 0-07-060725-7, New York.

Jitrapakdee, S., & Wallace, J.C. (1999). Structure, function and regulation of pyruvate carboxylase. Biochem J. Vol.340, pp.1–16, ISSN 0264-6021.

Kelly, A., Ng D., Ferry, R.J.Jr., Grimberg, A., Koo-McCoy, S., Thornton, P.S., & Stanley, C.A. (2001). Acute Insulin Responses to Leucine in Children with the Hyperinsulinism/Hyperammonemia Syndrome. *J Clin Endocrinol & Metab.* Vol.86, No.8, pp.3724-3728, ISSN 0021-972X.

King, M.W. (2011). In: *The medical biochemisty page,* March 31, 2011, Available at: http://themedicalbiochemistrypage.org/.html.

Kojima, M., & Kangawa, K. (2005). Ghrelin: Structure and Function. *Physiol Rev.* Vol.85, pp.495–522, ISSN 0031-9333.

Korner, J., & Leibel, R.L. (2003). To Eat or Not to Eat - How the Gut Talks to the Brain *N Engl J Med,* Vol.349, pp.926-928, ISSN 0090-3493.

Krinsley, J.S., & Grover, A. (2007). Severe hypoglycemia in critically ill patients: risk factors and outcomes. *Crit Care Med.* Vol.35, No.10, (Oct 2007), pp.2262-2267, ISSN 0090-3493.

Kogut, M.D. (1982). Idiopathic leucine-sensitive hypoglycemia syndrome: insulin and glucagon responses and effects of diazoxide. *Pediatr Res.* Vol.16, No.1, (Jan 1982), pp.1-4, ISSN 0031-3998.

Lehninger, A.L. (1977). Organ interrelationships in the metabolism of mammals. In. *Biochemistry,* 2nd edition, Leninger, A.L. (ed), pp.829-852, Worth Publications Inc, ISNB: 0-87901-047-9, New York.

Litwak, G. & Schmidt TJ. (1997)b. Biochemistry of Hormones I: Polypeptide hormones . Chapter 20, In: *Textbook of biochemistry with clinical correlations.* Devlin, T.M. (ed), pp.839-891, Wiley-Liss, ISBN 0-471-15451-2, New York.

Litwak, G. & Schmidt TJ. (1997)a. Biochemistry of hormones II: steroid hormones. Chapter 21, In: *Textbook of biochemistry with clinical correlations.* Devlin, T.M. (ed), pp.893-918, Wiley-Liss, ISBN 0-471-15451-2, New York.

MacMullen, C., Fang, J., Hsu, B.Y.L., Kelly, A., de Lonlay-Debeney, P., Saudubray, J.M., Ganguly, A., Smith, T.J., & Stanley, C.A. (2001). Hyperinsulinism/Hyperammonemia Syndrome in Children with Regulatory Mutations in the Inhibitory Guanosine Triphosphate-Binding Domain of Glutamate Dehydrogenase. *J Clin Endocrinol Metab.* Vol.86, pp.1782–1787, ISSN 0021-972X.

Maxton, D.G., Catt, S.D., & Menzies, I.S. (1989). Intestinal disaccharidases assessed in congenital asucrasia by differential urinary disaccharide excretion. *Dig Dis Sci.* Vol.34, No.1, (Jan 1989), pp.129-131, ISSN 0163-2116.

Mayatepek, E., Hoffmann, B., &, Meissner, T. (2010). Inborn errors of carbohydrate metabolism. *Best Pract Res Clin Gastroenterol.* Vol.24, No.5, (Oct 2010), pp.607-618, ISSN 1521-6918.

Mayer, P. (1975). Metabolism of Carbohydrate, In: *Rewiew of Physiological Chemistry,* 15th edition, Harper, H.A. (ed), pp 243-278, Lange Medical Publications, ISNB:0-87041-033-4, Los Altos, California.

Mithieux, G. (1996). Role of glucokinase and glucose-6 phosphatase in the nutritional regulation of endogenous glucose production. *Reprod Nutr Dev,* Vol.36,No.4, pp .357- 362, ISSN 0181-1916.

Mokán, M. (2008). Hypoglycaemia. *Vnitr Lek.* Vol.54, No.4, (Apr 2008), pp.387-394, ISSN 0042-773X.

Moss, D.W., Henderson, A.R., & Kachmar, J.F. (1986). Enzymes. In: *Textbook of Clinical Chemistry*, Tietz, N.W. (ed.), pp. 619-674, WB Saunders Company, ISBN 0-7216-8886-1, Philadelphia, London, Toronto.

Neary, N.M., Goldstone, A.P., & Bloom, S.R. (2004). Appetite regulation: from the gut to the hypothalamus. *Clin Endocrinol*, Vol.60, No.2, pp.153–160, ISSN 0300-0664.

Nordlie, R.C., Foster, J.D., & Lange, A.J. (1999). Regulation of glucose production by the liver. *Annu Rev Nutr*, Vol.19, pp.379-406, ISSN 0199-9885.

Odièvre, M., Gentil, C., Gautier, M., & Alagille, D. (1978). Hereditary fructose intolerance in childhood. Diagnosis, management, and course in 55 patients. *Am J Dis Child*, Vol.132, No.6, (Jun 1978), pp.605-608. 0096-8994

Ohro, M., Bosshard, N.U., Buist, N.R., Gitzelmann, R., Aynsley-Green, A., Blumel, P., Gannon, M.C., Nuttall, F.Q., & Groop, L.C. (1998). Mutations in the liver glycogen synthase gene in children with hypoglycemia due to glycogen storage disease type 0. J. *Clin Invest* Vol.102, No.3, 507-512, ISSN 0021-9738.

Pascual, J.M., Wang, D., Lecumberri, B., Yang, H., Mao, X., Yang, R., & De Vivo, D.C. (2004). GLUT1 deficiency and other glucose transporter diseases. *Eur J Endocrinol.* Vol.150, pp.627–633, ISSN 0804-4643.

Postic, C., Dentin, R., & Girard, J. (2004). Role of the liver in the control of carbohydrate and lipid homeostasis. *Diabetes Metab.* Vol.30, No.5, (Nov 2004), pp.398-408, ISSN 2233-6079.

Raddatz, D., & Ramadori, G. (2007). Carbohydrate metabolism and the liver: Actual aspects from physiology and disease. *Z Gastroenterol*, Vol.45, No.1, pp.51-62, ISSN 0044-2771.

Radziuk, J., & Pye, S. (2001). Hepatic glucose uptake, gluconeogenesis and the regulation of glycogen synthesis. *Diabetes Metab Res Rev.* Vol.17, No.4, (Jul 2001), pp.250-272, ISSN 1520-7552.

Rahib, L., MacLennan, N.K., Horvath, S., Liao, J.C., & Dipple, KM. (2007). Glycerol kinase deficiency alters expression of genes involved in lipid metabolism, carbohydrate metabolism, and insulin signaling. *Eur J Hum Genet*, Vol.15, (April 2007), pp.646–657, ISSN 1018-4813.

Rattarasarn, C. (1997). Hypoglycemia in sepsis: risk factors and clinical characteristics. *J Med Assoc Thai.* Vol.80, No.12, (Dec 1997), pp.760-766, ISSN 0125-2208.

Rivera, N., Ramnanan, C.J., An, Z., Farmer, T., Smith, M., Farmer, B., Irimia, J.M., Snead, W., Lautz, M., Roach P.J., & Cherrington, P.D. (2010). Insulin-induced hypoglycemia increases hepatic sensitivity to glucagon in dogs. *J Clin Invest.* Vol.120, No.12, (Dec 2010), pp.4425–4435, ISSN 0021-9738.

Roe, T.F., & Kogut, M.D. (1982). Idiopathic leucine-sensitive hypoglycemia syndrome: insulin and glucagon responses and effects of diazoxide. *Pediatr Res.* Vol.16, No.1, (Jan 1982), pp.1-4, ISSN 0031-3998.

Rutsky, E.A., McDaniel, H.G., Tharpe, D.L., Alred, G., & Pek, S. (1978). Spontaneous hypoglycemia in chronic renal failure. *Arch Intern Med*, Vol.138, No.9, (Sep 1978), pp.1364-1368.

Sarkar, M., Bose, S.S., Mondal, G., & Chatterjee, S. (2010). Generalized Epimerase Deficiency Galactosemia. *Indian J Pediatr* Vol.77, No.8, pp.909-910, ISSN 0019-5456.

Schaftingen, E.V., & Gerin, I. (2002) The glucose-6-phosphatase system. *Biochem J.* Vol.362, pp.513-532, ISSN 0264-6021.

Segal, S. (1989). Disorders of Galactose Metabolism, Chapter 13, In: *The Metabolic Basis of Inherited diseases I*, 6th Edition, Scriver, C.R., Beaudet, A.L., Sly, W.S., Valle, D. (eds), pp.453-480, McGraw-Hill Information Services Company, ISBN 0-07-060726-1, New York.

Segal, S. (1992). Disorders of catbohydrate metabolism. 168.Galactosemia.pp. In: *Cecil Textbook of Medicine*. Wyngaarden, B.J., Smith, H.L., & Bennett W.B. (ed), pp.1076-1081, W.B Saunders Company, ISBN 0-721608886-1, Phyladelphia, London, Toronto, Montreal, Sydney, Tokyo.

Service, F.J. (1992). Hypoglycemic Disorders. In: *Cecil Textbook of Medicine*. Wyngaarden, B.J., Smith, H.L., & Bennett W.B. (ed), pp.1310-1320, W.B Saunders Company, ISBN 0-721608886-1, Phyladelphia, London, Toronto, Montreal, Sydney, Tokyo.

Silvestre, R.A., Rodríguez-Gallardo, J., Jodka, C., Parkes, D.G., Pittner, R.A., Young, A.A., & Marco, J. (2001). Selective amylin inhibition of the glucagon response to arginine is extrinsic to the pancreas. *Am J Physiol Endocrinol Metab*. Vol.280, No.3, (Mar 2001), pp.E443-449, ISSN 0193-1849.

Sinclair, L. (1979). Hypoglycaemia, In. *Metabolic disease in childhood*. pp.97-131, Balckwell Scientific Publications, ISBN 0-632-00248-4, Oxford, London.

Sjarif, D.R., Hellerud, C., Ploos van Amstel, JK., Kleijer, W.J., Sperl, W., Lacombe, D., Sass, J.O., Beemer, F.A., Duran, M., & Poll-The, B.T. (2004) Glycerol kinase deficiency: residual activity explained by reduced transcription and enzyme conformation. *Eur J Hum Genet*, Vol.12, No.6, (March 2004), pp. 424–432, ISSN 1018-4813.

Smith-Laing, G. (1979). The glucoregulatory hormones in cirrhosis of the liver. *Z Gastroenterol*. Vol.17, No.7, (Jul 1979), 462-468, ISSN 0044-2771.

Song, K.H. (2011). Novel compound heterozygous mutations in the fructose-1,6-bisphosphatase gene cause hypoglycemia and lactic acidosis. Metabolism: clinical and experimental. *Metabolism*, Vol.60, No.1, (Jan 2011), pp.107-113, ISSN 0026-0495.

Sorlini, M., Benini, F., Cravarezza, P., & Romanelli, G. (2010). Hypoglycemia, an atypical early sign of hepatocellular carcinoma. *Gastrointest Cancer*, Vol.41, No.3, (Sep 2011), pp. 209-211, ISSN 1934-7820.

Stanley, C.A. (1997). Hyperinsulinism in infants and children. *Pediatr Clin North Am*. Vol.44, No.2, (Apr 1997), 363-374, ISSN 0031-3955.

Tappy, L., & Minehira, K. (2001). New data and new concepts on the role of the liver in glucose homeostasis. *Curr Opin Clin Nutr Metab Care*, Vol.4, No.4, (Jul 2001), 273-277. ISSN 1363-1950.

Thipaporn, T., Bubpha, P., & Varaphon, V. (2005). Hepatocellular Carcinoma with Persistent Hypoglycemia: Successful Treatment with Corticosteroid and Frequent High Carbohydrate Intake. *J Med Assoc Thai*, Vol. 88, No.12, pp 1941-1946. ISSN 0125-2208.

Tietz, N.W., Rinkler, A.D., & Henderson, R.A. (1986). Gastric, pancreatic, and intestinal function, Chapter 14, In: *Textbook of Clinical Chemistry*, Tietz, N.W. (ed.), pp.1434-1493, WB Saunders Company, ISBN 0-7216-8886-1, Philadelphia, London, Toronto.

Tyrrell, J.B. (1992). Adrenociortical hypofunction. 217.6 Disorders of adrenal cortex. In: *Cecil Textbook of Biochemistry*, 19th edition, Wingaarden, J.B., Smith, L.H., Bennett, J.C. (eds). pp.1281-1284, W.B Saunders Company, ISBN 0-721608886-1, Phyladelphia, London, Toronto, Montreal, Sydney, Tokyo.

van den Berghe, G. (1996). Disorders of gluconeogenesis. *J Inherit Metab Dis*. Vol.19, No.4, pp.470-477. ISSN 0141-8955.

Vidnes, J., & Sovik, O. (1976). Gluconeogenesis in infancy and childhood. III. Deficiency of the extramitochondrial form of hepatic phosphoenolpyruvate carboxykinase in a case of persistent neonatal hypoglycaemia. *Acta Paediatr Scand*, Vol.65, No.3, (May 1976), pp.307-312, ISSN 0001-656X.

Voet , D., & Voet, J.G. (2004). Sugar and polysaccharides, In: *Biochemistry*, 3rd edition, Wiley & Sons, pp 356–381, ISBN 0-471-19350-x, New York.

Voet ,D.& Voet, J.G. (2004). Glycogen Metabolism, Chapter 18, In: *Biochemistry*, 3rd edition, pp.626–656, Wiley & Sons INC, ISBN 0-471-19350-x, New York.

Voet, D. & Voet ,JG, b (2004) Signal transduction. Chapter.19.1.Hormones. In: *Biochemistry*, 3rd edition, pp.657-673, Wiley & Sons INC, ISBN 0-471-19350-x, New York.

Walter, J.H., Roberts, R.E.P., Besley, G.T.N., Wraith, J.E., Cleary, M.A., Holton, J.B., & MacFaul, R. (1999). Generalised uridine diphosphate galactose-4-epimerase deficiency. *Arch Dis Child*. Vol.80, pp.374–376. ISSN 0003-9888.

Weinstein, D.A., Correia, C.E., Saunders, A.C., &,Wolfsdorf, J.I. (2006). Hepatic glycogen synthase deficiency: an infrequently recognized cause of ketotic hypoglycemia. *Mol Genet Metab*, Vol.87, No.4, pp.284-288. ISSN 1096-7192.

Woerle, H.J., & Stumvoll, M. (2001). Renal Gluconeogenesis. Its importance in human glucose homeostasis. *Diabetes Care*, Vol.24, No.2, (Feb 2001), pp.382-391. ISSN 0149-5992.

Wolinsky, J.S. (1992). Neurologic disorders associated with altered immunity or unexplained host-parasite alteration. 480 Reye Syndrome, In *Cecil Textbook of Biochemistry*, 19th edition, Wingaarden, J.B., Smith, L.H., Bennett, J.C. (eds). pp.2194-2195, W.B Saunders Company, ISBN 0-721608886-1, Phyladelphia, London, Toronto, Montreal, Sydney, Tokyo.

Wolfsdorf, J.I., & Weinstein, D.A. (2003). Glycogen storage diseases. *Rev Endocr Metab Disord*. Vol.4, pp.95–102. ISSN 1389-9155.

Wright, E.M.I. (1998). Glucose galactose malabsorption. *Am J Physiol*. Vol.275, No.5(Pt 1), (Nov 1998), pp.G879-882. ISSN 0193-1849.

Wright E.M., Loo, D.D.F., Hirayama, B.A. & Turk, E. (2004). Surprising Versatility of Na+-Glucose Cotransporters: SLC5. *Physiology*, Vol.19, No.6, (Dec 2004),pp.370-376, ISSN 1548-9213.

Wright, E.M., Martín, M.G., & Turk, E. (2003). Intestinal absorption in health and disease--sugars. *Best Pract Res Clin Gastroenterol*. Vol.17, No.6, (Dec 2003), pp.943-956. ISSN 1521-6918.

Wright, E.M., Turk, E., & Martin, M.G. (2002). Molecular basis for glucose-galactose malabsorption. *Cell Biochem Biophys*. Vl.36, No.2-3:115-121. ISSN 1085-9195.

Yamashita, H., Takenoshita, M., Sakurai, M., Bruick, R.K., Henzel, W.J., Shillinglaw, W., Arnot, D., & Uyeda K. (2001) A glucose-responsive transcription factor that regulates carbohydrate metabolism in the liver. *Proc Natl Acad Sci USA*, Vol.98 ,No.16, pp. 9116-9121. ISSN 0027-8424.

Young, A. (2005). Inhibition of glucagon secretion. *Adv Pharmacol*. Vol.52, pp.151-171. ISSN 0568-0123.

Zaidi, S.H. (2009). Novel FBP1 gene mutations in Arab patients with fructose-1,6-bisphosphatase deficiency. *Eur J Pediatr*. Vol.168, No.12, (Dec 2009), pp.1467-1471. ISSN 0340-6199.

Zmire, J., Colak, B., & Cvitkovic, P. (1999) Glycemia regulation in diabetic patients with thyroid disease. *Diabetologia Croatica*, pp. 28-32. ISSN 0351-0042.

6

Autoimmune Associated Diseases in Pediatric Patients with Type 1 Diabetes Mellitus According to HLA-DQ Genetic Polymorphism

Miguel Ángel García Cabezas and Bárbara Fernández Valle
Servicio de Pediatría. Hospital General de Ciudad Real,
Spain

1. Introduction

Diabetes mellitus type 1 is the most common endocrine metabolic disorder in childhood and adolescence. In this condition there is an absolute insulin deficiency secondary to progressive destruction of pancreatic beta cells, causing severe alterations in the metabolism of all essential elements (carbohydrates, lipids and proteins).

The most obvious alteration is chronic hyperglycemia, which is essential to diagnose the disease, and moreover, is the main responsible of many vascular and neurological complications that diabetic patients may develop long-term.

In the development of diabetes mellitus type 1 involving both genetic and environmental factors. The traditional concept is that environmental factors may act as triggers of the immune response against β of Langerhans cell phenotype in a genetically predisposed to the development of diabetes mellitus type 1.

Autoimmune diseases are syndromes caused by activation of T cells or B or both, without evidence of other causes such as infection or cancer. When dendritic cells expressing self-antigens in the context of HLA molecules stimulate peripheral T cells, they do so that they remain alive but anergic, no response until they contact a dendritic cell with multiple moleculescostimulatory expressing microbial antigens.

Although many autoinmunes diseases characterized by abnormal production of pathogenic autoantibodies, most of it is caused by an overreaction, combined T and B cells. In animal models of type 1 diabetes mellitus have demonstrated the high expression of MAdCAM-1 and GlyCAM-1 on HEV (high endothelial venules) of the inflamed pancreatic islets and the treatment of animals with inhibitors of the L-function selectin and α4 integrin, blockeddevelopment of type 1 diabetes mellitus.

The American Diabetes Association divides the type 1 diabetes mellitus in two subgroups: 1A is the result of autoimmune destruction of beta cells and the 1B subtype, which do not immunomarkers indicating a destructive autoimmune process of beta cellspancreas. However develop insulin deficiency by unidentified mechanisms and are prone to ketosis. It has been a predominance of African Americans and Asians in the 1B subtype.

Genetic studies have shown that it is an inherited disease with polygenic trait. Genome wide studies have indicated the presence of at least 20 chromosomal regions that may contribute to genetic predisposition to type 1 diabetes mellitus. The most important genes that influence susceptibility to type 1 diabetes are located in the HLA complex located on the short arm of chromosome 6 (6p21.3).

The HLA-DQ is the locus that confers the major genetic susceptibility to develop type 1 diabetes in humans. DQ molecules have two chains, alpha and beta, encoded by the DQA and DQB genes. Susceptibility to type 1 diabetes mellitus has been described by combining alpha-beta chains with no amino acid aspartic acid at position 57 of beta chain (DQB1*0302 linked to DR4 and DQB1*0201 linked to DR3) and the presence of the amino acid arginine at position 52 of the alpha chain (DQA1*0301 linked to DR4 and DQA1*0501 linked to DR3).

Based on these findings have been described both genotypes DQA/DQB disease associated with DQA1*0501/DQB1*0201 and DQA1*0301/DQB1*0302, which is more specific than DR3/DR4 genotype.

Although other types of islet cells and α cells (glucagon producing), delta cells (somatostatin producing) cells or PP (pancreatic polypeptide-producing) are functionally and embryologically similar to beta cells and express the most same. These proteins, inexplicably are free of autoimmune process.

From the pathological standpoint, the cells of the pancreatic islets are infiltrated by lymphocytes (a process called insulitis). After the destruction of beta cells, the inflammatory process forwards, the islets are atrophic and disappear immunomarkers.

Insulitis studies in humans and in animal models of type 1 diabetes mellitus (NOD mouse and BB rat) have identified the following abnormalities in both humoral branch as in the immune system cells:

1.   Autoantibodies against cell islet.
2.   Activated lymphocytesin islets, peripancreatic lymph nodes and widespread circulation.
3.   T lymphocytes that proliferate when stimulated with islet proteins.
4.   Release of cytokines within the insulitis.

The beta cells appear to be particularly vulnerable to the toxic effect of some cytokines (tumor necrosis factor), interferon gamma and interleukin 1. Precise mechanisms are unknown the death of beta cells, but may involve formation of nitric oxide metabolites, apoptosis and direct cytotoxic effects of CD8+ T cells. It is believed that the destruction process does not involve autoantibodies against islet cells, since these antibodies do not react in general to the surface of islet cells and are capable of transferring diabetes mellitus in animals.

Among islet molecules that are targets of the autoimmune process are insulin, glutamic acid decarboxylase (glutamic acid decarboxylase, GAD), the biosynthetic enzyme of the neurotransmitter gamma aminobutyric acid (gamma-aminobutyric acid,GABA), ICA-512/IA-2 (with homology to tyrosine phosphatases, and fogrina (protein in secretory granules of insulin). Other less precisely defined autoantigens are islet ganglioside and carboxypeptidase H. Except none of the insulin-specific autoantigens are beta cells, which makes us wonder how these are destroyed selectively.

Current theories favor the onset of an autoimmune process directed against beta cell molecule, which then spreads to other islet molecules as the autoimmune process destroys the beta cells and creates a series of secondary autoantigens. Beta cells of individuals with type 1 diabetes mellitus do not differ from the beta cells of normal people, because the transplanted islets are destroyed by the recurrence of autoimmune process of type 1 diabetes mellitus.

Autoimmune Associated Diseases in Pediatric Patients with Type 1 Diabetes Mellitus According to HLA-DQ
Genetic Polymorphism

145

Autoantibodies against islet cells (ICA) is a combination of several different antibodies directed against islet molecules such as GAD, insulin, IA-2/ICA-512 and islet ganglioside and serve as a marker of the autoimmune process of type 1 diabetes mellitus. The determination of the ICA may be useful to classify as type 1 diabetes mellitus and nondiabetic individuals identify risk. The ICA is present in most (> 75%) of individuals newly diagnosed with type 1 diabetes mellitus in a significant minority of diabetics newly diagnosed type 2 (5-10%) and sometimes, in pregnant women with gestational diabetes (<5%).

In 3-4% of first-degree relatives of individuals with type 1 diabetes mellitus ICA exist. Along with the presence of a disorder of insulin secretion in the proof of intravenous glucose tolerance predict a 50% higher risk of developing type 1 diabetes mellitus in the next 5 years. Without this disorder of insulin secretion, the presence of ICA predicts a five-year risk <25%. After this it follows that the risk of a first degree relative of type 1 diabetes mellitus is low. Today no approved treatment to prevent development of type 1 diabetes mellitus, so the detection of ICA in non-diabetic population has not been established as screening.

There is another theory that talks about environmental factors as triggers of the autoimmune process in genetically vulnerable patients, but it is difficult to find an environmental trigger, since the event may precede by several years the development of the disease. Among the hypothetical environmental triggers include viruses (coxsackie and rubella), proteins early exposure to cow's milk and nitrosoureas.

A major advance would get delay or prevent diabetes, there have been some intervention in animal models, whose main objective has been the immune system (immunosuppression, selective deletion of T cell subsets, immune tolerance induction to proteinsisland), while others avoid the death of islet cells by blocking the cytotoxic cytokines or increasing islet resistance to the destruction process.

Type 1 diabetes mellitus is often associated with autoimmune diseases. Thus, there has been an increased prevalence of autoantibodies related to celiac disease and many other autoantibodies against endocrine and nonendocrine organs. Not infrequently, these diseases manifest themselves associated paucisymptomatic and are diagnosed late. Despite this apparent relationship between type 1 diabetes mellitus and these autoimmune diseases has not been shown that the degree of glycemic control influence the likelihood of developing or subsequent developments. We must not forget that many of these clinical situations produce per se a decrease in the expectancy and quality of life of patients, another reason to actively pursue and establish treatment as soon as detected.

Autoantibodies can be found in up to 25% of children and adolescents with diabetes, but only 3-5% have hypothyroidism. Hyperthyroidism is less common, but more often than children without diabetes.

Autoimmune hypothyroidism may be associated with goitre (Hashimoto's thyroiditis or goiter), or in later stages of the disease, minimal residual thyroid tissue (atrophic thyroiditis). Because the autoimmune process gradually reduces thyroid function, there is a compensatory phase during which thyroid hormone levels are maintained by an elevated TSH.

Although some patients may have mild symptoms, this phase is called subclinical or mild hypothyroidism. Later, T4 levels fall and TSH levels increase even more, the symptoms become more obvious at this stage (usually TSH> 10 mU/L) is called clinical hypothyroidism.

In Hashimoto's thyroiditis, there is a marked lymphocytic infiltration of the thyroid with germinal center formation, atrophy of thyroid follicles accompanied by oxyphil metaplasia, absence of colloid and mild or moderate fibrosis. As with most autoimmune disorders, susceptibility to this type of hypothyroidism depends on a combination of genetic and environmental factors and is increased sibling risk of autoimmune hypothyroidism or Graves disease.

Genetic risk factors for this type of hypothyroidism in subjects caucasians are HLA-DR polymorphisms, specifically the HLA-DR3, HLA-DR4 and HLA-DR5. There is also a weak relationship between polymorphism of CTLA-4, a gene regulating T cells and autoimmune hypothyroidism. HLA-DR polymorphisms and CTLA-4 constitute about half of cases hipotiroidsimo autoimmune susceptibility. It is still necessary to identify other contributing loci. A gene located on chromosome 21 could be the cause of the relationship between autoimmune hypothyroidism and Down syndrome.

The lymphocytic infiltrate thyroid autoimmune hypothyroidism is composed of CD4+ T cells and activated CD8+ and B cells. It is believed that the destruction of thyroid cells is mediated in a primary CD8+ T cells cytotoxic, which destroy their targets by perforin that cause cellular necrosis or through granzyme B, which induces apoptosis.

Addition, cytokine production by local T cells, such as tumor necrosis factor, IL-1 and interferon gamma, can return to thyroid cells more susceptible to apoptosis mediated by death receptors such as Fas, which activate their ligands respective T cellIn addition, these cytokines directly disrupt the function of thyroid cells, and induce the expression of other proinflammatory molecules by thyroid cells themselves, such as cytokines, molecules of HLA class I and II, adhesion molecules, CD40 and nitric oxide.

The administration of high concentrations for therapeutic cytokines (notably IFN alpha) is associated with enhancement of autoimmune thyroid disease, possibly by mechanisms similar to those involved in sporadic disease.

The Tg and TPO antibodies are markers of thyroid autoimmunity with clinical utility, but their pathogenic effect is limited to a secondary role in the amplification of a developing immune response. TPO antibodies fix complement and are complex to the complement membrane attack the thyroid gland in case of autoimmune hypothyroidism. However, the transplacental passage of anti-Tg antibodies or anti-TPO has no effect on fetal thyroid gland, indicating that it takes an injury mediated by T cells to initiate autoimmune injury of the gland.

Although it has been associated with the presence of subclinical hypothyroidism with an increased risk of symptomatic hypoglycemia and hipocrecimiento, it is quite common for thyroid dysfunction clinically pass unnoticed, so you must determine the levels of thyrotropic hormone (TSH) annually in those without autoantibodies or more often if there are or the patient has any symptoms.

Celiac disease is 10 times more common in diabetics than in the general population and may affect up to 1-10% of diabetic patients. Also known as celiac sprue or gluten sensitive enteropathy is an autoimmune disorder triggered by ingestion of gliadin fractions present in the gluten and similar proteins of rye and barley in genetically predisposed individuals.

Gluten is the main protein component of wheat, rye and barley. In celiac disease is triggered by an immune reaction that leads to inflammation of the small intestine mediated by T lymphocytes, with the development of hyperplastic crypts, intraepithelial lymphocytes and villous atrophy, causing a chronic enteropathy with a broad range of manifestations, which make a systemic disease of varying severity.

Adherence to a gluten-free diet is followed by clinical and histological improvement in these patients, with normalization of long-term intestinal architecture, and the property of the recurrence of symptoms when gluten is reintroduced in the diet .

The presence of an immune component in the etiology of the disease was suspected for three reasons. First, no serum IgA antigliadin antibodies and endomysial, although it is unclear whether primary or secondary to tissue injury. Endomysial antibody has a sensitivity of 90 and specificity 95%, and its antigen is tissue transglutaminase. Secondly, treatment with prednisolone for four weeks in a celiac patient who continues to eat gluten induces remission and duodenal epithelium gives a more normal level. Finally, the gliadin peptides interact with gliadin-specific T cells, which in turn can act as mediators of tissue injury or cause the release of one or more cytokines that are responsible for tissue injury.

In celiac disease are also implicated genetic factors, its incidence varies widely among different population groups (high in Caucasians and low in color and eastern race) and is 10% in first degree relatives of patients with celiac disease. In addition, about 95% of celiac patients express the allele of the human leukocyte antigen DQ2, whereas only a minority of all people who express DQ2 have celiac disease.

Not forget that the diagnosis of celiac disease is made by biopsy of the small intestine. Is performed on patients with symptoms and laboratory findings suggestive of malabsorption or lack of nutrients.

Is often asymptomatic, but can cause gastrointestinal symptoms, short stature and anemia. This condition is also associated with an increased number of hypoglycemic episodes and a progressive decrease in insulin requirements in the year prior to diagnosis. It is also recommended measuring endomysial or tissue transglutaminase after diagnosis and every 2-3 years in post, in asymptomatic patients or whenever there is clinical suspicion, given the possibility of seroconversion over time in some patientsin which antibodies were initially detected.

Addison's disease, another autoimmune disease is present up to 2% of type 1 diabetes presenting autoantibodies against the enzyme 21-hydroxylase and the enzyme cleavage of the side chain, but it ignores the importance of these antincuerpos in the pathogenesis ofadrenal insufficiency. Some antibodies cause adrenal insufficiency by blocking the binding of ACTH to its receptors.

The appearance of two or more of these autoimmune endocrine same person characterized in a polyglandular autoimmune syndrome type II (thyroid, parathyroid and gonadal tissue), this syndrome has yet mutated gene on chromosome 6 and is associated with alleles B8 and HLA DR3.

The presence of adrenal insufficiency is rare, so it is recommended not look systematically. In addition to the classic symptoms for adrenal insufficiency are at risk of frequent hypoglycemia and reduced daily insulin requirements.

The 15-20% of adults have diabetes autoimmune gastropathy presenting autoantibodies to gastric parietal cells, and 50% have clinical or pathological signs of atrophic gastritis. Yet there are no recommendations regarding the detection of these antibodies, given the lower prevalence in childhood.

With respect to autoimmune diseases of the skin, vitiligo has been found up to 7% of children and adolescents with type 1 diabetes mellitus.

The objectives of this study are the following: make an epidemiological study of type 1 diabetes mellitus in childhood and adolescence, to study the HLA-DQ genetic group and general parameters in the onset of the disease, and the pursuit of development of autoimmune diseases.

Today diabetes education is fundamental and essential, in consultation diabetes control emphasizes good glycemic control in order to reduce microvascular complications, rare in children because their development is in adulthood. It also reports on the association with microvascular problems such as diabetic retinopathy, microalbuminuria leading to nephropathy, and diabetic neuropathy, as well as on macrovascular problems such as atherosclerosis.

Are known to coexist in these patients, with chronic hyperglycemia in cardiovascular risk otrosfactores. Diabetes education programs and health promotion should report on the harmful effects of some of them, such as smoking, overweight or sedentary. We should not forget the high prevalence of these diseases justifies the systematic implementation of its screening in the units of pediatric endocrinology. The early diagnosis of these can improve the control of type 1 diabetes mellitus.

2. Patient and methods

This study was carried out at the Department of Pediatrics, General Hospital of Ciudad Real. This work is a descriptive epidemiological study on 129 children and adolescents under age 16 with type 1 diabetes mellitus, studied in this hospital since 1990. With regard to epidemiological studies by our group in the province of Ciudad Real, with an estimated total of 423 patients with DM1, of which 204 are under 16 years, the size of the sample makes it representative of the distribution of type 1 diabetes mellitus population.

The analysis began in January 2003 starting with a retrospective study of patients and performing a 3-year prospective follow-up on these patients and patients who were going to the Department of Pediatrics at the start of his diabetes. The analysis and recruitment was completed in December 2007. This study was approved by the Research and Ethics Committee of the General Hospital of Ciudad Real. Reported and informed consent was obtained from parents or guardians.

In our study we asked whether there is a relationship between the occurrence of autoimmune diseases in pediatric patients with type 1 diabetes mellitus, with the HLA-DQ genetic group. Main objective genetic group analyzed HLA-DQ by molecular biology of our patients. According to these HLA-DQ haplotypes have organized groups I, II and III, considered by the usual bibliography and diabetogenic risk.

- **Group I:** HLA-DQA1*0501/DQB1*0201
- **Group II:** HLA-DQA1*0301/DQB1*0302
- **Group III:** HLA-DQA1*0501,*0301/HLA-DQB1*0201,*0302
- **Group IV:** No genetic group associated with DM1

As secondary objectives we analyzed the disease onset general parameters such as sex and age. We collected data on whether patients had autoimmune disease associated with type 1 diabetes mellitus, if the onset of the disease has been before or after the debut of type 1 diabetes mellitus and the median time to onset of the disease. These parameters are studied during a follow-up period of 3 years with updates every 6 months. All of these secondary objectives relate them to the diabetogenic risk group assigned to each of our patients.

The degree of innovation under our study was that the determination of HLA-DQ alleles was performed by molecular biology techniques, to avoid large differences, about 50% errors (58% according to the results of our group), which are generated if only theserological determinations. HLA-DQ alleles were determined by reaction polymerase chain, with allele specific amplification (PCR-SSP). We used specific primers for DQA1 and DQB1 genes (Protrans, Ger.) Amplified products were separated by agarose gel electrophoresis in 2% and were assigned allele specific amplification.

Determinations of antithyroid antibodies, and antithyroglobulin antimicrosomal performed by chemiluminescence, IMMULITE 2000 (Dipesa ®). Thyroid hormones: T4 and TSH by chemiluminescent immunoassay technology microparticles, ARCHITECT (Abbott ®).

As serologic marker in detecting celiac disease transglutaminase antibodies were analyzed by enzyme immunoassay with recombinant human tissue transglutaminase (Eurospital ®) with a sensitivity around 95% and a specificity above 95% for populationspediatric. Patients with positive markers underwent a biopsy of the duodenum and subsequent intestinal pathology.

For the analysis of the data is first created a database with Microsoft Access and have subsequently be exported for statistical analysis by SPSS for Windows, version 12.0. We conducted a 6x4 design. Each patient was studied in 6 different moments of its evolution, with 4 viable possibilities, different genetic risk groups.

Study possible changes in the variables under study during the monitoring period, if the changes are influenced by risk group HLA-DQ, and if it influenced other control variables such as sex, age, etc. All statistical tests were performed with a significance level of 95% and an alpha of 0.05%.

2.1 Results

According to the HLA-DQ haplotypes obtained, the distribution of diabetogenic risk groups was as follows: group I (HLA-DQA1*0501/DQB1*0201): 45 patients, accounting for 34.9%, group II (HLA-DQA1*0301/DQB1*0302): 38 patients, representing 29.5%, group III (HLA-DQA1*0501,*0301/HLA-DQB1*0201,*0302): 38 patients, representing 29.5%, and group IV (no gene associated with DM1 group): 8 patients, representing 6, 2% (Figure 1).

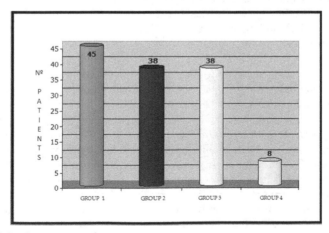

Fig. 1. HLA-DQ Diabetogenic risk groups

The gender distribution of our study population of 129 patients was as follows: males 67 patients representing 51.9% and women 62 patients representing 48.1%, with a ratio child of 1,08.

The distribution of patients by age at onset was as follows: 0 to 4 years 32 patients representing 24.8%, between 5 and 9 years 67 patients, representing 51.9%, between 10 and 14 years 29 patients who account for 22.4% and between 15 and 16 years 1 patientrepresents 0.8%. The mean age of patients, whose mean values (mean ± SD), expressed in years, diabetogenic risk groups were as follows: Group I (8.6 ± 3.4), Group II (7 ± 3), Group III (6.1 ± 2.7) and Group IV (6.8 ± 2.6). In our study found significant differences in age at debut by diabetogenic risk groups, age at onset being significantly lower in group III with group I (Figure 2).

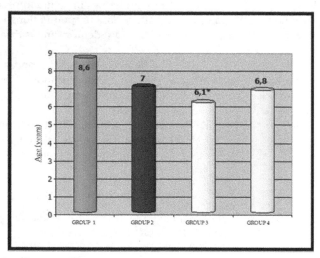

Fig. 2. Distribution of patients by age at onset

The incidence of patients with autoimmune thyroiditis in our series is 15.5%, representing a total of 20 patients. At the time of diagnosis of thyroiditis, 85% were euthyroid autoimmune thyroiditis and 15% had undergone an underactive thyroid. In the euthyroid, 17.6% (n = 3) associated with thyroid hypofunction later.

The sex distribution is as follows: 55% (n = 11) were women and 45% (n = 9) were male. No significant differences were observed in the distribution of autoimmune thyroiditis by sex.

Distribution diabetogenic risk groups was as follows: Group I: 6 patients, Group II: 5 patients, Group III: 8 patients, and Group IV: 1 patient. No significant differences were found in the diagnosis of autoimmune thyroiditis diabetogenic risk groups (Figure 3).

When analyzing patients with autoimmune thyroiditis, it was observed that 76.4% started after the debut of type 1 diabetes mellitus, whereas 23.6% were diagnosed simultaneously with the debut of it. By contrast patients with underactive thyroiditis, 28.6% presented prior to the commencement of type 1 diabetes mellitus, 42.8% thereafter, and 28.6% to debut simultaneously do the same.

In our series we found a case of hyperthyroidism in a 11-year-old was diagnosed with type 1 diabetes three years ago. The frequency of patients with celiac disease associated with type 1 diabetes mellitus in our series is 6.2%, which corresponds to 8 patients. The sex distribution is as follows: 75% (n = 6) are women and 25% (n = 2) are male. We found significant differences in favor of women (p <0.001).

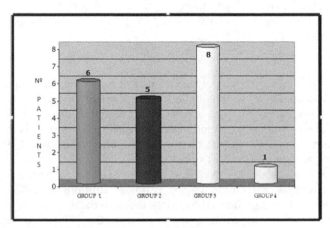

Fig. 3. Autoimmune thyroiditis by diabetogenic risk groups

Distribution diabetogenic risk groups was as follows: Group I: 2 patients, Group II: 2 patients, Group III: 3 patients, and Group IV: 1 patient. No significant differences were found in the diagnosis of celiac disease by diabetogenic risk groups (Figure 4).

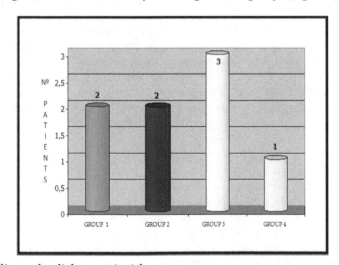

Fig. 4. Celiac disease by diabetogenic risk groups

As for the timing of the debut has been observed that in 75% (n = 6), the debut of celiac disease after debut of type 1 diabetes mellitus, and 25% (n = 2) the onset is earlier. In most cases of celiac disease were asymptomatic at diagnosis and only observed the existence of signs of malabsorption in 1 patient, abdominal distention and diarrhea. The average time between debut and diagnosis was 22 months with a minimum of 6 months and a maximum of 34 months.

In our series, 2 patients are associated with type 1 diabetes mellitus, celiac disease and autoimmune thyroiditis (1 patient 1 patient euthyroid and hypothyroid).

In 13 patients (10.1%) were type allergic processes associated allergic rhinitis and conjunctivitis, 8 patients (6.2%) had asthma, 8 patients (6.2%) were diagnosed with atopic dermatitis and 1 patient (0.7%) of vitiligo.

2.1.1 Discussion

In type 1 diabetes mellitus there is a polygenic susceptibility. The most important genes that influence human susceptibility to type 1 diabetes mellitus are located in the complex HLA class II. In our series, these data are corroborated, and that these associations are most common. 93.8% of our patients with type 1 diabetes mellitus corresponds to the genetic risk groups as has been described elsewhere, so a 6.2% suffer from type 1 diabetes mellitus without belonging to a group of HLA-DQ risk.

Our results agree with others, as published by the EURODIAB indicating that in most mediterranean countries the male/female ratio is around 1, with a slight male predominance, but with no significant differences between them.

The period of highest incidence in the study is between 5 and 9 years. These findings are consistent with studies in other countries, which show a tendency for the disease much earlier debut. In our study found significant differences in age at debut by diabetogenic risk groups, age at onset being significantly lower in group III with group I. These results indicate that the combination of different molecules in susceptibility, heterozygous in group III, accelerating the destruction of beta cells by promoting an early onset of type 1 diabetes mellitus.

Autoimmune disease most often associated to type 1 diabetes mellitus is an autoimmune thyroid disease. Our results, 15.5% compared to the percentage of subjects who agree thyroiditis associated with many studies, such as in Spain by Roland and cols (1999) or made in Italy by Lorini and cols (1996). However, some international studies show higher prevalence, such as that conducted by Lindberg et al (1997), with a prevalence of 38%.

As in other studies in our series of cases in which thyroiditis manifested clinically, it is in the form of an underactive thyroid. Although thyroid status of the majority of subjects with positive markers is euthyroid.

In our series we found a case of hyperthyroidism in a 11-year-old was diagnosed with type 1 diabetes three years ago. Hyperthyroidism is associated with type 1 diabetes mellitus present in 1% of cases, most often in adults. Other studies indicate that hyperthyroidism is usually diagnosed before or while type 1 diabetes mellitus.

Studies show that thyroiditis is more prevalent in diabetic girls than in boys. However, our results do not indicate such a difference, matching other studies.

The prevalence of celiac disease associated with children with type 1 diabetes mellitus varies between 1-16%. In our series, we found a total of 8 patients under 6.2% of all patients. These results are consistent with those of Vitoria et al. However, some studies show minor incidents, such as by Barera and colleagues (2002) with a prevalence of 3.9%. In some other series have reported higher frequencies, between 8 and 12.3%.

As for the timing of the debut our results coincide with those published by Barera et al, and Holmes et al (2002), in which the majority of patients the diagnosis of celiac disease is posterior to that of type 1 diabetes mellitus. The time elapsed since the debut of the type 1 diabetes mellitus and identification of antibodies in our series are consistent with the results of Saukkonen et al (1996), which are located around the 2 years following the onset of type 1 diabetes mellitus. Other studies such as Maki and colleagues (1995), who observed a lower average interval around 13 months. Our results on the significant association in women are endorsed by other studies in this regard, as published in Spain by Roldan et al (1998).

Most patients were asymptomatic at the time of his presentation and noted that there were no signs of frank malnutrition. Were diagnosed by serological screening and subsequent confirmation with intestinal biopsy. Our results are consistent with those of Barrera et al.

Not found in our series more partnerships with other autoimmune diseases such as pernicious anemia, Addison's disease, Sjögren syndrome, alopecia areata, and rheumatoid arthritis.

Among the background approximately 10% of the patients had atopy and bronchial asthma. These data are consistent with those reported by Lopez Medina et al in their series. The presence of vitiligo in our series (0.7%) is lower than that observed in other studies like the one made in Italy by Romano et al (1998), showing a prevalence of 9%.

3. Conclusion

The major autoimmune diseases, autoimmune thyroiditis and celiac disease are more prevalent in our diabetic patients than in the nondiabetic population. Although we found more patients in risk group III, no significant differences with other groups.

In conclusion, these data support the recommendation that from the moment of diagnosis of type 1 diabetes mellitus regular determination of thyroid antibodies and celiac disease related. Current recommendations are vague as to what should be the most appropriate timing for this in pediatric patients. We must try to detect such diseases early, but that does not justify excessive and unnecessary repetition of diagnostic tests. The use of standardized monitoring protocols is becoming increasingly necessary to ensure better health care for children and adolescents with type 1 diabetes mellitus.

4. References

Green, A.; Gale, EA. & Patterson, CC for the EURODIAB ACE Study Group (1992) Incidence of childhood-onset insulin-dependent diabetes mellitus: the EURODIAB ACE study. *Lancet* 1992; 339: 905-909.

Roldan, MB.; Alonso M.; Barrio R.; (1999) Thyroid autoimmunity in children and adolescents with type 1 diabetes mellitus. *Diabetes Nutr Metab* 1999; 12:27-31.

Lorini, R; Scaramuzza, A; Vitali, L; d'Annunzio, G; Avanzini, MA; De Giacomo, C et al. (1996) Clinical aspects of celiac disease in children with insulin-dependent diabetes mellitus. *J Pediatr Endocrinol Metab* 1996;(Suppl 1):101-11.

Lindberg, B.; Ericsson, UB.; Ljung, R.; (1997) High prevalence of thyroid autoantibodies at diagnosis of insulin-dependent diabetes mellitus in Sweden children. *J Lab Clin Med* 1997; 130: 585-589.

Holmes GTK. (2002). Screening for coeliac disease in type 1 diabetes. *Arch Dis Child* 2002;87:495-8.

Barera, G.; Bonfanti, R.; Viscardi, M et al.(2002) Ocurrence of celiac disease alter onset of type 1 diabetes: a six-year prospective longitudinal study. *Pediatrics* 2002; 109: 261-267.

Romano, G.; Moretti, G.; Di Benedetto, A.; Ruso, G et al. (1998) Skin lesion in diabetes mellitus: prevalence and clinical correlations. *Diabetes Res Clin Pract* 1998; 39(2): 101-106.

Saukkonen, T.; Savilahti, E.; Reijonen, H.; Ilonen, J.; Tuomilehto-Wolf, E.; Akerblom, HK. (1996) Celiac disease: Frequent occurrence after clinical onset of insulin-dependent diabetes mellitus: Childhood Diabetes in Finland Study Group. *Diabet Med* 1996; 13:464-70.

Maki, M.; Holm, K.; Hallstrom, O.; (1995) Seroconversion of reticulin autoahmtibodies predios coeliac disease in insulin dependent diabetes mellitus. *Gut* 1995; 36: 239-42.

Roldan, MB.; Barrio, R.; Roy, G.; Parra, C.; Alonso, M et al. (1998) Diagnostic value of serological markers for celiac disease in diabetic children and adolescent. *J Pediatr Endocrinol Metab* 1998; 11: 751-756.

Part 2

Cardiovascular Complications

7

Etiopathology of Type 1 Diabetes: Focus on the Vascular Endothelium

Petru Liuba and Emma Englund
Division of Paediatric Cardiology, Pediatric Heart Center,
Lund University and Skåne University Hospital Lund
Sweden

1. Introduction

Type 1, or insulin-dependent diabetes results from the destruction of insulin-producing β-cells in the pancreas. It typically occurs in previously healthy children, being one of the most common childhood diseases in modern time. Intriguingly, the diabetes morbidity continues to rise in most parts of the world, but the causes of this development remain elusive (the Diabetes Mondial (DIAMOND) Project Group, 2006).

Many of the patients with type 1 diabetes may develop particularly in adult life severe complications encompassing both the microvascular (retinopathy, nephropathy, and neuropathy) and macrovascular (myocardial infarction, stroke and peripheral artery disease) system. The main underlying mechanism in the large vessels is represented by accelerated atherosclerosis with subsequent narrowing of the vessels and potential risk for plaque rupture. In smaller, as in the large vessels, severely impaired function of the inner layer (so-called endothelium) has been detected, and correlated with the risk of developing vascular complications, suggesting it to play a major role in precipitating the vascular disease.

It is now well established that this widespread vasculopathy develop many years before the onset of vascular complications, perhaps even before the outbreak of diabetic hyperglycemia. What exactly drives this process remains speculative, but increasing evidence suggest that factors thought to trigger type 1 diabetes may as well be harmful for the vessels. Furthermore, as delineated below, the microvascular network surrounding the islets in the pancreas appears to have important contribution to the injury process that ultimately leads to type 1 diabetes. Further multidisciplinary efforts are warranted in order to better understand the mechanism of this disease and its complications.

2. Epidemiology and pathogenesis of type 1 diabetes

There is a widespread global variation in the incidence and prevalence of type 1 diabetes. In a report by Karvonen et al. from 2000, age-adjusted incidences ranged from a low of <1/100,000 per year in China and South America to a high of >20/100,000 per year in Sardinia, Finland, Sweden, Norway, Portugal, the United Kingdom, Canada, and New Zeeland. The incidence increased with age in most of the populations with the highest incidence observed in children 10-14 years of age. An updated report from 2006 (the

DIAMOND Project Group, 2006) showed trends of increased incidence annually across the world in the populations studied (4.0% in Asia, 3.2% in Europe, and 5.3% in North America) with the exception of Central America and the West Indies were the trend was a decrease of 3.6%. The rate of increase in incidence cannot be explained by genetic shift in such a short period of time. An increasing burden of environmental factors, probably along with increased immune-mediated sensitivity of pancreatic cells to gene-environment interaction, could account at least in part for the rising prevalence of type 1 diabetes.

Traditionally, interplay between genetic susceptibility and environmental factors is thought to provide the fundamental element for the disease. The major genetic susceptibility for developing type 1 diabetes is located on the human leukocyte antigen (HLA)-DQ region on chromosome 6. Two HLA-DQ haplotypes, DQA1*0301-DQB1*0302 (DQ8) and DQA1*0501-DQB1*0201 (DQ2) are associated with high risk for developing diabetes. Almost 90% of patients with type 1 diabetes have at least one of these two haplotypes, compared to 20% of the general population (Redondo et al., 2001). These susceptibility genes are important regulators of the immune response; the molecules they encode reside on the cell surface and have the ability to process and present antigens to autoreactive T-cells.

In genetically susceptible individuals there is a pathological presentation of autoantigens on the cell surface of the pancreatic islet cells. This, in combination with a failing negative selection of the T-cells in the thymus and decreased regulatory capacity of regulatory T-cells in peripheral blood (Lindley et al., 2005), leads to an inflammatory response within the pancreatic islets as well as to the production of antibodies against β-cell antigens. Islet cell antibodies were the first ones described, but we now also recognize autoantibodies to insulin, glutamic acid decarboxylase and protein tyrosine phosphatase. Up to 90% of the patients with new onset type 1 diabetes have autoantibodies directed against one or more of these autoantigens It is yet to prove if the autoantibodies have an active role in the pathogenesis of type 1 diabetes but the presence and persistency of autoantibodies appear to increase the likelihood of developing type 1 diabetes. The inflammatory response leads to destruction of the pancreatic β-cells and progressive loss of insulin secretion until reaching critically low levels or even complete insulin deficiency.

3. Vascular endothelium in type 1 diabetes

In children with diabetes risk HLA, signs of systemic endothelial cell activation can be seen already before the clinical onset of diabetes (Toivonen et al, 2004), suggesting it to be an early event in the disease process. Postmortem studies near the onset of type 1 diabetes have shown that class II HLA molecules may be abundantly expressed on vascular endothelial cells lining the capillaries and capillary sinusoids in the islets (Itoh et al., 1993). The upregulation of HLA is paralleled by strong expression of adhesion molecules (i.e. ICAM-1) in the same endothelial areas (Hanninen et al., 1992). These events, seemingly induced by circulating proinflammatory mediators, facilitate homing and migration of inflammatory cells such as T cells across the dysfunctional endothelium . Interaction between antigen-specific T-cells and antigen/HLA complexes on the endothelial cells surface induced a rapid transmigration of the T-cells across the endothelial cell layer (Greening et al., 2003). Similar changes may be found on the surface of endothelial cells of other vascular beds (Greening et al., 2003).This fits well with the clinical observation that type 1 diabetes is often comorbid with chronic autoimmune diseases in other organs such as gut (celiac disease) and thyroid gland (autoimmune thyroiditis). These disorders also share some of the HLA DQ diabetes risk alleles. An activated endothelium could be the link.

It is well known that long-term exposure to hyperglycemia, hyperlipidemia and inflammation, all of which being important features of type 1 diabetes, is harmful to the endothelial cells, causing further endothelial dysfunction, and in the long run, accelerated atherosclerosis. Lymphocyte accumulation within the arterial wall is an important mechanistic component in the atherosclerotic process and contributes to endothelial cell injury and dysfunction. The endothelial injury, in turn, promotes additional immune events, including release of different chemokines and cytokines resulting in further transmigration of immune cells, and synthesis of C-reactive protein via liver activation by interleukin-6.

Recent study, assessing the relationship of genetic susceptibility with endothelial dysfunction in young patients with type 1 diabetes, found significant correlation between HLA-DQ 2/8, which confers the highest risk for developing type 1 diabetes, and cutaneous microvascular dysfunction (Odermarsky et al., 2007). This could imply, although its does not prove, a role for HLA in the pathogenesis of type 1 diabetes. Further studies at our center are under way to investigate whether such changes could be present already before the clinical onset of type 1 diabetes.

4. Exogenous risk factors and type 1 diabetes: Is vascular endothelium a link?

Putative environmental triggers include viruses, environmental toxins and foods, but it has been difficult to demonstrate a reproducible correlation between them and the development of type 1 diabetes (The environmental determinants of diabetes in the young (TEDDY) Study Group, 2008). Although appealing, there is no evidence to date of a direct interplay between infections and genetics in the causation of type 1 diabetes. the risk of developing T1D seems to increase with the number of infections experienced by an individual during the year preceding the onset of T1D. Although we currently lack the knowledge of the precise underlying mechanisms, there are other reports on similar associations between infectious recurrence and chronic diseases such as multiple sclerosis or rheumatoid arthritis. In some animal studies, the development of atherosclerotic plaque was accelerated by repeated infection. One possible mechanistic link between these chronic inflammatory diseases (e.g. atherosclerosis and T1D) and infection might be endothelial injury. Infections cause vascular endothelial dysfunction, which may persist for up to 1 year after the infectious illness. Mild respiratory infections ("common cold") seem to aggravate arterial endothelial dysfunction in young patients with T1D. Those with increased recurrence of infections of this type are more susceptible to decreased carotid artery elasticity. The latter was earlier shown to be in part dependent on the functional integrity of endothelial cells. In atherosclerosis-susceptible mice, the degree of endothelial vasomotor dysfunction in skin microcirculation correlates with the number of pathogen inoculations (Odermarsky M, Liuba P unpublished data).

It has been shown that even mild viral infection causes vascular endothelial dysfunction, which may persist for up to 1 year after the infectious illness (Charakida et al., 2005). Infections promote the inflammatory environment needed for endothelial cell activation and upregulation of HLA. These changes could, if genetic susceptibility is present, contribute to homing, transmigration, and accumulation of inflammatory cells in certain tissues. In the pancreas these microcirculatory changes could perhaps have a role in the pathogenesis of type 1 diabetes, but this is still hypothetical.

5. Endothelial function and dysfunction

The endothelial cells line the inner surface of all blood vessels, providing a metabolically active interface between blood and tissue. These cells modulate blood flow, nutrient delivery, coagulation and thrombosis, and leukocyte diapedesis. The endothelium synthesizes important bioactive substances. Of these, nitric oxide is the most potent vasodilator and protector of vascular function, inhibiting platelet activation and aggregation, preventing leukocyte adhesion and migration through the vessel wall, diminishing smooth muscle cell proliferation and migration, and counteracting adhesion molecule expression (Beckman et al., 2002). Nitric oxide is synthezised by the endothelial isoform of nitric oxide synthase. The process involves enzymatic conversion of L-arginine into nitric oxide and L-citrulline. The release of nitric oxide can be up- or downregulated by different factors. The hormone estrogen, physical exercise, and certain dietary factors are examples of upregulators, whereas smoking and oxidized low-density lipoproteins, via oxidative stress, are examples of downregulators (Michel & Vanhoutte, 2010).

Endothelial dysfunction is considered to be the first step in a long-lasting and complex development that leads to atherosclerosis. The dysfunction is a result of an imbalance in the redox-equilibrium towards oxidative stress leading to impaired nitric oxide bioavailability, either caused by its reduced synthesis or by increased breakdown via reactive oxygen species. (Versari et al., 2009). The dysfunctioning endothelium may produce other substances and mediators such as endothelin 1, thromboxane A_2, prostaglandin H and reactive oxygen species, with vasoconstricting, pro-inflammatory, and proatherosclerotic effects (Virdis et al., 2010).

Given the excess of inflammatory and oxidative stress in type 1 diabetes, the endothelium in individuals with type 1 diabetes is continually exposed to factors promoting the development of endothelial dysfunction. The hyperglycemia, excess free fatty acid release, and insulin resistance leads to adverse events within the endothelial cell (Beckman et al., 2002). Recent findings support the concept that genetically susceptible individuals, i.e. diabetes high-risk HLA, are more prone to develop endothelial dysfunction (Odermarsky et al., 2007) and ongoing studies are investigating whether this dysfunction in fact may precede the clinical onset of type 1 diabetes.

The generalized microvascular dysfunction in type 1 diabetes is an important mechanism in the development of these microvascular complications. Nephropathy, retinopathy and neuropathy are all related to damage to the small vessels of the kidney, retina and nerves. Significant associations have been reported between the different microvascular complications of type 1 diabetes; patients with one complication often develops a second one, suggesting common risk factors and pathogenetic mechanisms (Girach & Vignati, 2006).

Overt microvascular disease is however rare during childhood and adolescence. Early signs, such as increases in albumin excretion rates and glomerular filtration rates, renal hypertrophy, changes in retinal microvasculature and impaired autonomic nervous system function may be detectable in kids with type 1 diabetes and often progress during puberty. Microalbuminuria is the earliest stage of clinical nephropathy and is predictive of progression to overt diabetes nephropathy and, notably, of cardiovascular disease (Rossing et al., 1996).

6. Methods for evaluating endothelial function

The ability to detect endothelial dysfunction, before it progresses to overt vasculopathy, could facilitate the early diagnosis and management of high-risk individuals in childhood. There are several techniques that can be used, though they are not in clinical use to any higher extent. Here we will present two methods; flow-mediated dilatation and laser doppler flowmetry with iontophoresis, which are the ones used in our research.

6.1 Assessment of arterial dysfunction via flow-mediated dilatation of the brachial artery

Blood vessels respond to an increase in blood flow, or more precisely shear stress, by dilating. This phenomenon is called flow-mediated dilatation. The principal mediator for this is endothelium-derived nitric oxide. Assessment of flow-mediated dilatation of the brachial artery safely and non-invasively provides a measure of the systemic endothelial function. The brachial artery response to increased shear stress has been shown to correlate significantly with invasive testing of brachial (Irace et al., 2001) and coronary endothelial function (Andersson et al., 1995), as well as with the extent and severity of coronary atherosclerosis (Neunteufl et al., 1997), and carotid artery intima-media thickness (Gaeta et al., 2000).

Several factors affect the response to the increase in shear stress, including temperature, food, drugs and sympathetic stimuli, female hormonal status, among others, and when conducting a study using this technique you must take these confounding factors into consideration. Ultra sound systems used must be equipped with software for two-dimensional imaging, colour and spectral Doppler, an internal electrocardiogram monitor and a high-frequency vascular transducer. A straight segment of the brachial artery above the antecubital fossa is imaged in the longitudinal plane with the ultrasound probe securely fixed using a stereotactic clamp. A blood pressure cuff is then placed on the forearm and inflated to supra-systolic pressure. After cuff release, reactive hyperaemia results and is quantified using Doppler. The arterial diameter is recorded at end diastole using electrocardiographic gating to determine the response of the brachial artery to increase in flow. The flow-mediated dilatation is expressed as a percentage change of the arterial diameter from the baseline vessel size (Corretti et al., 2002; Thijssen et al., 2011). To control the smooth muscle cells ability to dilate the vessel, independently of the endothelium, and to determine maximum obtainable vasodilatation a dose of nitro-glycerine is administrated via spray or sublingual tablet.

6.2 Assessment of microvascular dysfunction via laser doppler flowmetry with iontophoresis in the skin

Iontophoresis is a non-invasive method of introducing charged substances across the surface of the skin by means of a small electric charge. The basic principle is that molecules of drugs in a solution that are positively or negatively charged will migrate across the skin under influence of an applied current according to the rule that like charges repel each other. The amount of drug delivered is dependent on the magnitude and duration of the current applied. The response in the skin vasculature is measured via a laser doppler device (Morris & Shore, 1996). The coherent light directed at the skin changes when it comes in contact with moving tissues (red blood cells) and the emerged light, i.e. skin perfusion, is measured by a photodiode.

Acetylcholine is the standard test drug for the assessment of endothelial function. The response to acetylcholine, using iontophoresis, correlates with diabetes duration and level of glycosylated haemoglobin (Khan et al., 2000). The mechanisms of acetylcholine-induced vasodilatation via ionphoresis remain debatable. In humans, nitric oxide appears to be the main mediator, but other endothelium-dependent vasodilators may contribute as well (Turner et al., 2008).

Sodium nitroprusside is a nitric oxide donor and acts directly, i.e. endothelium-independent, as a control on the smooth muscle cells causing vasodilatation. Cathodal current is used for delivering sodium nitroprusside.

The current for both substances is set to 100 µA for 20 seconds. For each of the substances to be tested five consecutive and equal doses are applied to generate dose-response curves. Baseline perfusion and changes in response to the substance are expressed as area under the curve.

7. The "common soil" hypothesis-is this applicable in type 1 diabetes?

In 1995, Michael Stern put forward the "common soil" hypothesis, which suggests a shared genetic and environmental origin for type 2 diabetes and atherosclerosis (Stern, 1995). According to this hypothesis, infections leading to chronic inflammation could pertain to the group of environmental etiological factors. Indeed, the risk of developing type 1 diabetes – a condition associated with significant morbidity in cardiovascular diseases in adult life – could rise during viral infections (Blom et al., 1991). Moreover, the risk for childhood diabetes seems to increase in accordance with a higher number of infections during the year preceding diagnosis. Studies in rodent models of atherosclerosis suggest similar dose-dependent association between infection and vascular changes (Liuba et al., 2000; Tormakangas et al., 2005). Furthermore, diabetic patients are more vulnerable to viral infections due to defective lymphocyte-related immunity. In a previous cross-sectional study on diabetic children, we found that recurrent viral infections in the upper airways ("common cold") during the past year had cumulative adverse effects on the elastic properties (i.e. compliance) of carotid arteries. In a multivariate analysis, the number of viral infections, along with age and plasma levels of glycosylated hemoglobin, significantly and independently predicted the decrease in carotid artery compliance (Odermarsky et al., 2008a). Although impaired carotid elasticity is generally regarded as a marker of early atherosclerosis, these findings do not necessarily imply causality to accelerated atherosclerosis. Prospective studies in children are currently in progress.

8. Prevention strategies in type 1 diabetes via vascular pathways?

Should vascular endothelial dysfunction prove to play a pivotal role in the pathogenesis of both type 1 diabetes and its associated vascular disease, it is then conceivable that combined endothelium-targeting and immunoregulatory strategies already in diabetes-risk individuals without overt type 1 diabetes (i.e. diabetes high-risk HLA individuals) might reduce not only the cardiovascular burden but also the prevalence of type 1 diabetes later in life. Dietary supplementation with L-arginine (substrate for nitric oxide synthesis via nitric oxide synthase), or antioxidants, in order to improve nitric oxide bioactivity, could for instance be relatively simple, risk-free strategy with potential benefit on endothelial dysfunction. Further studies are needed to provide additional mechanistic insights into the gene-environment interaction on vascular endothelium and the timing and role of endothelial dysfunction in the development of type 1 diabetes and associated cardiovascular disease.

9. References

Aburawi, E., Liuba, P., Pesonen, E., Ylä-Herttuala, S. & Sjoblad, S. (2004). Acute respiratory viral infections aggravate endothelial dysfunction in children with type 1 diabetes. Diabetes care, Vol. 27, No. 11, (November 2004), pp. 2733-5, ISSN 1935-5548

Akerblom, HK., Vaarala, O., Hyöty, H., Ilonen, J. & Knip, M. (2002). Environmental factors in the etiology of type 1 diabetes. Am J Med Genet, Vol. 115, No. 1, (May 2002), pp. 18-29, ISSN 1552-4833

Anderson, TJ., Uehata, A., Gerhard, MD., Meredith, IT., Knab, S., Delagrange, D., Lieberman, EH., Ganz, P., Creager, M., Yeung, A. & Selwyn, AP. (1995). Close relation of endothelial function in the human coronary and peripheral circulations. J Am Coll Cardiol, Vol. 26, No. 5, (November 1995), pp. 1235-41, ISSN 0735-1097

Beckman, JA., Creager, MA. & Libby, P. (2002). Diabetes and atherosclerosis: epidemiology, patophysiology, and management. JAMA, Vol. 287, No. 19, (May 2002), pp. 2570-81, ISSN 1528-0020

Blom, L., Nyström, L. & Dahlquist, G. (1991). The Swedish childhood diabetes study. Vaccinations and infections as risk determinants for diabetes in childhood. Diabetologia, Vol. 34, No. 3, (March 1991), pp. 176-81, ISSN 0012-186X

Charakida, M., Donald, AE., Terese, M., Leary, S., Halcox, JP., Ness, A., Davey Smith, G., Golding, J., Friberg, P., Klein, NJ. & Deanfield JE. for the Avon Longitudinal Study of Parents and Children study team. (2005). Endothelial dysfynction in childhood infection. Circulation, Vol. 111, No. 13, (March 2005), pp. 1660-65, ISSN 1524-4539

Cines, DB., Pollak, ES., Buck, CA., Loscalzo, J., Zimmerman, GA., McEver, RP., Pober, JS., Wick, TM., Konkle, BA., Schwartz, BS., Barnathan, ES., McCrae, KR., Hug, BA., Schmidt, A-M. & Stern, DM. (1998). Endothelial cells in physiology and in the pathophysiology of vascular disorders. Blood, Vol. 91, No. 10, (May 1998), pp. 3527-3561, ISSN 1528-0020

Corretti, MC., Anderson, TJ., Benjamin, EJ., Celermajer, D., Charbonneau, F., Creager, MA., Deanfield, J., Drexler, H., Gerhard-Herman, M., Herrington, D., Vallance, P., Vita, J. & Vogel, R. for the International Brachial Artery Reactivity Task Force. (2002). Guidelines for the ultrasound assessment of endothelial-dependent flow-mediated vasodilation of the brachial artery-a report from the International Brachial Artery Reactivity Task Force. J Am Coll Cardiol, Vol. 39, No. 2, (January 2002), pp. 257-65, ISSN 0735-1097

EURODIAB ACE Study group. (2000). Variations and trends in incidence of childhood diabetes in Europe. Lancet, Vol. 355, No. 9207, (March 2000), pp. 873-876, ISSN 0140-6736

Gaeta, G., Di Michele, M., Cuomo, S., Guarini, P., Foglia, MC., Gene Bond, M. & Trevisan, M. (2000). Arterial abnormalities in the offspring of patients with premature myocardial infarction. N Engl J Med, Vol. 343, No. 12, (September 2000), pp. 840-6, ISSN 1533-4406

Girach, A. & Vignati, L. (2006). Diabetic microvascular complications – can the presence of one predict the development of another? J Diabetes Complications, Vol. 20, No. 4, (July-August 2006), pp. 228-37, ISSN 1056-8727

Greening, JE., Tree, TIM., Kotowicz, K., Halteren, AG., Roep, BO., Klein, NJ., & Peakman, M. (2003). Processing and presentation of the islet autoantigen GAD by vascular endothelial cells promotes transmigration of autoreactive T-cells. Diabetes, Vol. 52, No. 3, (2003), pp. 717-25, ISSN 1939-327X

Hanninen, A., Jalkanen, S., Salmi, M., Toikkanen, S., Nikolakaros, G. & Simell, O. (1992). Macrophages, T cell receptor usage, and endothelial cell activation in the pancreas at the onset of insulin-dependent diabetes mellitus. J Clin Invest, Vol. 90, No. 5, (1992), pp. 1901-1910, ISSN 1558-8238

Irace, C., Ceravolo, R., Notarangelo, L., Crescenzo, A., Ventura, G., Tamburrini, O., Perticone, F. & Gnasso, A. (2001). Comparison of endothelial function evaluated by strain gauge pletysmography and brachial artery ultrasound. Atherosclerosis, Vol. 158, No. 1, (September 2001), pp. 53-9, ISSN 0021-9150

Itoh N, Hanafusa T, Miyazaki A, et al.. Mononuclear cell infiltration and its relation to the expression of major histocompatibility complex antigens and adhesion molecules in pancreas biopsy specimens from newly diagnosed insulin-dependent diabetes mellitus patients.(1993). J Clin Invest, (1993)92: 2313-2322.

Karvonen, M., Viik-Kajander, M., Moltchanova, E., Libman, I., LaPorte, R. & Toumilehto, J. (2000). Incidence of childhood type 1 diabetes worldwide. Diabetes Care, Vol. 23, No. 11, (October 2000), pp. 1516-1526, ISSN 1935-5548

Khan, F., Elhadd, TA., Greene, SA. & Belch, JJF. (2000). Impaired skin microvascular functions in children, adolescents, and young adults with type 1 diabetes. Diabetes Care, Vol. 23, No. 2, (February 2000), pp. 215-20, ISSN 1935-5548

Lammi, N., Karvonen, M. & Tuomilehto, J. (2005). Do microbes have a causal role in type 1 diabetes? Med Sci Monit, Vol. 11, No. 3, (March 2005), pp. RA63-69, ISSN 1643-3750

Liuba, P., Karnani, P., Pesonen, E., Paakkari, I., Forslid, A., Johansson, L., Persson, K., Wadstrom, T. & Laurini, R. (2000). Endothelial dysfunction after repeated Chlamydia pneumoniae infection in apolipoprotein E-knockout mice. Circulation, Vol. 102, No. 9, (August 2000), pp. 1039–44, ISSN 0009-7322

Lindley, S., Dayan, CM., Bishop, A., Roep, BO., Peakman, M. & Tree, TIM. (2005). Defective suppressor function in CD4+CD25+ T-cells from patients with type 1 diabetes. Diabetes, Vol. 54, No. 1, (January 2005), pp. 92-9, ISSN 1939-327X

Michel, T. & Vanhoutte, PM. (2010). Cellular signalling and NO production. Pflugers Arch-Eur J Physiol, Vol. 459, No. 6, (May 2010), pp. 807-16, ISSN 1432-2013

Morris, SJ. & Shore, AC. (1996). Skin blood flow reponses to the iontophoresis of acetylcholine and sodium nitroprusside in man: possible mechanisms. J Physiol, Vol. 496, No. Pt 2, (October 1996), pp. 531-42, ISSN 1469-7793

Neunteufl, T., Katzenschlager, R., Hassan, A., Klaar, U., Schwarzacher, S., Glogar, D., Bauer, P. & Weidinger, F. (1997). Systemic endothelial dysfunction is related to the extent and severity of coronary artery disease. Atherosclerosis, Vol. 129, No. 1, (February 1997), pp. 111-8, ISSN 0021-9150

Odermarsky, M., Nilsson, A., Lernmark, A., Sjoblad, S. & Liuba, P. (2007). Atherogenic vascular and lipid phenotypes in young patients with type 1 diabetes are associated with diabetes high-risk HLA genotype. Am J Physiol Heart Circ Physiol, Vol. 293, No. 5, (September 2007), pp. 3175-9, ISSN 1522-1539

Odermarsky, M., Lernmark, A., Truedsson, L. & Liuba, P. (2008b). Cutaneous microvascular dysfunction is associated with human leukocyte antigen-DQ in youths with type 1 diabetes. Pediatr Res, Vol. 63, No. 4, (April 2008), pp. 420-2, ISSN 0031-3998

Odermarsky, M., Andersson, S., Pesonen, E. Sjoblad, S., Ylä-Herttuala, S. & Liuba, P. (2008a). Respiratory infection recurrence and passive smoking in early atherosclerosis in children and adolescents with type 1 diabetes. Eur J Clin Invest, Vol. 38, No. 6, (June 2008), pp. 381-8, ISSN 1365-2362

Redondo, MJ., Fain, PR. & Eisenbarth, GS. (2001). Genetics of type 1A diabetes. Recent Prog Horm Res, Vol. 56, No. 1, (2001), pp. 69-89, ISSN 0079-9963

Rossing, P., Hougaard, P., Borch-Johnsen, K. & Parving, HH. (1996). Predictors of mortality in insulin dependent diabetes: 10 year observational follow up study. BMJ, Vol. 313, No. 7060, (September 1996), pp. 779-84, ISSN 0959-8146

Stern MP. (1995). Diabetes and cardiovascular disease. The "common soil" hypothesis. Diabetes, Vol. 44, No. 4, (April 1995), pp. 369-74, ISSN 0012-1797

TEDDY Study Group., (2008). The environmental determinants of diabetes in the young (TEDDY) study. Ann N Y Acad Sci, Vol. 1150, (December 2008), pp. 1-13, ISSN 1749-6632

The DIAMOND Project Group. (2006). Incidence and trends of childhood Type 1 diabetes worldwide 1990-1999. Diabet Med, Vol. 23, No. 8, (August 2006), pp. 857-866, ISSN 1464-5491

Thijssen, DHJ., Black, MA., Pyke, KE., Padilla, J., Atkinson, G., Harris, RA., Parker, B., Widlansky, ME., Tschakovsky, ME. & Green, DJ. (2011). Assessment of flow-mediated dilation in humans: a methodological physiological guideline. Am J Physiol Heart Circ Physiol, Vol. 300, No. 1, (January 2011), pp. H2-12, ISSN 1522-1539

Toivonen A, Kulmala P, Rahko J, Ilonen J, Knip M. (2004). Soluble adhesion molecules in Finnish schoolchildren with signs of preclinical type 1 diabetes. Diabetes Metab Res Rev, (2004), 20: 48-54.

Toivonen, A., Turner, J., Belch, JJF. & Khan, F. (2008). Current concepts in assessment of microvascular endothelial function using laser doppler imaging and iontophoresis. Trends Cardiovasc Med, Vol. 18, No. 4, (May 2008), pp. 109-16, ISSN 1050-1738

Tormakangas, L. ,Erkkila, L., Korhonen, T., Tiirola, T., Bloigu, A., Saikku, P. & Leinonen, O. Effects of repeated Chlamydia pneumoniae inoculations on aortic lipid accumulation and inflammatory response in C57BL/6J mice. Infect Immun,Vol. 73, No. 10, (October 2005), pp. 6458-66, ISSN 1098-5522

Versari, D., Daghini, E., Virdis, A., Ghiadoni, L. & Taddei, S. (2009). Endothelial dysfunction as a target for prevention of cardiovascular disease. Diabetes care, Vol. 32, No. suppl 2, (November 2009), pp. S314-21, ISSN 1935-5548

Virdis, A., Ghiadoni, L., Taddei, S. (2010). Human endothelial dysfunction: EDCFs. Pflugers Arch-Eur J Physiol, Vol. 459, No. 6, (May 2010), pp. 1015-23, ISSN 1432-2013

8

Cardiovascular Autonomic Dysfunction in Diabetes as a Complication: Cellular and Molecular Mechanisms

Yu-Long Li

Department of Emergency Medicine, University of Nebraska Medical Center
United States of America

1. Introduction

Diabetes is a major world health problem, which affects more than 23 million people in the US and an estimated 250 million worldwide. Diabetes mellitus is a metabolic disease characterized by high blood glucose levels resulted from an inability in pancreatic insulin secretion or insulin resistance. Usually diabetes mellitus is mainly divided into type 1 diabetes characterized by loss of the insulin production from beta cells of the pancreatic islets and type 2 diabetes characterized by insulin resistance (defective responsiveness of body tissues to insulin) and relatively reduced insulin secretion. Although type II diabetes is by far the most common affecting 90 to 95% of the US diabetic population, the studies focusing on the type 1 diabetes cannot be ignored because about 1 in every 400 to 600 children and adolescents has type 1 diabetes and about 2 million adolescents aged 12-19 have pre-diabetes in the US.

Diabetes mellitus is chronic progressive disease that usually cannot be cured. Following the natural progression of disease, diabetes without proper treatments can cause many severe complications including diabetic ketoacidosis, cardiovascular disease, chronic renal failure, retinal damage. These complications obviously enhance the risk for diabetic patients. In these complications of the diabetes mellitus, cardiovascular autonomic dysfunction is a serious although poorly understood long term diabetic complication. Indeed, diabetic patients with cardiovascular autonomic dysfunction have consistently been shown to have an enhanced risk of premature death (Rosengard-Barlund et al., 2009). More importantly, the age-adjusted relative risk for cardiovascular disease in type 1 diabetes far exceeds that of type 2 diabetes (Krolewski et al., 1987; Libby et al., 2005). Therefore, exploring the mechanisms responsible to the cardiovascular autonomic dysfunction can provide an important and new pharmacological and genetic target for improving the prognosis and reducing the mortality in diabetic state.

2. Baroreflex dysfunction in type 1 diabetes and the contribution of the baroreflex dysfunction in prognosis and mortality of the type 1 diabetes

Cardiovascular autonomic function is the autonomic neural regulation of cardiovascular function, which presents the balance between sympathetic and parasympathetic innervation resulting in periodic fluctuation in heart rate and rhythm. Although there are many invasive and non-invasive methods to evaluate the cardiovascular autonomic function in diverse clinical and research settings, cardiovascular autonomic function typically is measured by a short-term evoked cardiovascular reflex, especially arterial baroreflex.

2.1 Baroreflex dysfunction

The arterial baroreflex normally acts to prevent wide oscillations in blood pressure and heart rate, acting on both sympathetic and parasympathetic limbs of the cardiovascular autonomic nervous system. Dysfunction of the arterial baroreflex control on the blood pressure and heart rate has been described in many studies not only in the type I diabetic patients, but also in experimental models of the type I diabetes.

In the diabetic patients, heart rate variability is the most widely used index of the arterial baroreflex function. Some studies in more heterogeneous groups of patients with type 1 diabetes have indicated that: (1) showing lower global heart rate variability; (2) relative increase in the low-frequency component (sympathetic activity) of the heart rate variability; (3) relative reduction in the high-frequency component (parasympathetic activity) of the heart rate variability; and (4) higher ratio of the low frequency to the high-frequency (Lishner *et al.*, 1987; Rosengard-Barlund *et al.*, 2009; Ziegler *et al.*, 2001). Clinical research data have confirmed that arterial baroreflex sensitivity is reduced in type 1 diabetic patients with a wide range of age and diabetic duration (Lefrandt *et al.*, 1999; Weston *et al.*, 1996;Weston *et al.*, 1998; Dalla *et al.*, 2007). More importantly, this attenuated arterial baroreflex function was found in the type 1 diabetic patients without the clinical complications, the alterations of the other autonomic function tests, or the overt autonomic neuropathy (Lefrandt *et al.*, 1999; Rosengard-Barlund *et al.*, 2009). Therefore, it is of note that the reduced arterial baroreflex sensitivity can be an earlier sensitive marker of the cardiovascular autonomic dysfunction in the type 1 diabetic patients.

In order to obtain new insights into human type 1 diabetes, animal models of the type 1 diabetes have been widely used in the biomedical studies focusing on the type 1 diabetes, such as alloxan-induced diabetic rabbits (McDowell *et al.*, 1994b), streptozotocin-induced diabetic rats (Hicks *et al.*, 1998; Maeda *et al.*, 1995; Van *et al.*, 1998; Chen *et al.*, 2008), and calmodulin transgenic OVE26 diabetic mice (Gu *et al.*, 2008). Streptozotocin (STZ)-induced diabetic rat is an animal model of insulin-dependent diabetes usually used to study the cardiovascular alterations including cardiovascular autonomic dysfunction caused by diabetes even if the changes of cardiovascular function in this animal model don't fully match the alterations observed under the clinical type 1 diabetic states (Hicks *et al.*, 1998). In the STZ-induced diabetic rats, the arterial baroreflex dysfunction is presented as early as 5 days after the STZ administration (Maeda *et al.*, 1995). Much evidence has documented that the arterial baroreflex is decreased in all kinds of type 1 diabetic models (Chen *et al.*, 2008; Dall'Ago *et al.*, 1997; De Angelis *et al.*, 2000; Gu *et al.*, 2008; Maliszewska-Scislo *et al.*, 2003; McDowell *et al.*, 1994b; Van *et al.*, 1998).

2.2 Association of cardiovascular autonomic dysfunction with mortality rate

30 years ago, Ewing et al (Ewing *et al.*, 1980) first reported that there was a mortality rate of 53% after 5 years in diabetic patients with abnormal autonomic function, compared with a mortality rate of about 15% over the 5 year period among diabetic patients without abnormal autonomic function. Thereafter the growing evidence has confirmed that

cardiovascular autonomic dysfunction is associated with a high risk of cardiac arrhythmias and with sudden death in the diabetic state. A longitudinal study by O'Brien et al (O'Brien *et al.*, 1991) has investigated 5-year survival in 506 randomly selected patients with insulin-dependent diabetes mellitus. In this study, the cumulative 5-year mortality rate in the diabetic patients with cardiovascular autonomic dysfunction (27%) is about 5-fold more than in the diabetic patients with normal cardiovascular autonomic function (5%). However, there is no difference in duration of diabetes between the deceased diabetic patients with and without cardiovascular autonomic dysfunction (O'Brien *et al.*, 1991). A meta-analysis (Maser *et al.*, 2003) and the epidemiology of diabetes complication study (Orchard *et al.*, 1996) also showed that cardiovascular autonomic dysfunction could contribute to the increased risk of mortality rate in the individuals with diabetes. In the recent EURODIAB prospective complications study, the researchers have found that cardiovascular autonomic dysfunction is an important risk marker for mortality rate, exceeding the effect of the traditional risk factors (such as age, waist-to-hip ratio, pulse pressure, and non-HDL cholesterol) (Soedamah-Muthu *et al.*, 2008).

Since the diabetic patients are more likely to have many known diabetes-associated risk factors besides cardiovascular autonomic dysfunction (Soedamah-Muthu *et al.*, 2008), the question is whether cardiovascular autonomic dysfunction is an independent risk factor to predict the mortality rate of the diabetic patients. Some studies have addressed this question to minimize the potential interference of other risk factors (for example age, sex, height, smoking, diabetes duration, etc) by matching these variables in the diabetic patients with and without cardiovascular autonomic dysfunction (O'Brien *et al.*, 1991; Orchard *et al.*, 1996; Rathmann *et al.*, 1993). In Rathmann's study (Rathmann *et al.*, 1993), diabetic patients with and without cardiovascular autonomic dysfunction were matched for age, sex, and duration of diabetes. The 8-year survival rate estimate in patients with cardiovascular autonomic dysfunction was 77% compared with 97% in those with normal cardiovascular autonomic function in this study (Rathmann *et al.*, 1993). O'Brien et al. have also matched age, sex, and duration of diabetes in the diabetic patients with and without cardiac autonomic dysfunction in their study (O'Brien *et al.*, 1991). They found that the cardiovascular autonomic dysfunction was associated with the mortality rate of the type 1 diabetic patients (O'Brien *et al.*, 1991).

2.3 Potential mechanisms responsible for cardiovascular autonomic dysfunction-increased mortality rate

Although many studies mentioned above have confirmed that the cardiovascular autonomic dysfunction is involved in increasing mortality rate of type 1 diabetic patients, we really don't know whether cardiovascular autonomic dysfunction is directly or indirectly responsible for the increased mortality rate. It is possible that several possible mechanisms are involved in this clinical phenomenon.

First, a few clinical studies have reported that some type 1 diabetic patients in good health the previous day are found dead in the morning in an undisturbed bed with no sign of the symptoms (such as sweating and struggle) and negative autopsy results, which is named as the 'dead in bed' syndrome (Tattersall & Gill, 1991; Weston & Gill, 1999). One recent clinical study has found that ECG abnormalities including QT prolongation, cardiac rhythm disturbance, and subsequent ventricular tachyarrhythmia appear in the ambulant patients with type 1 diabetes (Gill *et al.*, 2009). The ECG abnormalities can serve as principal underlying causes of the 'dead in bed' syndrome (Gill *et al.*, 2009). Cardiovascular autonomic dysfunction itself can link to the QT prolongation and sudden death (Weston & Gill, 1999). In another study, type 1 diabetic adolescents with impaired cardiovascular autonomic function are associated with the possible development of cardiac arrhythmias and left-ventricular hypertrophy (Karavanaki *et al.*, 2007). In addition, decreased heart rate variability is also a predictive risk factor for ventricular arrhythmia and sudden cardiac death (Kleiger *et al.*, 1987). Loss of cardiac vagal drive combined with loss of baroreceptor reflex sensitivity is thought to mediate the decreased heart rate variability and autonomic instability that exacerbate arrhythmia susceptibility (Binkley *et al.*, 1991). These studies indicate that cardiovascular autonomic dysfunction (decreased heart rate variability and loss of baroreceptor reflex sensitivity) is correlated with the prognosis and mortality in patients with type 1 diabetes via increasing the susceptibility to the lethal arrhythmias.

Second, although cardiovascular autonomic dysfunction is an independent risk factor to predict the mortality rate of the diabetic patients described above, other abnormalities (such as increased stiffness of the vascular walls at the site of the arterial baroreceptors, left ventricular hypertrophy, endothelial dysfunction, renal failure, peripheral neuropathy, etc) usually coexist with cardiovascular autonomic dysfunction in type 1 diabetic patients (Toyry *et al.*, 1997; Lluch *et al.*, 1998; Lefrandt *et al.*, 2010). Therefore, it is possible that the interaction between cardiovascular autonomic dysfunction and other concomitant abnormalities is responsible for the increased mortality rate in type 1 diabetic patients. It has been shown that cardiovascular autonomic function is easily impaired in type 1 diabetic patients with microalbuminuria (renal dysfunction) (Lefrandt *et al.*, 1999; Clarke *et al.*, 1999). O'Brien et al have reported that renal failure-induced mortality rate is higher in type 1 diabetic patients with cardiovascular autonomic dysfunction than in those without cardiovascular autonomic dysfunction (O'Brien *et al.*, 1991). In a 23 year follow-up study, cardiovascular autonomic dysfunction may be involved in a higher mortality rate induced by microalbuminuria in type 1 diabetic patients (Messent *et al.*, 1992). Similarly, renal disease also can partially explicate the cardiovascular autonomic dysfunction-increased mortality rate in patients with diabetes mellitus (Weinrauch *et al.*, 1998; Kim *et al.*, 2009). In addition, using logistic regression analysis, one recent study has addressed the relationship between cardiovascular autonomic dysfunction and other abnormalities in 684 type 1 diabetic patients (Pavy-Le *et al.*, 2010). The research data have shown that retinopathy, peripheral neuropathy, and erectile dysfunction are closely correlated to the severity of the cardiovascular autonomic dysfunction (Pavy-Le *et al.*, 2010). Furthermore, some studies have also found a consistent association between cardiovascular autonomic dysfunction and silent myocardial ischemia, in which the patient's risk coefficient related to the cardiovascular autonomic dysfunction is higher in asymptomatic diabetic patients with silent myocardial ischemia than in those without silent myocardial ischemia (Valensi *et al.*, 2001; Vinik & Ziegler, 2007; Katz *et al.*, 1999).

Finally, several studies reported the involvement of cardiorespiratory arrest in the mortality of the diabetic patients with cardiovascular autonomic dysfunction (Page & Watkins, 1978; Bergner & Goldberger, 2010; Douglas *et al.*, 1981). The research data from Page et al. (Page & Watkins, 1978) have demonstrated that young diabetic patients with severe cardiovascular autonomic dysfunction can appear to have cardiorespiratory arrest due to the impairment of cardiorespiratory function. The cardiorespiratory arrest may be responsible for the mortality of these diabetic patients (Page & Watkins, 1978).

3. Mechanisms responsible for the reduced baroreflex function in type 1 diabetes

The arterial baroreflex is a homeostatic mechanism that alters heart rate and blood pressure in response to changes in arterial wall tension detected by the baroreceptors in the carotid sinus and aortic arch. The arterial baroreflex arc includes an afferent limb, a central neural component and autonomic neuroeffector components. As the primary afferent limb of the baroreceptor reflex, baroreceptor neurons sense blood pressure by increasing their discharge (excitation) when arterial blood pressure rises. This excited signal in baroreceptor neurons reaches to the dorsal medial nucleus tractus solitarii (NTS, the first site of baroreceptor neuron contacting with central nervous system), in which the integrated input signal inhibits the efferent sympathetic outflow to the heart and peripheral vascular, and activates efferent parasympathetic activity to the heart those decrease peripheral vascular resistance, heart rate, and arterial blood pressure. Conversely, the baroreceptor afferent signal decreases when arterial blood pressure falls, which reflexly induces an increase in heart rate and arterial blood pressure.

As mentioned above, blunted arterial baroreflex sensitivity is observed in type 1 diabetic patients and animal models. What are the mechanisms responsible for the attenuated arterial baroreflex sensitivity in type 1 diabetes? Every site within the baroreflex arc may be responsible for the depressed baroreflex sensitivity in type 1 diabetes. Therefore, we will discuss the fact that the reduced baroreflex sensitivity results from functional and/or structural changes in the baroreceptors (including nerve terminals and neuron somata), central neural integration, and autonomic efferent component.

3.1 Role of baroreceptor in the blunted arterial baroreflex in type 1 diabetes

As the primary afferent limb of the arterial baroreceptor reflex, baroreceptor neurons are pseudo-unipolar neurons (T-shaped neurons) consisting of a cell body existing in the nodose or petrosal ganglia and an initial axon segment. This axon segment bifurcates near the soma into a peripheral process innervating aortic arch and carotid sinus for sensing the alteration of the arterial blood pressure and a central process terminating in the NTS for conveying the afferent signals to the central nervous system. The mechanisms responsible for mediating afferent sensitivity of barosensitive neurons to pressure are complex and not thoroughly understood. The process of translating changes in arterial wall tension into impulse traffic to the NTS involves 2 broad functional steps: 1) mechanotransduction which is governed by the properties of mechanosensitive ion channels in the nerve terminal and the mechanical properties of the coupling of the arterial wall to the sensory terminal; and 2) spike initiation which is governed by the excitability of membrane voltage sensitive ion channels that influence the electrical (cable) properties of the axonal process and cell body. All of these factors could be (and likely are) altered in type 1 diabetes, which can directly affect the arterial baroreflex function.

3.1.1 Changes of baroreceptor afferent nerve and terminal in type 1 diabetes

Although some studies have suggested that diabetes-induced postural hypotension results from impairments of afferent baroreceptors and of sympathetic neurons innervating the vascular wall and heart in diabetic patients (Low et al., 1975; Iovino et al., 2011), there is only fragmentary evidence to support this assumption because of the inability of clinical cardiovascular autonomic function tests to separate the role of the afferent, central, and efferent components of the arterial baroreflex. In general, the function of the baroreceptor afferent nerve and terminal is investigated by recording the single fiber or multifiber activity of the aortic depressor nerve or carotid sinus nerve in a perfused isolated aortic arch/carotid sinus preparation (do Carmo *et al.*, 2007; Doan *et al.*, 2004; Fazan, Jr. *et al.*, 1997; McDowell *et al.*, 1994b; Reynolds *et al.*, 1994; Reynolds *et al.*, 1999; Xiao *et al.*, 2007; Zhang *et al.*, 2004). However, the baroreceptor function in the diabetic state is studied only in the aortic depressor nerve (Fazan, Jr. *et al.*, 1997; Fazan, Jr. *et al.*, 1999; McDowell *et al.*, 1994b; Reynolds *et al.*, 1999) but not in the carotid sinus nerve (Salgado *et al.*, 2001). This may be because there are only baroreceptor afferent fibers and no chemoreceptor afferent fibers in rat aortic depressor nerve unlike the carotid sinus nerve (Fan *et al.*, 1996; Kobayashi *et al.*, 1999; Sapru & Krieger, 1977; Sapru *et al.*, 1981). Based on the results from some studies, there is no evidence to show the changes of the aortic depressor nerve activity in STZ-induced type 1 diabetic rats (Fazan, Jr. *et al.*, 1997; Reynolds *et al.*, 1999; Dall'Ago *et al.*, 2002) and alloxan-induced diabetic rabbits (McDowell *et al.*, 1994b), compared to the sham animals. In addition, Gu *et al* (Gu *et al.*, 2008) have found that the baroreceptor function of the aortic depressor nerve is preserved in the ascending phase of the arterial blood pressure but is blunted in the descending phase of the arterial blood pressure in type 1 diabetic mice. Nevertheless, the results obtained by a new approach, named as cross-spectral analysis, indicate that a significant decrease of the aortic baroreceptor nerve function is observed in anesthetized rats with either short term (10-20 days) or long term (12-18 weeks) STZ-induced diabetes (Fazan, Jr. *et al.*, 1999). This new approach uses the magnitude of the transfer function obtained by analyzing the relationship between beat-by-beat time series of mean arterial blood pressure and aortic depressor nerve activity as the index of the aortic baroreceptor nerve function, whose advantage is to evaluate the aortic baroreceptor nerve function under more physiological conditions (Salgado *et al.*, 2001; Fazan, Jr. *et al.*, 1999; deBoer *et al.*, 1987) compared to the arterial blood pressure/aortic depressor nerve activity curve used in other studies (Dall'Ago *et al.*, 2002; Fazan, Jr. *et al.*, 1997; Gu *et al.*, 2008; McDowell *et al.*, 1994b; Reynolds *et al.*, 1999). In addition, Fazan et al have found that the morphological change in the aortic depressor nerve, an afferent arm of the baroreflex may result in the arterial baroreflex impairment in the STZ-induced diabetic rats (Fazan *et al.*, 2006). Therefore, the functional and structural alterations of the baroreceptor afferent nerve in type 1 diabetes still need to be further clarified in future study.

By light, electron, and confocal microscopies, some researchers have identified the aortic baroreceptor terminals in the adventitia of the aortic arch from dogs, rabbits, cats, rats, and mice (Aumonier, 1972; Cheng *et al.*, 1997; Krauhs, 1979; Li *et al.*, 2010). More importantly, Li et al have demonstrated that diabetes induces morphological atrophy of the aortic baroreceptor terminals in type 1 diabetic mice (Li *et al.*, 2010). However, there is no report on the functional role of the aortic baroreceptor terminals in sham and type 1 diabetic animals because it is difficult to separate aortic baroreceptor terminals to other tissues (such as smooth muscle and endothelium) in the aortic arch. It is possible that using gene and short hairpin RNA (shRNA) transfection can solve this problem in future study.

3.1.2 Role of aortic baroreceptor neurons in the arterial baroreflex in the type 1 diabetes

Many studies have used the responses of blood pressure and heart rate to electrical stimulation of baroreceptor-containing nerve (aortic depressor nerve) for the evaluation of the baroreflex sensitivity in rats (Fan & Andresen, 1998; Salgado *et al.*, 2007; Tang &

Dworkin, 2007). The aortic depressor nerves (the peripheral process of the aortic baroreceptor neuron) are composed of both afferent A-type (myelinated) axons (about 25%) and C-type (unmyelinated) axons (about 75%) (Yamasaki et al., 2004). There are very different dynamic sensory discharge characteristics between A-type and C-type baroreceptor afferents. C-type afferents are activated mainly at very high pressure and have lower firing frequencies, irregular discharge patterns (Thoren et al., 1999), and appear to be the primary regulators of tonic baseline levels of arterial blood pressure besides regulating the baroreflex sensitivity (Seagard et al., 1993). A-type afferents have lower pressure thresholds with very stable, proportional firing patterns (Thoren et al., 1999), which are thought to regulate the baroreflex sensitivity but not baseline levels of arterial blood pressure (Seagard et al., 1993). Electrical Stimulation of the rat aortic depressor nerve has several advantages to examine the baroreflex function. First, the rat aortic depressor nerve contains only baroreceptor afferent fibers and no chemoreceptor afferent fibers to transmit the chemoreceptor information (Fan et al., 1996; Kobayashi et al., 1999; Sapru & Krieger, 1977; Sapru et al., 1981). Second, the baroreflex induced by stimulating rat aortic depressor nerve is measured without the aortic baroreceptor terminals in the reflex arc, which allows us to specifically examine the role of electrical excitability of aortic baroreceptor in the baroreflex function (second process mentioned above). Third, by varying the frequency of stimulus, one can differentially activate A- and C- afferent fibers, and thus evaluate the relative contribution of each to the altered aortic baroreceptor excitability and baroreflex function in STZ-induced diabetes. In our preliminary study, the baroreflex responses of blood pressure and heart rate to the electrical stimulation of the aortic baroreceptor nerve are significantly depressed in STZ-induced diabetic rats (Fig. 1). In addition, our study also found that microinjection of angiotensin II type 1 (AT_1) receptor antagonist (20 μM L158,809) into the nodose ganglia significantly improved the baroreflex sensitivity induced by aortic depressor nerve stimulation in STZ-induced diabetic rats (Fig. 1). Simultaneously, AT_1 receptor antagonist also normalized the depressed cell excitability in the aortic baroreceptor neurons of STZ-induced diabetic rats (Li & Zheng, 2011). The fact is that nodose neurons are found to influence the conduction and frequency of the electrical impulses in the baroreceptor central axons projecting to the central nervous system when electrical signals in the baroreceptor peripheral axons reach the nodose neurons (Ducreux et al., 1993). One review paper has concluded that the excitability of vagal afferent neurons has dramatic consequences for the regulation and modulation of vago-vagal reflex (Browning, 2003). Furthermore, Devor (Devor, 1999) has reported that electrical excitability of the soma in the dorsal root ganglia may be required to insure the reliable afferent electrical impulses transmitted to the spinal cord. These results, taken together, demonstrate that the reduced cell excitability of the aortic baroreceptor neurons contributes to the blunted baroreflex sensitivity in STZ-induced diabetic rats.

However, results from reflex experiments evoked by the electrical stimulation need to be tempered because the electrical stimulation technique does not represent a physiological substrate for baroreceptor activation. Thus, arterial baroreflex evoked by changes in arterial blood pressure should be done to further address the role of the aortic baroreceptor neurons in the arterial baroreflex in the type 1 diabetes. Of course, in this approach (blood pressure-mediated baroreflex sensitivity), possible alterations in the mechanotransduction process at the baro-sensory nerve terminal may also play a role in the suppressed baroreceptor function in response to pressure changes.

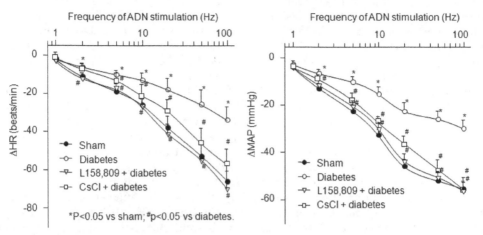

Fig. 1. Reflex ΔMAP and ΔHR in response to different frequencies of ADN stimulation in anesthetized sham and STZ-induced diabetic rats (n=8 in each group). L158,809: AT₁ receptor antagonist; CsCl: HCN channel blocker. MBP, mean blood pressure; HR, heart rate; ADN, aortic depressor nerve.

3.1.3 Contribution of the HCN channel to the cell excitability of aortic baroreceptor neuron in the type 1 diabetes

Until now it is controversial whether either severe degenerative changes or neuronal cell loss in sensory and autonomic nervous tissues are found in STZ-induced diabetic animals (Yagihashi, 1997). Apoptotic cell death was reported in the sensory neurons, satellite cells, and Schwann cells from dorsal root ganglia (DRG) of STZ-induced diabetic rats (Russell *et al.*, 1999; Srinivasan *et al.*, 2000). Kogawa et al. also found that apoptotic cell death of DRG neurons and impaired sensory nerve regeneration were induced by sciatic nerve crush in STZ-induced diabetic rats (Kogawa *et al.*, 2000). On the other hand, the findings from Sango et al (Sango *et al.*, 1991; Sango *et al.*, 1995; Sango *et al.*, 1997) indicated no difference in the dissociated neurons from DRG between sham and STZ-induced diabetic mice. Furthermore, some studies have demonstrated that there are no morphological changes of the peripheral nerves (Sharma & Thomas, 1987) and cell death of the nodose afferent neurons (Sango *et al.*, 2002) in STZ-induced diabetic animals. Our recent study (Tu *et al.*, 2010) also suggests that STZ-induced diabetes does not change the total cell number of the nodose afferent neurons and the ratio of A-/C-type neurons (Fig. 2). These results provide an important piece of information that the parasympathetic reflex dysfunction (Li *et al.*, 2008b; Thomas & Tomlinson, 1993; Ziegler, 1994) in STZ-induced diabetes might be not due to the structural changes in the nodose afferent neurons but most likely due to the functional changes at the cellular and molecular levels.

As everyone knows, many ion channels (such as sodium channels, calcium channels, potassium channels, etc) are responsible for the cell excitation in the excitable cells such as cardiac/skeletal myocytes and neurons including aortic baroreceptor neurons. However, much evidence has indicates that Hyperpolarization-activated cyclic nucleotide-gated (HCN) channels play an important role in the cell excitability of the aortic baroreceptor neurons from sham and STZ-induced diabetic rats.

HCN channels have been found in various types of cells including cardiac and neuronal cells (DiFrancesco, 1985; DiFrancesco, 1993; Pape, 1996). In these spontaneously exciting cells, HCN channels normally associate to the cardiac pacemaker activity and the neuronal oscillatory behavior (Brown et al., 1979; DiFrancesco, 1993; Kaupp & Seifert, 2001; Notomi & Shigemoto, 2004; Pape, 1996; Robinson & Siegelbaum, 2003). However, HCN channels may have a different role in the nodose ganglion neurons (the non-oscillatory and non-automatic exciting cells) because the nodose neurons are inactive except in response to a depolarizing stimulus generated by their peripheral sensory terminals (Doan & Kunze, 1999; Li et al., 2008a). In the nodose neurons, the resting membrane potential is about -50 to -65 mV, in which voltage-dependent sodium, calcium, and potassium channels are almost inactivated (Robinson & Siegelbaum, 2003). The inactivation of these voltage-dependent channels can be recovered to the activation state during the hyperpolarization of the resting membrane potential, which means the number of available voltage-dependent channels for activation is increased if the nodose neurons receive the depolarizing stimulus (Doan & Kunze, 1999). Inhibition of HCN channels has been shown to hyperpolarize the nodose neurons (increasing the resting membrane potential) and to reduce action potential threshold in response to a depolarizing current stimulation, which suggests that HCN channels are involved in the cell excitability of the nodose neurons (Doan et al., 2004; Li et al., 2008a). Results from our recent studies (Li et al., 2008a; Li & Zheng, 2011; Tu et al., 2010) confirm that the HCN current density in A- and C-type aortic baroreceptor neurons from STZ-induced diabetic rats is larger than that from the sham rats (Fig. 3). In addition, the resting membrane potential is depolarized and the current threshold induced the action potentials was elevated in the A-/C-type aortic baroreceptor neurons from STZ-induced diabetic rats, compared with that in sham rats (Li et al., 2008a; Li & Zheng, 2011). Furthermore, HCN channel blockers (CsCl and ZD-7288) lowered the HCN current density, hyperpolarized the resting membrane potential, and raised the cell membrane excitability in A-/C-type aortic baroreceptor neurons from sham and STZ-induced diabetic rats (Li et al., 2008a; Zhang et al., 2010). These results clearly indicate that the HCN channels are involved in the regulation of aortic baroreceptor neuron excitability. The enhancement of HCN currents can contribute to the blunted aortic baroreceptor neuron excitability, and subsequently attenuate the arterial baroreflex sensitivity in STZ-induced diabetic rats. This is true because microinjection of HCN channel blocker (5 mM CsCl) improves the arterial baroreflex sensitivity induced by the electrical stimulation of the aortic depressor nerve (Fig. 1) (Li et al., 2008b).

Four mammalian genes encoding HCN channel isoforms (HCN1, HCN2, HCN3, and HCN4) have been identified (Doan et al., 2004; Ishii et al., 1999; Ludwig et al., 1998; Santoro et al., 1998; Vaccari et al., 1999). In cell lines transfected HCN isoform cDNA, electrophysiological studies have shown that each channel isoform is activated by membrane hyperpolarization with distinct activation kinetics (Ludwig et al., 1999; Moosmang et al., 2001; Qu et al., 2002; Santoro et al., 1998). Activation of the HCN channels is also directly modulated by cAMP, which is dependent on the HCN channel isoform (Stieber et al., 2003; Wainger et al., 2001; Wang et al., 2002). HCN channels are activated with the different activation rates in this order: HCN1>HCN2>HCN3>HCN4 (Accili et al., 2002; Altomare et al., 2001; Moosmang et al., 2001; Stieber et al., 2003; Stieber et al., 2005). HCN1 and HCN3 are only weakly affected by cAMP whereas HCN2 and HCN4 are very sensitive to cAMP (Accili et al., 2002; Stieber et al., 2005; Wahl-Schott & Biel, 2009; Wang et al., 2001). Our studies (Li et al., 2008a; Tu et al., 2010) have found that a fast-activated and cAMP-

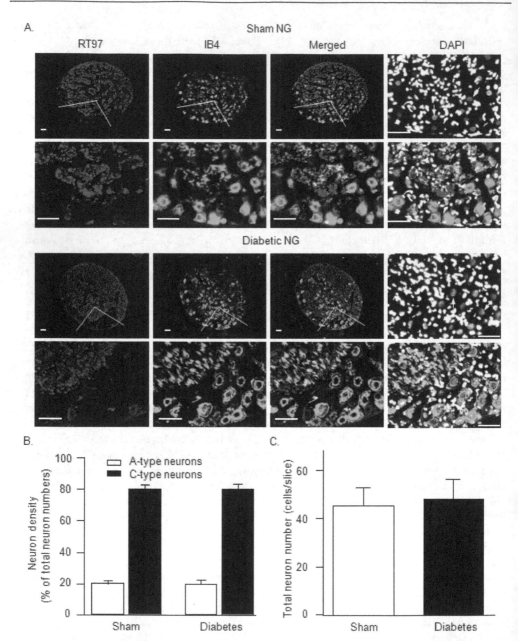

Fig. 2. Ratio of A-type/C-type neurons (A and B) and total neuron number (C) in nodose ganglia from sham and STZ-induced diabetic rats. Calibration bar: 100 μm. RT97, A-type neuron marker; IB4, C-type neuron marker; DAPI, cell nucleus marker. Yellow arrows indicate nodose neurons in DAPI staining (Adapted and reprinted from Tu *et al.*, 2010, page 42, with permission from Elsevier)

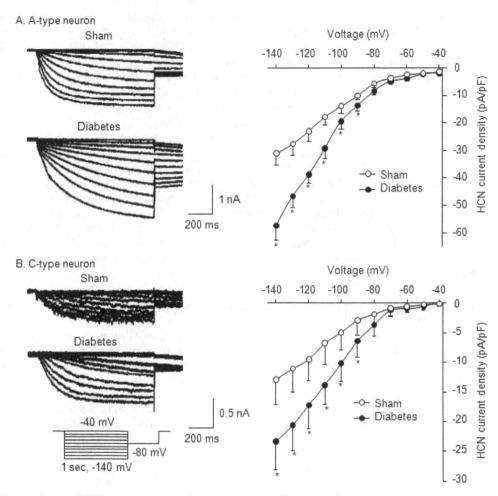

Fig. 3. Original HCN current recording and current density-voltage curves in A- and C-type neurons from sham and STZ-induced diabetic rats. *P<0.05 vs. sham rats (Reprinted from Tu *et al.*, 2010, page 48, with permission from Elsevier).

insensitive HCN current is induced in sham A-type aortic baroreceptor neurons whereas a slow-activated and cAMP-sensitive HCN current is induced in sham C-type aortic baroreceptor neurons. From these electrophysiological results, we can imagine that there is a differential distribution of the HCN channel isoforms in the A- and C-type aortic baroreceptor neurons. Data from immunofluorescent double staining also show that HCN1, HCN3, and HCN4 are expressed in sham A-type nodose neurons, whereas HCN2, HCN3, and HCN4 are expressed in sham C-type nodose neurons (Li *et al.*, 2008a; Tu *et al.*, 2010). Based on these results, it is reasonable to assume that there are marked different activation kinetics and cAMP sensitivity of HCN channels between A-fiber neurons and C-fiber neurons, which might be due to the neuron cell-specific expression of HCN channel isoforms.

Our studies further demonstrate that diabetes enhances the HCN currents and the expression of HCN1, HCN2, and HCH 3 channel proteins in A-type aortic baroreceptor neurons (Li et al., 2008a; Tu et al., 2010). Overexpression of HCN1, HCN2, and HCN3 but not HCN4 channel isoforms can link to the enhanced HCN currents, the slow-activated HCN channel kinetics, and the increased cAMP-sensitivity of HCN channels in diabetic A-type aortic baroreceptor neurons (Li et al., 2008a; Tu et al., 2010). Although diabetes also increases the HCN currents and the expression of HCN2 and HCN3 channel proteins in C-type aortic baroreceptor neurons, diabetes does not change the activation kinetics and the cAMP sensitivity of the HCN channels in C-type aortic baroreceptor neurons due to no expression of HCN1 channel in diabetic C-type aortic baroreceptor neurons (Li et al., 2008a; Tu et al., 2010). From these results, we propose that HCN currents are markedly enhanced via increasing the numbers of HCN channels and sensitivity of HCN channels to cAMP in the aortic baroreceptor neurons. The enhanced HCN currents can contribute to the depressed neuron excitability in diabetic aortic baroreceptor neurons. However, we do realize that these data cannot explain why diabetes induces the different changes of HCN channel protein expression and cannot identify the contribution of the various HCN channel isoforms to the enhanced HCN currents in diabetic A- and C-type aortic baroreceptor neurons.

3.1.4 Regulation of the angiotensin II-superoxide signaling on the HCN channel in the type 1 diabetes

Angiotensin II, an endogenous peptide, has been thought to be a prime candidate in the regulation of the HCN channel function and cell excitability in the diabetic state. It is known that circulating and tissue angiotensin II concentrations are elevated in human and animals with diabetes (Frustaci et al., 2000; Sechi et al., 1994; Shimoni & Liu, 2004). Previous autoradiographic study has identified a high density of angiotensin II receptor binding sites over the nodose neurons (Allen et al., 1988). Widdop, et al. provided evidence for the direct neuronal effects of angiotensin II on the vagal afferent neurons (Widdop et al., 1992). Indeed, our research data not only confirm AT_1 and AT_2 receptors exist in nodose neuronal cells, but also indicate that exogenous angiotensin II enhances the HCN currents and subsequently reduces cell excitability in the aortic baroreceptor neurons from normal rats (Zhang et al., 2010). This is via NADPH oxidase-derived superoxide because a specific HCN channel blocker blunts the inhibitory effect of the exogenous angiotensin II on action potentials (Zhang et al., 2010). More importantly, angiotensin II concentration and protein expression of AT_1 receptors are increased in the nodose neuronal cells from STZ-induced diabetic rats (Li & Zheng, 2011). At the same time, mRNA expression of AT_1 receptors measured by single cell real-time PCR technique is enhanced in the aortic baroreceptor neuron cells from the STZ-induced diabetic rats (Li & Zheng, 2011). In addition, AT_1 receptor antagonist (losartan) significantly normalizes the enhanced HCN currents and the attenuated cell excitability (including depolarization of the resting membrane potential, fall in the input resistance, and decrease in the action potential number) in the aortic baroreceptor neurons induced by diabetes (Li & Zheng, 2011) or exogenous angiotensin II (Zhang et al., 2010). Furthermore, angiotensin II-AT_1 receptor is also involved in the attenuated arterial baroreflex sensitivity in STZ-induced diabetic rats (Fig. 1) (Li et al., 2008b). Based on these results, it is reasonable to assume that elevation of local angiotensin II level can blunt the membrane excitability of the aortic baroreceptor neurons via enhancement of the HCN currents, and consequently attenuate the aortic baroreflex function in the type 1 diabetes.

Above results suggest that elevation of local tissue angiotensin II plays an important role on the enhanced HCN channel activity and the blunted cell excitability in the AB neurons in diabetes. However, it is unclear how angiotensin II and its antagonist within an isolated aortic baroreceptor neuron from diabetic rat interact with AT_1 receptor to affect the HCN channel activity and cell excitability. Classical viewpoint about the effects of angiotensin II binding with AT_1 receptor is that angiotensin II binds with AT_1 receptor at the cell membrane, and following the phosphorylation of the AT_1 receptor, angiotensin II induces intracellular responses via activating intracellular downstream signal transduction. However, Zhuo, et al. (Zhuo *et al.*, 2002) have found that there is substantial intracellular accumulation of angiotensin II in renal cortical endosomes during angiotensin II-dependent hypertension via an AT_1 receptor-mediated process. Recent studies have shown that intracellular administration of angiotensin II increases the peak inward calcium current density and decreases the junctional conductance via intracellular angiotensin II receptors in cardiac myocytes (De Mello, 2003; De Mello & Monterrubio, 2004). Intracellular treatment of losartan (a selective AT_1 receptor antagonist) abolishes the effect of intracellular angiotensin II (Allen *et al.*, 1988; Bacal & Kunze, 1994). Based on these studies, we reason that diabetes-induced elevation of intracellular angiotensin II concentration in the nodose neurons contributes to the enhanced HCN channel activity and the blunted cell excitability in the AB neurons in diabetes. This viewpoint is confirmed by our observation that intracellular administration of losartan (added to the recording pipette solution) decreased the HCN current density and increased the cell excitability in the AB neurons from diabetic rats (Li & Zheng, 2011). Therefore, it is possible there is an intracellular angiotensin II production system in the nodose ganglion tissue. Of course, it would be optimal to measure intracellular angiotensin II concentration in the aortic baroreceptor neurons, but there is no appropriate measurement for it so far due to insufficient cellular material of tiny nodose ganglia. This issue needs to be confirmed by further study.

Growing evidence has shown that the AT_1 and AT_2 receptors are defined on the basis of their opposite pharmacological and biochemical effects (Levy, 2004). Activation of AT_1 receptors mainly results in vasoconstriction, augmentation of cardiac contractility, cell proliferation, vascular and cardiac hypertrophy, oxidative stress, and inhibition of the neuronal potassium currents (Gelband *et al.*, 1999; Levy, 2004; Sumners *et al.*, 1996). On the other hand, stimulation of AT_2 receptors induces vasodilation, anti-growth, anti-hypertrophy, and enhancement of the neuronal potassium currents (Horiuchi *et al.*, 1999; Kang *et al.*, 1995; Martens *et al.*, 1996; Matsubara, 1998; Siragy, 2000). Although AT_2 receptors are expressed in the rat nodose neurons, activation of AT_2 receptors does not affect the activation of HCN channels because AT_2 receptor antagonist (PD123,319) does not alter the effect of angiotensin II on the HCN currents (Zhang *et al.*, 2010). Until now there is no study to explain this result, but it is possible that many factors (such as species, tissue, channel sensitivity, etc) are responsible for this discrepancy.

Now the question is how angiotensin II regulates the activation of HCN channels and what is the downstream of angiotensin II-AT_1 receptor. NADPH oxidase has been considered as a main source of intracellular superoxide in many tissues (Cifuentes *et al.*, 2000; Franco *et al.*, 2003; Gao *et al.*, 2004; Griendling *et al.*, 2000; Li *et al.*, 2007; Schieffer *et al.*, 2000). NADPH oxidase is a multicomponent enzyme composed of three cytosolic subunits (p40[phox], p47[phox], and p67[phox]), two membrane-associated subunits (gp91[phox] and p22[phox]), and the small G-proteins (Rac and Rap1a) (Kim & Iwao, 2000; Lassegue & Clempus, 2003). Angiotensin II significantly activates NADPH oxidase via AT_1 receptors, resulting in the superoxide production (Touyz & Berry, 2002). In the nodose ganglia from STZ-induced diabetic rats, the protein expression of the NADPH oxidase components (gp91phox, p22phox, p40phox, p47phox, and p67phox) is elevated, compared to sham rats (Li & Zheng, 2011). In addition, NADPH oxidase inhibitor or superoxide scavenger significantly improves the superoxide over-production, the enhanced HCN currents, and the lowered membrane excitability induced by exogenous angiotensin II (Zhang *et al.*, 2010) or diabetes (Li & Zheng, 2011). These results strongly indicate that NADPH-derived superoxide can mediate the effect of endogenous angiotensin II on the HCN channels and membrane excitability in diabetic rat aortic baroreceptor neurons.

3.1.5 Role of other channels in the aortic baroreceptor neuron in the type 1 diabetes

Using patch-clamp technique, all major voltage-gated ion channels including channels subunits are recorded in the nodose neurons, such as sodium channels (tetrodotoxin-sensitive and tetrodotoxin-resistant sodium channels), calcium channels (N-type, L-type, T-/R-type, and other type calcium channels), and potassium channels (4-aminopyridine-sensitive, tetraethylammonium-sensitive, and calcium-activated potassium channels) (Lancaster *et al.*, 2002; Li *et al.*, 2005; Li & Schild, 2006; Schild & Li, 2001). These channels all are involved in the initiation and formation of the action potential and affect the nodose neuron excitability. Angiotensin II is known to modulate the calcium channel kinetics in the nodose neurons (Bacal & Kunze, 1994; Moreira *et al.*, 2005). However, until now we did not obtain any information about the changes of these channels in the aortic baroreceptor neurons in the type 1 diabetes. Therefore, the role of these channels in the diabetic baroreceptor neurons remains to be revealed.

3.2 Involvement of the central neural component in the blunted arterial baroreflex in type 1 diabetes

Central neural integration of the input signals from the baroreceptors usually occurs at the level of nucleus tractus solitarii and rostral ventrolateral medulla (Spyer *et al.*, 1997). Although many studies have shown that diabetes causes a variety of functional and morphological disorders in the central nervous system (including hippocampus, cortex, and cerebellum) (Biessels *et al.*, 1999; Selvarajah & Tesfaye, 2006; Mooradian, 1997a; Mooradian, 1997b; Guven *et al.*, 2009), the role of the central neural component in the blunted arterial baroreflex in type 1 diabetes is less well documented. One recent study from Gu, et al (Gu *et al.*, 2008) suggests that a deficit of the central neural component contributes to the attenuation of arterial baroreflex in OVE26 type 1 diabetic mice. This is because they found that stimulation of the aortic depressor nerve induced a lesser magnitude of bradycardia in OVE26 type 1 diabetic mice as compared to sham mice, but the bradycardic response to vagal efferent stimulation was enhanced (Gu *et al.*, 2008). Immunoreactive study has shown that reduced c-Fos expression (an indicator of early cellular response to many extracellular signals) in the nucleus tractus solitarii links to the attenuated arterial baroreflex sensitivity in STZ-induced diabetic rats (Gouty *et al.*, 2001). In addition, Chen, et al (Chen *et al.*, 2008) have reported that neural firing activity of the nucleus tractus solitarii in STZ-induced diabetes is reduced, which is involved in the impaired arterial baroreflex function in STZ-induced diabetic rats. Furthermore, a chronic intracerebroventricular infusion of leptin (a hormone produced by fat cells and improving glucose utilization, Minokoshi *et al.*, 1999; Wang *et al.*, 1999) totally normalizes the impaired arterial baroreflex sensitivity in STZ-induced diabetic rats (do Carmo *et al.*, 2008), which indirectly suggests that impairment of the central neural system is associated with the arterial baroreflex dysfunction in type 1 diabetes. These findings allow us to assume the involvement of the impaired central neural integration in the blunted arterial baroreflex in type 1 diabetes even though there is no report focusing on the mechanisms responsible for the impairment of the central neural component of the arterial baroreflex.

3.3 Participation of autonomic neuroeffector component in the blunted arterial baroreflex in type 1 diabetes

The autonomic neuroeffector component of the arterial baroreflex includes intracardiac ganglia, parasympathetic efferents, and sympathetic efferents. Morphological studies have shown that there is a remarkable structural remodeling of the intracardiac ganglia (such as cellular contraction, cytoplasmic condensation, degenerated axons, reduced cell size and number) in STZ-induced diabetic rats (Kamal *et al.*, 1991; Lund *et al.*, 1992), mice (Lin *et al.*, 2010), and diabetic patients (Tsujimura *et al.*, 1986). Biochemical studies also found a decrease in acetylcholine (a neurotransmitter in both the central and parasympathetic nervous system) concentration in alloxan-induced diabetic rats (Kuntscherova & Vlk, 1970) and a reduced choline acetyltransferase activity (an enzyme producing acetylcholine) in the hearts of the STZ-induced diabetic rats (Lund *et al.*, 1992). In addition, the function of the parasympathetic (vagal) efferent is reduced in STZ-induced diabetic rats (Maeda *et al.*, 1995; Yagihashi, 1995). However, functional studies have reported normal, reduced, or enhanced heart rate response to vagal efferent nerve stimulation in diabetic animal models (Dall'Ago *et al.*, 2007; de *et al.*, 2002; Lin *et al.*, 2010; Maeda *et al.*, 1995; McDowell *et al.*, 1994a). This discrepancy might be due to different animal species, experimental diabetic animal models, and time course of development of diabetes. Therefore, further studies are needed to explore whether the altered efferent component of the arterial baroreflex is responsible for the arterial baroreflex dysfunction in type 1 diabetes besides the arterial baroreceptor and central integration.

4. Conclusion

As a homeostatic mechanism, the arterial baroreflex normally alters heart rate and blood pressure in response to changes in arterial wall tension detected by the baroreceptors in the carotid sinus and aortic arch. As illustrated by the above evidence, arterial baroreflex impairment, a characteristic of the autonomic cardiovascular dysfunction is a frequent complication in type 1 diabetic patients and animal models. The arterial baroreflex dysfunction not only is an independent predictor for mortality of the type 1 diabetic patients, but also is associated with a poor prognosis and bad quality of life in the type 1 diabetic patients.

Although the mechanisms responsible for attenuated arterial baroreflex function in the type 1 diabetes are not yet fully understood, any part of the arterial baroreflex arc including an afferent limb, a central neural component, and an autonomic neuroeffector component can contribute to the arterial baroreflex dysfunction in the type 1 diabetic state. Especially at the level of the afferent limb, recent studies have revealed that aortic depressor nerve discharge and excitability of aortic baroreceptor neurons are blunted in the type 1 diabetic animals. HCN channels are significantly suppressed in the aortic baroreceptor neurons and are involved in the blunted baroreceptor neuron excitability in the type 1 diabetes. Angiotensin

II/AT$_1$ receptor-NADPH oxidase-superoxide signaling regulates this alteration of the HCN channels in the aortic baroreceptor neurons and consequently decreases the arterial baroreflex function. In addition, we also consider that angiotensin II/AT$_1$ receptor-NADPH oxidase-superoxide signaling affects the changes in the central neural and autonomic neuroeffector components beyond the afferent limb of the arterial baroreflex arc. These studies provide new information on the mechanisms underlying the impaired arterial baroreflex in the type 1 diabetes and unveil important pharmacological and genomic targets for improving the arterial baroreflex function and reducing the mortality in the type 1 diabetes.

5. Acknowledgments

This work was supported by a Scientist Development Grant from American Heart Association National Center (award no. 0730108N) to Yu-Long Li.

6. References

Accili, E.A.; Proenza, C.; Baruscotti, M. & DiFrancesco, D. (2002). From funny current to HCN channels: 20 years of excitation. *News in Physiological Sciences*, Vol.17, No. 1, (February, 2002), pp. 32-37, ISSN 1548-9213

Allen, A.M.; Lewis, S.J.; Verberne, A.J. & Mendelsohn, F.A. (1988). Angiotensin receptors and the vagal system. *Clinical & Experimental Hypertension. Part A*, Vol.10, No. 6, (August, 1988), pp. 1239-1249, ISSN 1064-1963

Altomare, C.; Bucchi, A.; Camatini, E.; Baruscotti, M.; Viscomi, C.; Moroni, A. & DiFrancesco, D. (2001). Integrated allosteric model of voltage gating of HCN channels. *Journal of General Physiology*, Vol. 117, No. 6, (June, 2001), pp. 519-532, ISSN 0022-1295

Aumonier, F.J. (1972). Histological observations on the distribution of baroreceptors in the carotid and aortic regions of the rabbit, cat and dog. *Acta Anatomica (Basel)*, Vol. 82, No. 1, pp. 1-16, ISSN 0001-5180

Bacal, K. & Kunze, D.L. (1994). Dual effects of angiotensin II on calcium currents in neonatal rat nodose neurons. *Journal of Neuroscience*, Vol. 14, No. 11, (Novermber, 1994), pp. 7159-7167, ISSN 0270-6474

Bergner, D.W. & Goldberger, J.J. (2010). Diabetes mellitus and sudden cardiac death: what are the data? *Cardiology Journal*, Vol. 17, No. 2, (March, 2010), pp. 117-129, ISSN 1897-5593

Biessels, G.J.; Cristino, N.A.; Rutten, G.J.; Hamers, F.P.; Erkelens, D.W. & Gispen, W.H. (1999). Neurophysiological changes in the central and peripheral nervous system of streptozotocin-diabetic rats. Course of development and effects of insulin treatment. *Brain*, Vol. 122, No. 4, (April, 1999), pp. 757-768, ISSN 0006-8950

Binkley, P.F.; Nunziata, E.; Haas, G.J.; Nelson, S.D. & Cody, R.J. (1991). Parasympathetic withdrawal is an integral component of autonomic imbalance in congestive heart failure: demonstration in human subjects and verification in a paced canine model of ventricular failure. *Journal of the American College of Cardiology*, Vol. 18, No. 2, (August, 1991), pp. 464-472, ISSN 0735-1097

Brown, H.F.; DiFrancesco, D. & Noble, S.J. (1979). How does adrenaline accelerate the heart? *Nature*, Vol. 280, No. 5719, (July, 1979), pp. 235-236, ISSN 0028-0836

Browning, K.N. (2003). Excitability of nodose ganglion cells and their role in vago-vagal reflex control of gastrointestinal function. *Current Opinion in Pharmacology*, Vol. 3, No. 6, (December, 2003) pp. 613-617, ISSN 1471-4892

Chen, H.Y.; Wu, J.S.; Chen, J.J. & Cheng, J.T. (2008). Impaired regulation function in cardiovascular neurons of nucleus tractus solitarii in streptozotocin-induced diabetic rats. *Neuroscience Letters*, Vol. 431, No. 2, (January, 2008), pp. 161-166, ISSN 0304-3940

Cheng, Z.; Powley, T.L.; Schwaber, J.S. & Doyle, F.J. (1997). A laser confocal microscopic study of vagal afferent innervation of rat aortic arch: chemoreceptors as well as baroreceptors. *Journal of the Autonomic Nervous System*, Vol. 67, No. 1-2, (December, 1997), pp. 1-14, ISSN 0165-1838

Cifuentes, M.E.; Rey, F.E.; Carretero, O.A. & Pagano, P.J. (2000). Upregulation of p67(phox) and gp91(phox) in aortas from angiotensin II-infused mice. *American Journal of Physiology Heart and Circulatory Physiology*, Vol. 279, No. 5, pp. (November, 2000), H2234-H2240, ISSN 0363-6135

Clarke, C.F.; Eason, M.; Reilly, A.; Boyce, D. & Werther, G.A. (1999). Autonomic nerve function in adolescents with Type 1 diabetes mellitus: relationship to microalbuminuria. *Diabetic Medicine*, Vol. 16, No. 7, (July, 1999), pp. 550-554, ISSN 0742-3071

Dall'Ago, P.; D'Agord, S.B., Da, S.V.O.; Werner, J.; da Silva Soares, P.P.; de, A.K. & Irigoyen, M.C. (2007). Parasympathetic dysfunction is associated with baroreflex and chemoreflex impairment in streptozotocin-induced diabetes in rats. *Autonomic Neuroscience*, Vol. 131, No. 1-2, (January, 2007), pp. 28-35, ISSN 1566-0702

Dall'Ago, P.; Fernandes, T.G.; Machado, U.F.; Bello, A.A. & Irigoyen, M.C. (1997). Baroreflex and chemoreflex dysfunction in streptozotocin-diabetic rats. *Brazilizan Journal of Medical Biological Research*, Vol. 30, No. 1, (January, 1997), pp. 119-124, ISSN 0100-879X

Dall'Ago, P.; Silva, V.O.; De Angelis, K.L.; Irigoyen, M.C.; Fazan, R.Jr. & Salgado, H.C. (2002). Reflex control of arterial pressure and heart rate in short-term streptozotocin diabetic rats. *Brazilizan Journal of Medical Biological Research*, Vol. 35, No. 7, (July, 2002), pp. 843-849, ISSN 0100-879X

Dalla, P.R.; Bechtold, S.; Bonfig, W.; Putzker, S.; Kozlik-Feldmann, R.; Schwarz, H.P. & Netz, H. (2007). Impaired short-term blood pressure regulation and autonomic dysbalance in children with type 1 diabetes mellitus. *Diabetologia*, Vol. 50, No. 12, (December, 2007), pp. 2417-2423, ISSN 0012-186X

De Angelis, K.L.; Oliveira, A.R.; Dall'Ago, P.; Peixoto, L.R.; Gadonski, G.; Lacchini, S.; Fernandes, T.G. & Irigoyen, M.C. (2000). Effects of exercise training on autonomic and myocardial dysfunction in streptozotocin-diabetic rats. *Brazilizan Journal of Medical Biological Research*. Vol. 33. No. 6, (June, 2000), pp. 635-641, ISSN 0100-879X

De Mello, W.C. (2003). Further studies on the effect of intracellular angiotensins on heart cell communication: on the role of endogenous angiotensin II. *Regulatory Peptides*, Vol. 115, No. 1, (August, 2003), pp. 31-36, ISSN 0167-0115

De Mello, W.C. & Monterrubio, J. (2004). Intracellular and extracellular angiotensin II enhance the L-type calcium current in the failing heart. *Hypertension*, Vol. 44, No. 3, (September, 2004), pp. 360-364, ISSN 0194-911X

De, A.K.; Schaan, B.D.; Maeda, C.Y.; Dall'Ago, P.; Wichi, R.B. & Irigoyen, M.C. (2002). Cardiovascular control in experimental diabetes. *Brazilizan Journal of Medical Biological Research*, Vol. 35, No. 9, (September, 2002), pp. 1091-1100, ISSN 0100-879X

deBoer, R.W.; Karemaker, J.M. & Strackee, J. (1987). Hemodynamic fluctuations and baroreflex sensitivity in humans: a beat-to-beat model. *American Journal of Physiology*, Vol. 253, No. 3, (September, 1987), pp. H680-H689, ISSN 0002-9513

Devor, M. (1999). Unexplained peculiarities of the dorsal root ganglion. *Pain*, Vol. Suppl 6, (August, 1999), pp. S27-S35, ISSN 0304-3959

DiFrancesco, D. (1985). The cardiac hyperpolarizing-activated current, if. Origins and developments. *Progress in Biophysics and Molecular Biology*, Vol. 46, No. 3, pp. 163-183, ISSN 0079-6107

DiFrancesco, D. (1993). Pacemaker mechanisms in cardiac tissue. *Annual Review of Physiology*, Vol. 55, pp. 455-472, ISSN 0066-4278

do Carmo, J.M.; Hall, J.E. & da Silva, A.A. (2008). Chronic central leptin infusion restores cardiac sympathetic-vagal balance and baroreflex sensitivity in diabetic rats. *American Journal of Physiology Heart and Circulatory Physiology*, Vol. 295, No. 5, (November, 2008), pp. H1974-H1981, ISSN 0363-6135

do Carmo, J.M., Huber, D.A.; Castania, J.A.; Fazan, V.P.; Fazan, R.Jr. & Salgado, H.C. (2007). Aortic depressor nerve function examined in diabetic rats by means of two different approaches. *Journal of Neuroscience Methods*, Vol. 161, No. 1, (March, 2007), pp. 17-22, ISSN 0165-0270

Doan, T.N. & Kunze, D.L. (1999). Contribution of the hyperpolarization-activated current to the resting membrane potential of rat nodose sensory neurons. *Journal of Physiology*, Vol. 514, No. 1, (January, 1999), pp. 125-138, ISSN 0022-3751

Doan, T.N.; Stephans, K.; Ramirez, A.N.; Glazebrook, P.A.; Andresen, M.C. & Kunze, D.L. (2004). Differential distribution and function of hyperpolarization-activated channels in sensory neurons and mechanosensitive fibers. *Journal of Neuroscience*, Vol. 24, No. 13, (March, 2004), pp. 3335-3343, ISSN 0270-6474

Douglas, N.J.; Campbell, I.W.; Ewing, D.J.; Clarke, B.F. & Flenley, D.C. (1981). Reduced airway vagal tone in diabetic patients with autonomic neuropathy. *Clinical Science (London)*, Vol. 61, No. 5, (November, 1981), pp. 581-584, ISSN 0143-5221

Ducreux, C.; Reynaud, J.C. & Puizillout, J.J. (1993). Spike conduction properties of T-shaped C neurons in the rabbit nodose ganglion. *Pflugers Archive*, Vol. 424, No. 3-4, (August, 1993), pp. 238-244, ISSN 0031-6768

Ewing, D.J.; Campbell, I.W. & Clarke, B.F. (1980). The natural history of diabetic autonomic neuropathy. *Quarterly Journal of Medicine*, Vol. 49, No. 1, pp. 95-108, ISSN 0033-5622

Fan, W. & Andresen, M.C. (1998). Differential frequency-dependent reflex integration of myelinated and nonmyelinated rat aortic baroreceptors. *American Journal of Physiology*, Vol. 271, No. 2, (August, 1998), pp. H632-H640, ISSN 0002-9513

Fan, W.; Reynolds, P.J. & Andresen, M.C. (1996). Baroreflex frequency-response characteristics to aortic depressor and carotid sinus nerve stimulation in rats. *American Journal of Physiology*, Vol. 271, No. 6, (December, 1996), pp. H2218-H2227, ISSN 0002-9513

Fazan, R.Jr.; Ballejo, G.; Salgado, M.C.; Moraes, M.F. & Salgado, H.C. (1997). Heart rate variability and baroreceptor function in chronic diabetic rats. *Hypertension*, Vol. 30, No. 3, (September, 1997), pp. 632-635, ISSN 0194-911X

Fazan, R.Jr.; Dias da Silva, V.J. & Salgado, H.C. (1999). Baroreceptor function in streptozotocin-induced diabetes in rats: a spectral analysis approach. *Journal of Hypertension*, Vol. 18, pp. S136, ISSN 0263-6352

Fazan, V.P.; Salgado, H.C. & Barreira, A.A. (2006). Aortic depressor nerve myelinated fibers in acute and chronic experimental diabetes. *American Journal of Hypertension*, Vol. 19, No. 2, (February, 2006), pp. 153-160, ISSN 0895-7061

Franco, M.C.; Akamine, E.H.; Di Marco, G.S.; Casarini, D.E.; Fortes, Z.B.; Tostes, R.C.; Carvalho, M.H. & Nigro, D. (2003). NADPH oxidase and enhanced superoxide generation in intrauterine undernourished rats: involvement of the renin-angiotensin system. *Cardiovascular Research*, Vol. 59, No. 3, (September, 2003), pp. 767-775, ISSN 0008-6363

Frustaci, A.; Kajstura, J.; Chimenti, C.; Jakoniuk, I.; Leri, A.; Maseri, A.; Nadal-Ginard, B. & Anversa, P. (2000). Myocardial cell death in human diabetes. *Circulation Research*, Vol. 87, No. 12, (December, 2000), pp. 1123-1132, ISSN 0009-7330

Gao, L.; Wang, W.; Li, Y.L.; Schultz, H.D.; Liu, D.; Cornish, K.G. & Zucker, I.H. (2004). Superoxide mediates sympathoexcitation in heart failure: roles of angiotensin II and NAD(P)H oxidase. *Circulation Research*, Vol. 95, No. 9, (October, 2004), pp. 937-944, ISSN 0009-7330

Gelband, C.H.; Warth, J.D.; Mason, H.S.; Zhu, M.; Moore, J.M.; Kenyon, J.L.; Horowitz, B. & Sumners, C. (1999). Angiotensin II type 1 receptor-mediated inhibition of K+ channel subunit kv2.2 in brain stem and hypothalamic neurons. *Circulation Research*, Vol. 84, No. 3, (February, 1999), pp. 352-359, ISSN 0009-7330

Gill, G.V.; Woodward, A.; Casson, I.F. & Weston, P.J. (2009). Cardiac arrhythmia and nocturnal hypoglycaemia in type 1 diabetes--the 'dead in bed' syndrome revisited. *Diabetologia*, Vol. 52, No. 1, (January, 2009), pp. 42-45, ISSN 0012-186X

Gouty, S.; Regalia, J. & Helke, C.J. (2001). Attenuation of the afferent limb of the baroreceptor reflex in streptozotocin-induced diabetic rats. *Autonomic Neuroscience*, Vol. 89, No. 1-2, (June, 2001), pp. 86-95, ISSN 1566-0702

Griendling, K.K.; Sorescu, D. & Ushio-Fukai, M. (2000). NAD(P)H oxidase: role in cardiovascular biology and disease. *Circulation Research*, Vol. 86, No. 5, (March, 2000), pp. 494-501, ISSN 0009-7330

Gu, H.; Epstein, P.N.; Li, L.; Wurster, R.D. & Cheng, Z.J. (2008). Functional changes in baroreceptor afferent, central and efferent components of the baroreflex circuitry in type 1 diabetic mice (OVE26). *Neuroscience*, Vol. 152, No. 3, (March, 2008), pp. 741-752, ISSN 0306-4522

Guven, A.; Yavuz, O.; Cam, M.; Comunoglu, C. & Sevi'nc, O. (2009). Central nervous system complications of diabetes in streptozotocin-induced diabetic rats: a histopathological and immunohistochemical examination. *International Journal of Neuroscience*, Vol. 119, No.8, (August, 2009), pp. 1155-1169, ISSN 1563-5279

Hicks, K.K.; Seifen, E.; Stimers, J.R. & Kennedy, R.H. (1998). Effects of streptozotocin-induced diabetes on heart rate, blood pressure and cardiac autonomic nervous control. *Journal of the Autonomic Nervous System*, Vol. 69, No. 1, (March, 1998), pp. 21-30, ISSN 0165-1838

Horiuchi, M.; Akishita, M. & Dzau, V.J. (1999). Recent progress in angiotensin II type 2 receptor research in the cardiovascular system. *Hypertension*, Vol. 33, No. 2, (February, 1999), pp. 613-621, ISSN 0194-911X

Iovino, M.; Triggiani, V.; Licchelli, B.; Tafaro, E.; Giagulli, V.; Sabba, C.; Resta, F.; Sciannimanico, S.V.; Panza, R. & Guastamacchia, E. (2011). Vasopressin release induced by hypotension is blunted in patients with diabetic autonomic neuropathy. *Immunopharmacology and Immunotoxicology*, Vol. 33, No. 1, (March, 2011), pp. 224-226, ISSN 0892-3973

Ishii, T.M.; Takano, M.; Xie, L.H.; Noma, A. & Ohmori, H. (1999). Molecular characterization of the hyperpolarization-activated cation channel in rabbit heart sinoatrial node. *Journal of Biological Chemistry*, Vol. 274, No. 18, (April, 1999), pp. 12835-12839, ISSN 0021-9258

Kamal, A.A.; Tay, S.S. & Wong, W.C. (1991). The cardiac ganglia in streptozotocin-induced diabetic rats. *Archives of Histology and Cytology*, Vol. 54, No. 1, (March, 1991), pp. 41-49, ISSN 0914-9465

Kang, J.; Richards, E.M.; Posner, P. & Sumners, C. (1995). Modulation of the delayed rectifier K+ current in neurons by an angiotensin II type 2 receptor fragment. *American Journal of Physiology*, Vol. 268, No. 1, (January, 1995), pp. C278-C282, ISSN 0002-9513

Karavanaki, K.; Kazianis, G.; Kakleas, K.; Konstantopoulos, I. & Karayianni, C. (2007). QT interval prolongation in association with impaired circadian variation of blood pressure and heart rate in adolescents with Type 1 diabetes. *Diabetic Medicine*, Vol. 24, No. 11, (November, 2007), pp. 1247-1253, ISSN 0742-3071

Katz, A.; Liberty, I.F.; Porath, A.; Ovsyshcher, I. & Prystowsky, E.N. (1999). A simple bedside test of 1-minute heart rate variability during deep breathing as a prognostic index after myocardial infarction. *American Heart Journal*, Vol. 138, No. 1, (July, 1999), pp. 32-38, ISSN 0002-8703

Kaupp, U.B. & Seifert, R. (2001). Molecular diversity of pacemaker ion channels. *Annual Review of Physiology*, Vol. 63, pp. 235-257, ISSN 0066-4278

Kim, S. & Iwao, H. (2000). Molecular and cellular mechanisms of angiotensin II-mediated cardiovascular and renal diseases. *Pharmacological Reviews*, Vol. 52, No. 1, (March, 2000), pp. 11-34, ISSN 0031-6997

Kim, Y.K.; Lee, J.E.; Kim, Y.G.; Kim, D.J.; Oh, H.Y.; Yang, C.W.; Kim, K.W. & Huh, W. (2009). Cardiac autonomic neuropathy as a predictor of deterioration of the renal function in normoalbuminuric, normotensive patients with type 2 diabetes mellitus. *Journal of Korean Medical Science*, Vol. 24, No. suppl, (January, 2009), pp. S69-S74, ISSN 1011-8934

Kleiger, R.E.; Miller, J.P.; Bigger, J.T.Jr. & Moss, A.J. (1987). Decreased heart rate variability and its association with increased mortality after acute myocardial infarction. *American Journal of Cardiology*, Vol. 59, No. 4, (February, 1987), pp. 256-262, ISSN 0002-9149

Kobayashi, M.; Cheng, Z.B.; Tanaka, K. & Nosaka, S. (1999). Is the aortic depressor nerve involved in arterial chemoreflexes in rats? *Journal of the Autonomic Nervous System*, Vol. 78, No. 1, (October, 1999), pp. 38-48, ISSN 0165-1838

Kogawa, S.; Yasuda, H.; Terada, M.; Maeda, K. & Kikkawa, R. (2000). Apoptosis and impaired axonal regeneration of sensory neurons after nerve crush in diabetic rats. *Neuroreport*, Vol. 11, No. 4, (March, 2000), pp. 663-667, ISSN 0959-4965

Krauhs, J.M. (1979). Structure of rat aortic baroreceptors and their relationship to connective tissue. *Journal of Neurocytology*, Vol. 8, No. 4, (August, 1979), pp. 401-414, ISSN 0300-4864

Krolewski, A.S.; Kosinski, E.J.; Warram, J.H.; Leland, O.S.; Busick, E.J.; Asmal, A.C.; Rand, L.I.; Christlieb, A.R.; Bradley, R.F. & Kahn, C.R. (1987). Magnitude and determinants of coronary artery disease in juvenile-onset, insulin-dependent diabetes mellitus. *American Journal of Cardiology*, Vol. 59, No. 8, (April, 1987), pp. 750-755, ISSN 0002-9149

Kuntscherova, J. & Vlk, J. (1970). Influence of alloxan diabetes on acetylcholine synthesis in tissues of the albino rat. *Physiologia Bohemoslovaca*, Vol. 19, No. 5, pp. 431-434, ISSN 0369-9463

Lancaster, E.; Oh, E.J.; Gover, T. & Weinreich, D. (2002). Calcium and calcium-activated currents in vagotomized rat primary vagal afferent neurons. *Journal of Physiology*, Vol. 540, No. 2, (April, 2002), pp. 543-556, ISSN 0022-3751

Lassegue, B. & Clempus, R.E. (2003). Vascular NAD(P)H oxidases: specific features, expression, and regulation. *American Journal of Physiology Regulatory, Integrative and Comparative Physiology*, Vol. 285, No. 2, (August, 2003), pp. R277-R297, ISSN 0363-6119

Lefrandt, J.D.; Hoogenberg, K.; van Roon, A.M.; Dullaart, R.P.; Gans, R.O. & Smit, A.J. (1999). Baroreflex sensitivity is depressed in microalbuminuric Type I diabetic patients at rest and during sympathetic manoeuvres. *Diabetologia*, Vol. 42, No. 11, (November, 1999), pp. 1345-1349, ISSN 0012-186X

Lefrandt, J.D.; Smit, A.J.; Zeebregts, C.J.; Gans, R.O. & Hoogenberg, K.H. (2010). Autonomic dysfunction in diabetes: a consequence of cardiovascular damage. *Current Diabetes Reviews*, Vol. 6, No. 6, (November, 2010), pp. 348-358, ISSN 1875-6417

Levy, B.I. (2004). Can angiotensin II type 2 receptors have deleterious effects in cardiovascular disease? Implications for therapeutic blockade of the renin-angiotensin system. *Circulation*, Vol. 109, No. 1, (January, 2004), pp. 8-13, ISSN 0009-7322

Li, B.Y.; Alfrey, K.D. & Schild, J.H. (2005). Correlation between the activation and inactivation gating profiles of the TTX-resistant Na$^+$ current from fluorescently identified aortic baroreceptor neurons of the adult rat. *FASEB Journal*, Vol. 19, No. 4, (March, 2005), pp. A606, ISSN 0892-6638

Li, B.Y. & Schild, J.H. (2006). Differential distribution of voltage-gated K$^+$ ion channels in adult rat aortic baroreceptor neurons with myelinated and unmyelinated afferent fibre. *FASEB Journal*, Vol. 20, No. 4, (March, 2006), pp. A775, ISSN 0892-6638

Li, L.; Huang, C.; Ai, J.; Yan, B.; Gu, H.; Ma, Z.; Li, A.Y.; Xinyan, S.; Harden, S.W.; Hatcher, J.T.; Wurster, R.D. & Cheng, Z.J. (2010). Structural remodeling of vagal afferent innervation of aortic arch and nucleus ambiguus (NA) projections to cardiac ganglia in a transgenic mouse model of type 1 diabetes (OVE26). *Journal of Comparative Neurology*, Vol. 518, No. 14, (July, 2010), pp. 2771-2793, ISSN 0021-9967

Li, Y.L.; Gao, L.; Zucker, I.H. & Schultz, H.D. (2007). NADPH oxidase-derived superoxide anion mediates angiotensin II-enhanced carotid body chemoreceptor sensitivity in heart failure rabbits. *Cardiovascular Research*, Vol. 75, No. 3, (August, 2007), pp. 546-554, ISSN 0008-6363

Li, Y.L.; Tran, T.P.; Muelleman, R. & Schultz, H.D. (2008a). Blunted excitability of aortic baroreceptor neurons in diabetic rats: involvement of hyperpolarization-activated channel. *Cardiovascular Research*, Vol. 79, No. 4, (September, 2008), pp. 715-721, ISSN 0008-6363

Li, Y.L.; Tran, T.P.; Muelleman, R. & Schultz, H.D. (2008b). Elevated angiotensin II in rat nodose ganglia mediates diabetes-blunted arterial baroreflex sensitivity. *Circulation*, Vol. 118, No. 18, (Vovember, 2008), pp. S360, ISSN 0009-7322

Li, Y.L. & Zheng, H. (2011). Angiotensin II-NADPH oxidase-derived superoxide mediates diabetes-attenuated cell excitability of aortic baroreceptor neurons. *Cardiovascular Research*, In press, ISSN 0008-6363

Libby, P.; Nathan, D.M.; Abraham, K.; Brunzell, J.D.; Fradkin, J.E.; Haffner, S.M.; Hsueh, W.; Rewers, M.; Roberts, B.T.; Savage, P.J.; Skarlatos, S.; Wassef, M. & Rabadan-Diehl, C. (2005). Report of the National Heart, Lung, and Blood Institute-National Institute of Diabetes and Digestive and Kidney Diseases Working Group on Cardiovascular Complications of Type 1 Diabetes Mellitus. *Circulation*, Vol. 111, No. 25, (June, 2005), pp. 3489-3493, ISSN 0009-7322

Lin, M.; Ai, J.; Harden, S.W.; Huang, C.; Li, L.; Wurster, R.D. & Cheng, Z.J. (2010). Impairment of baroreflex control of heart rate and structural changes of cardiac ganglia in conscious streptozotocin (STZ)-induced diabetic mice. *Autonomic Neuroscience*, Vol. 155, No. 1-2, (June, 2010), pp. 39-48, ISSN 1566-0702

Lishner, M.; Akselrod, S.; Avi, V.M.; Oz, O.; Divon, M. & Ravid, M. (1987). Spectral analysis of heart rate fluctuations. A non-invasive, sensitive method for the early diagnosis of autonomic neuropathy in diabetes mellitus. *Journal of the Autonomic Nervous System*, Vol. 19, No. 2, (May, 1987), pp. 119-125, ISSN 0165-1838

Lluch, I.; Hernandez, A.; Real, J.T.; Morillas, C.; Tenes, S.; Sanchez, C. & Ascaso, J.F. (1998). Cardiovascular autonomic neuropathy in type 1 diabetic patients with and without peripheral neuropathy. *Diabetes Research and Clinical Practice*, Vol. 42, No. 1, (October, 1998), pp. 35-40, ISSN 0168-8227

Low, P.A.; Walsh, J.C.; Huang, C.Y. & McLeod, J.G. (1975). The sympathetic nervous system in alcoholic neuropathy. A clinical and pathological study. *Brain*, Vol. 98, No. 3, (September, 1975), pp. 357-364, ISSN 0006-8950

Ludwig, A.; Zong, X.; Jeglitsch, M.; Hofmann, F. & Biel, M. (1998). A family of hyperpolarization-activated mammalian cation channels. *Nature*, Vol. 393, No. 6685, (June, 1998), pp. 587-591, ISSN 0028-0836

Ludwig, A.; Zong, X.; Stieber, J.; Hullin, R.; Hofmann, F. & Biel, M. (1999). Two pacemaker channels from human heart with profoundly different activation kinetics. *EMBO Journal*, Vol. 18, No. 9, (May, 1999), pp. 2323-2329, ISSN 0261-4189

Lund, D.D.; Subieta, A.R.; Pardini, B.J. & Chang, K.S. (1992). Alterations in cardiac parasympathetic indices in STZ-induced diabetic rats. *Diabetes*, Vol. 41, No. 2, (February, 1992), pp. 160-166, ISSN 0012-1797

Maeda, C.Y.; Fernandes, T.G.; Timm, H.B. & Irigoyen, M.C. (1995). Autonomic dysfunction in short-term experimental diabetes. *Hypertension*, Vol. 26, No. 6, (December, 1995), pp. 1100-1104, ISSN 0194-911X

Maliszewska-Scislo, M.; Scislo, T.J. & Rossi, N.F. (2003). Effect of blockade of endogenous angiotensin II on baroreflex function in conscious diabetic rats. *American Journal of Physiology Heart and Circulatory Physiology*, Vol. 284, No. 5, (May, 2003), pp. H1601-H1611, ISSN 0363-6135

Martens, J.R.; Wang, D.; Sumners, C.; Posner, P. & Gelband, C.H. (1996). Angiotensin II type 2 receptor-mediated regulation of rat neuronal K^+ channels. *Circulation Research*, Vol. 79, No. 2, (August, 1996), pp. 302-309, ISSN 0009-7330

Maser, R.E.; Mitchell, B.D.; Vinik, A.I. & Freeman, R. (2003). The association between cardiovascular autonomic neuropathy and mortality in individuals with diabetes: a meta-analysis. *Diabetes Care*, Vol. 26, No. 6, (June, 2003), pp. 1895-1901, ISSN 0149-5992

Matsubara, H. (1998). Pathophysiological role of angiotensin II type 2 receptor in cardiovascular and renal diseases. *Circulation Research*, Vol. 83, No. 12, (December, 1998), pp. 1182-1191, ISSN 0009-7330

McDowell, T.S.; Chapleau, M.W.; Hajduczok, G. & Abboud, F.M. (1994a). Baroreflex dysfunction in diabetes mellitus. I. Selective impairment of parasympathetic control of heart rate. *American Journal of Physiology*, Vol. 266, No. 1, (January, 1994), pp. H235-H243, ISSN 0002-9513

McDowell, T.S.; Hajduczok, G.; Abboud, F.M. & Chapleau, M.W. (1994b). Baroreflex dysfunction in diabetes mellitus. II. Site of baroreflex impairment in diabetic rabbits. *American Journal of Physiology*, Vol. 266, No. 1, (January, 1994), pp. H244-H249, ISSN 0002-9513

Messent, J.W.; Elliott, T.G.; Hill, R.D.; Jarrett, R.J.; Keen, H. & Viberti, G.C. (1992). Prognostic significance of microalbuminuria in insulin-dependent diabetes mellitus: a twenty-three year follow-up study. *Kidney International*, Vol. 41, No. 4, (April, 1992), pp. 836-839, ISSN 0085-2538

Minokoshi, Y.; Haque, M.S. & Shimazu, T. (1999). Microinjection of leptin into the ventromedial hypothalamus increases glucose uptake in peripheral tissues in rats. *Diabetes*, Vol. 48, No. 2, (February, 1999), pp. 287-291, ISSN 0012-1797

Mooradian, A.D. (1997a). Central nervous system complications of diabetes mellitus--a perspective from the blood-brain barrier. *Brain Research Reviews*, Vol. 23, No. 3, (April, 1997), pp. 210-218, ISSN 0165-0173

Mooradian, A.D. (1997b). Pathophysiology of central nervous system complications in diabetes mellitus. *Clinical Neuroscience*, Vol. 4, No. 6, pp. 322-326, ISSN 1065-6766

Moosmang, S.; Stieber, J.; Zong, X.; Biel, M.; Hofmann, F. & Ludwig, A. (2001). Cellular expression and functional characterization of four hyperpolarization-activated pacemaker channels in cardiac and neuronal tissues. *European Journal of Biochemistry*, Vol. 268, No. 6, (March, 2001), pp. 1646-1652, ISSN 0014-2956

Moreira, T.H.; Rodrigues, A.L.; Beirao, P.S.; dos Santos, R.A. & Santos, C.J. (2005). Angiotensin II inhibition of Ca2+ currents is independent of ATR1 angiotensin II receptor activation in rat adult vagal afferent neurons. *Autonomic Neuroscience*, Vol. 117, No. 2, (February, 2005), pp. 79-86, ISSN 1566-0702

Notomi, T. & Shigemoto, R. (2004). Immunohistochemical localization of Ih channel subunits, HCN1-4, in the rat brain. *Journal of Comparative Neurology*, Vol. 471, No. 3, (April, 2004), pp. 241-276, ISSN 0021-9967

O'Brien, I.A.; McFadden, J.P. & Corrall, R.J. (1991). The influence of autonomic neuropathy on mortality in insulin-dependent diabetes. *Quarterly Journal of Medicine*, Vol. 79, No. 290, (June, 1991), pp. 495-502, ISSN 0033-5622

Orchard, T.J.; Lloyd, C.E.; Maser, R.E. & Kuller, L.H. (1996). Why does diabetic autonomic neuropathy predict IDDM mortality? An analysis from the Pittsburgh Epidemiology of Diabetes Complications Study. *Diabetes Research and Clinical Practice*, Vol. 34, No. suppl, (October, 1996), pp. S165-S171, ISSN 0168-8227

Page, M.M. & Watkins, P.J. (1978). Cardiorespiratory arrest and diabetic autonomic neuropathy. *Lancet*, Vol. 1, No. 8054, (January, 1978), pp. 14-16, ISSN 0140-6736

Pape, H.C. (1996). Queer current and pacemaker: the hyperpolarization-activated cation current in neurons. *Annual Review of Physiology*, Vol. 58, pp. 299-327, ISSN 0066-4278

Pavy-Le, T.A.; Fontaine, S.; Tap, G.; Guidolin, B.; Senard, J.M. & Hanaire, H. (2010). Cardiovascular autonomic neuropathy and other complications in type 1 diabetes. *Clinical Autonomic Research*, Vol. 20, No. 3, (June, 2010), pp. 153-160, ISSN 0959-9851

Qu, J.; Altomare, C.; Bucchi, A.; DiFrancesco, D. & Robinson, R.B. (2002). Functional comparison of HCN isoforms expressed in ventricular and HEK 293 cells. *Pflugers Archive*, Vol. 444, No. 5, (August, 2002), pp. 597-601, ISSN 0031-6768

Rathmann, W.; Ziegler, D.; Jahnke, M.; Haastert, B. & Gries, F.A. (1993). Mortality in diabetic patients with cardiovascular autonomic neuropathy. *Diabetic Medicine*, Vol. 10, No. 9, (November, 1993), pp. 820-824, ISSN 0742-3071

Reynolds, P.J.; Fan, W. & Andresen, M.C. (1999). Aortic baroreceptor function in long term streptozotocin diabetic rats. *Social Neuroscience*, Vol. 16, pp. 221, ISSN 1747-0919

Reynolds, P.J.; Yang, M. & Andresen, M.C. (1994). Contribution of potassium channels to the discharge properties of rat aortic baroreceptor sensory endings. *Brain Research*, Vol. 665, No. 1, (November, 1994), pp. 115-122, ISSN 0006-8993

Robinson, R.B. & Siegelbaum, S.A. (2003). Hyperpolarization-activated cation currents: from molecules to physiological function. *Annual Review of Physiology*, Vol. 65, pp. 453-480, ISSN 0066-4278

Rosengard-Barlund, M.; Bernardi, L.; Fagerudd, J.; Mantysaari, M.; Af Bjorkesten, C.G.; Lindholm, H.; Forsblom, C.; Waden, J. & Groop, P.H. (2009). Early autonomic dysfunction in type 1 diabetes: a reversible disorder? *Diabetologia*, Vol. 52, No. , (June, 2009), pp. 1164-1172, ISSN 0012-186X

Russell, J.W.; Sullivan, K.A.; Windebank, A.J.; Herrmann, D.N. & Feldman, E.L. (1999). Neurons undergo apoptosis in animal and cell culture models of diabetes. *Neurobiology of Disease*, Vol. 6, No. 5, (October, 1999), pp. 347-363, ISSN 0969-9961

Salgado, H.C.; Barale, A.R.; Castania, J.A.; Machado, B.H. Chapleau, M.W. & Fazan, R.Jr. (2007). Baroreflex responses to electrical stimulation of aortic depressor nerve in conscious SHR. *American Journal of Physiology Heart and Circulatory Physiology*, Vol. 292, No. 1, (January, 2007), pp. H593-H600, ISSN 0363-6135

Salgado, H.C.; Fazan, J.R.; Fazan, V.P. Da, S.V, & Barreira, A.A. (2001). Arterial baroreceptors and experimental diabetes. *Annals of the New York Academy of Sciences*, Vol. 940, (June, 2001), pp. 20-27, ISSN 0077-8923

Sango, K.; Horie, H. & Inoue, S. (1997). Biophysical and biochemical features of diabetic neurons in culture: what have we learned about diabetic neuropathy? *Journal of the Peripheral Nervous System*, Vol. 2, No. 3, pp. 203-211, ISSN 1085-9489

Sango, K.; Horie, H.; Okamura, A.; Inoue, S. & Takenaka, T. (1995). Diabetes impairs DRG neuronal attachment to extracellular matrix proteins in vitro. *Brain Research Bulletin*, Vol. 37, No. 5, pp. 533-537, ISSN 0361-9230

Sango, K.; Horie, H.; Saito, H.; Ajiki, K.; Tokashiki, A.; Takeshita, K.; Ishigatsubo, Y.; Kawano, H. & Ishikawa, Y. (2002). Diabetes is not a potent inducer of neuronal cell death in mouse sensory ganglia, but it enhances neurite regeneration in vitro. *Life Sciences*, Vol. 71, No. 20, (October, 2002), pp. 2351-2368, ISSN 0024-3205

Sango, K.; Horie, H.; Sotelo, J.R. & Takenaka, T. (1991). A high glucose environment improves survival of diabetic neurons in culture. *Neuroscience Letters*, Vol. 129, No. 2, (August, 1991), pp. 277-280, ISSN 0304-3940

Santoro, B.; Liu, D.T.; Yao, H.; Bartsch, D.; Kandel, E.R.; Siegelbaum, S.A. & Tibbs, G.R. (1998). Identification of a gene encoding a hyperpolarization-activated pacemaker channel of brain. *Cell*, Vol. 93, No. 5, (May, 1998), pp. 717-729, ISSN 0092-8674

Sapru, H.N.; Gonzalez, E. & Krieger, A.J. (1981). Aortic nerve stimulation in the rat: cardiovascular and respiratory responses. *Brain Research Bulletin*, Vol. 6, No. 5, (May, 1981), pp. 393-398, ISSN 0361-9230

Sapru, H.N. & Krieger, A.J. (1977). Carotid and aortic chemoreceptor function in the rat. *Journal of Applied Physiology*, Vol. 42, No. 3, (March, 1977), pp. 344-348, ISSN 8750-7587

Schieffer, B.; Luchtefeld, M.; Braun, S.; Hilfiker, A.; Hilfiker-Kleiner, D. & Drexler, H. (2000). Role of NAD(P)H oxidase in angiotensin II-induced JAK/STAT signaling and cytokine induction. *Circulation Research*, Vol. 87, No. 12, (December, 2000), pp. 1195-1201, ISSN 0009-7330

Schild, J.H. & Li, B.Y. (2001). The N-type Ca^{2+} current is not responsible for the repolarization 'hump' in the action potential of nodose sensory neurons. *FASEB Journal*, Vol. 15, No. 5, (March, 2001), pp. A1150, ISSN 0892-6638

Seagard, J.L.; Hopp, F.A.; Drummond, H.A. & Van Wynsberghe, D.M. (1993). Selective contribution of two types of carotid sinus baroreceptors to the control of blood pressure. *Circulation Research*, Vol. 72, No. 5, (May, 1993), pp. 1011-1022, ISSN 0009-7330

Sechi, L.A.; Griffin, C.A. & Schambelan, M. (1994). The cardiac renin-angiotensin system in STZ-induced diabetes. *Diabetes*, Vol. 43, No. 10, (October, 1994), pp. 1180-1184, ISSN 0012-1797

Selvarajah, D. & Tesfaye, S. (2006). Central nervous system involvement in diabetes mellitus. *Current Diabetes Report*, Vol. 6, No. 6, (December, 2006), pp. 431-438, ISSN 1534-4827

Sharma, A.K. & Thomas, P.K. (1987). Animal models: pathophysiology, In: *Diabetic Neuropathy*, Dyck, P.J.; Thomas, P.K.; Asbury, A.K.; Winegrad, A.I. & Porte, D. (Eds.), pp. 237-252. ISBN 0721621252, Saunders, Philadelphia

Shimoni, Y. & Liu, X.F. (2004). Gender differences in ANG II levels and action on multiple K+ current modulation pathways in diabetic rats. *American Journal of Physiology Heart and Circulatory Physiology*, Vol. 287, No. 1, (July, 2004), pp. H311-H319, ISSN 0363-6135

Siragy, H.M. (2000). The role of the AT2 receptor in hypertension. *American Journal of Hypertension*, Vol. 13, No. 5, (May, 2000), pp. 62S-67S, ISSN 0895-7061

Soedamah-Muthu, S.S.; Chaturvedi, N.; Witte, D.R.; Stevens, L.K.; Porta, M. & Fuller, J.H. (2008). Relationship between risk factors and mortality in type 1 diabetic patients in Europe: the EURODIAB Prospective Complications Study (PCS). *Diabetes Care*, Vol. 31, No. 7, (August, 2008), pp. 1360-1366, ISSN 0149-5992

Spyer, K.M.; Lambert, J.H. & Thomas, T. (1997). Central nervous system control of cardiovascular function: neural mechanisms and novel modulators. *Clinical and Experimental Pharmacology and Physiology*, Vol. 24, No. 9-10, (September, 1997), pp. 743-747, ISSN 0305-1870

Srinivasan, S.; Stevens, M. & Wiley, J.W. (2000). Diabetic peripheral neuropathy: evidence for apoptosis and associated mitochondrial dysfunction. *Diabetes*, Vol. 49, No. 11, (November, 2000), pp. 1932-1938, ISSN 0012-1797

Stieber, J.; Stockl, G.; Herrmann, S.; Hassfurth, B. & Hofmann, F. (2005). Functional expression of the human HCN3 channel. *Journal of Biological Chemistry*, Vol. 280, No. 41, (October, 2005), pp. 34635-34643, ISSN 0021-9258

Stieber, J.; Thomer, A.; Much, B.; Schneider, A.; Biel, M. & Hofmann, F. (2003). Molecular basis for the different activation kinetics of the pacemaker channels HCN2 and HCN4. *Journal of Biological Chemistry*, Vol. 278, No. 36, (September, 2003), pp. 33672-33680, ISSN 0021-9258

Sumners, C.; Zhu, M.; Gelband, C.H. & Posner, P. (1996). Angiotensin II type 1 receptor modulation of neuronal K^+ and Ca^{2+} currents: intracellular mechanisms. *American Journal of Physiology*, Vol. 271, No. 1, (July, 1996), pp. C154-C163, ISSN 0002-9513

Tang, X. & Dworkin, B.R. (2007). Baroreflexes of the rat. V. Tetanus-induced potentiation of ADN A-fiber responses at the NTS. *American Journal of Physiology Regulatory, Integrative and Comparative Physiology*, Vol. 293, No. 6, (December, 2007), pp. R2254-R2259, ISSN 0363-6119

Tattersall, R.B. & Gill, G.V. (1991). Unexplained deaths of type 1 diabetic patients. *Diabetic Medicine*, Vol. 8, No. 1, (January, 1991), pp. 49-58, ISSN 0742-3071

Thomas, P.K. & Tomlinson, D.R. (1993). Diabetic and hypoglycemic neuropathy, In: *Peripheral neuropathy*, Dyck, P.J. & Thomas, P.K. (Eds.), pp. 1219-1250, ISBN 0721644317, Saunders, Philadelphia

Thoren, P.; Munch, P.A. & Brown, A.M. (1999). Mechanisms for activation of aortic baroreceptor C-fibres in rabbits and rats. *Acta Physiologica Scandinavica*, Vol. 166, No. 3, (July, 1999), pp. 167-174, ISSN 0001-6772

Touyz, R.M. & Berry, C. (2002). Recent advances in angiotensin II signaling. *Brazilizan Journal of Medical Biological Research*, Vol. 35, No. 9, (September, 2002), pp. 1001-1015, ISSN 0100-879X

Toyry, J.P.; Partanen, J.V.; Niskanen, L.K.; Lansimies, E.A. & Uusitupa, M.I. (1997). Divergent development of autonomic and peripheral somatic neuropathies in NIDDM. *Diabetologia*, Vol. 40, No. 8, (August, 1997), pp. 953-958, ISSN 0012-186X

Tsujimura, T.; Nunotani, H.; Fushimi, H. & Inoue, T. (1986). Morphological changes in autonomic ganglionic cells of the heart in diabetic patients. *Diabetes Research and Clinical Practice*, Vol. 2, No. 3, (June, 1986), pp. 133-137, ISSN 0168-8227

Tu, H.; Zhang, L.; Tran, T.P.; Muelleman, R.L. & Li, Y.L. (2010). Diabetes alters protein expression of hyperpolarization-activated cyclic nucleotide-gated channel subunits in rat nodose ganglion cells. *Neuroscience*, Vol. 165, No. 1, (January, 2010), pp. 39-52, ISSN 0306-4522

Vaccari, T.; Moroni, A.; Rocchi, M.; Gorza, L.; Bianchi, M.E.; Beltrame, M. & DiFrancesco, D, (1999). The human gene coding for HCN2, a pacemaker channel of the heart. *Biochimica et Biophysicac Acta*, Vol. 1446, No. 3, (September, 1999), pp. 419-425, ISSN 0006-3002

Valensi, P.; Sachs, R.N.; Harfouche, B.; Lormeau, B.; Paries, J.; Cosson, E.; Paycha, F.; Leutenegger, M. & Attali, J.R. (2001). Predictive value of cardiac autonomic neuropathy in diabetic patients with or without silent myocardial ischemia. *Diabetes Care*, Vol. 24, No. 2, (February, 2001), pp. 339-343, ISSN 0149-5992

Van, B.T.; Kasbergen, C.M.; Gispen, W.H. & De Wildt, D.J. (1998). In vivo cardiovascular reactivity and baroreflex activity in diabetic rats. *Cardiovascular Research*, Vol. 38, No. 3, (June, 1998), pp. 763-771, ISSN 0008-6363

Vinik, A.I. & Ziegler, D. (2007). Diabetic cardiovascular autonomic neuropathy. *Circulation*, Vol. 115, No. 3, (January, 2007), pp. 387-397, ISSN 0009-7322

Wahl-Schott, C. & Biel, M. (2009). HCN channels: structure, cellular regulation and physiological function. *Cellular and Molecular Life Sciences*, Vol. 66, No. 3, (February, 2009), pp. 470-494, ISSN 1420-682X

Wainger, B.J.; DeGennaro, M.; Santoro, B.; Siegelbaum, S.A. & Tibbs, G.R. (2001). Molecular mechanism of cAMP modulation of HCN pacemaker channels. *Nature*, Vol. 411, No. 6839, (June, 2001), pp. 805-810, ISSN 0028-0836

Wang, J.; Chen, S.; Nolan, M.F. & Siegelbaum, S.A. (2002). Activity-dependent regulation of HCN pacemaker channels by cyclic AMP: signaling through dynamic allosteric coupling. *Neuron*, Vol. 36, No. 3, (October, 2002), pp. 451-461, ISSN 0896-6273

Wang, J.; Chen, S.; & Siegelbaum, S.A. (2001). Regulation of hyperpolarization-activated HCN channel gating and cAMP modulation due to interactions of COOH terminus and core transmembrane regions. *Journal of General Physiology*, Vol. 118, No. 3, (September, 2001), pp. 237-250, ISSN 0022-1295

Wang, J.L.; Chinookoswong, N.; Scully, S.; Qi, M. & Shi, Z.Q. (1999). Differential effects of leptin in regulation of tissue glucose utilization in vivo. *Endocrinology*, Vol. 140, No. 5, (May, 1999), pp. 2117-2124, ISSN 0013-7227

Weinrauch, L.A.; Kennedym, F.P.; Gleason, R.E.; Keough, J. & D'Elia, J.A. (1998). Relationship between autonomic function and progression of renal disease in diabetic proteinuria: clinical correlations and implications for blood pressure control. *American Journal of Hypertension*, Vol. 11, No. 3, (March, 1998), pp. 302-308, ISSN 0895-7061

Weston, P.J. & Gill, G.V. (1999). Is undetected autonomic dysfunction responsible for sudden death in Type 1 diabetes mellitus? The 'dead in bed' syndrome revisited. *Diabetic Medicine*, Vol. 16, No. 8, (August, 1999), pp. 626-631, ISSN 0742-3071

Weston, P.J.; James, M.A.; Panerai, R.; McNally, P.G.; Potter, J.F.; Thurston, H. & Swales, J.D. (1996). Abnormal baroreceptor-cardiac reflex sensitivity is not detected by conventional tests of autonomic function in patients with insulin-dependent diabetes mellitus. *Clinical Science (London)* , Vol. 91, No. 1, (July, 1996), pp. 59-64, ISSN 0143-5221

Weston, P.J.; James, M.A.; Panerai, R.B.; McNally, P.G.; Potter, J.F. & Thurston, H. (1998). Evidence of defective cardiovascular regulation in insulin-dependent diabetic patients without clinical autonomic dysfunction. *Diabetes Research and Clinical Practice*, Vol. 42, No. 3, (December, 1998), pp. 141-148, ISSN 0168-8227

Widdop, R.E.; Krstew, E. & Jarrott, B. (1992). Electrophysiological responses of angiotensin peptides on the rat isolated nodose ganglion. *Clinical & Experimental Hypertension. Part A*, Vol. 14, No. 4, pp. 597-613, ISSN 1064-1963

Xiao, L.; Wu, Y.M.; Wang, R.; Liu, Y.X.; Wang, F.W. & He, R.R. (2007). Hydrogen sulfide facilitates carotid sinus baroreceptor activity in anesthetized male rats. *Chinese Medical Journal (English)* , Vol. 120, No. 15, (August, 2007), pp. 1343-1347, ISSN 0336-6999

Yagihashi, S. (1995). Pathology and pathogenetic mechanisms of diabetic neuropathy. *Diabetes/Metabolism Reviews*, Vol. 11, No. 3, (October, 1995), pp. 193-225, ISSN 0742-4221

Yagihashi, S. (1997). Pathogenetic mechanisms of diabetic neuropathy: lessons from animal models. *Journal of the Peripheral Nervous System*, Vol. 2, No. 2, (June, 1997), pp. 113-132, ISSN 1085-9489

Yamasaki, M.; Shimizu, T.; Katahira, K.; Waki, H.; Nagayama, T.; Ishi, H.; Katsuda, S.; Miyake, M.; Miyamoto, Y.; Wago, H.; Okouchi, T. & Matsumoto, S. (2004). Spaceflight alters the fiber composition of the aortic nerve in the developing rat. *Neuroscience*, Vol. 128, No. 4, pp. 819-829, ISSN 0306-4522

Zhang, H.; Liu, Y.X.; Wu, Y.M.; Wang, Z.M. & He, R.R. (2004). Capsaicin facilitates carotid sinus baroreceptor activity in anesthetized rats. *Acta Pharmacologica Sinica*, Vol. 25, No. 11, (November, 2004), pp. 1439-1443, ISSN 1671-4083

Zhang, L.; Tu, H. & Li, Y.L. (2010). Angiotensin II enhances hyperpolarization-activated currents in rat aortic baroreceptor neurons: involvement of superoxide. *American Journal of Physiology Cell Physiology*, Vol. 298, No. 1, (January, 2010), pp. C98-C106, ISSN 0363-6143

Zhuo, J.L.; Imig, J.D.; Hammond, T.G.; Orengo, S.; Benes, E. & Navar, L.G. (2002). Ang II accumulation in rat renal endosomes during Ang II-induced hypertension: role of AT(1) receptor. *Hypertension*, Vol. 39, No. 1, (January, 2002), pp. 116-121, ISSN 0194-911X

Ziegler, D. (1994). Diabetic cardiovascular autonomic neuropathy: prognosis, diagnosis and treatment. *Diabetes/Metabolism Reviews*, Vol. 10, No. 4, (December, 1994), pp. 339-383, ISSN 0742-4221

Ziegler D, Laude D, Akila F, & Elghozi JL (2001). Time- and frequency-domain estimation of early diabetic cardiovascular autonomic neuropathy. *Clinical Autonomic Research*, Vol. 11, No. 6, (December, 2001), pp. 369-376, ISSN 0959-9851

9

Microvascular and Macrovascular Complications in Children and Adolescents with Type 1 Diabetes

Francesco Chiarelli and M. Loredana Marcovecchio
Department of Paediatrics, University of Chieti,
Italy

1. Introduction

Diabetes mellitus is a serious chronic disorder of childhood and represents a major public health problem. Type 1 diabetes is the predominant form of diabetes during childhood and adolescence, accounting for about 90% of cases, although the growing epidemic of obesity has been associated with an increasing number of cases of childhood-onset type 2 diabetes (Craig et al., 2009; Patterson et al., 2009).

The global incidence of type 1 diabetes is increasing worldwide, at an annual rate of 3-5%, particularly in children under the age of 5 years, and this trend leads to a significant health burden (Patterson et al., 2009). Recent studies have shown that in European countries childhood-onset type 1 diabetes is associated with three to four fold increased mortality when compared with the general population (Asao et al., 2003; Skrivarhaug et al., 2006). Similar data emerged from a long-term study of a young cohort with type 1 diabetes in the USA, where mortality was 7 times higher than in the non-diabetic population (Secrest et al., 2010a). The high mortality reported for individuals with type 1 diabetes is mainly due to diabetes-related acute and chronic complications. As recently emerged from a large population-based cohort with long-standing childhood-onset type 1 diabetes, during the first decade of diabetes acute complications, such as diabetic ketoacidosis and hypoglycemia, are the main causes of death, being responsible for about 73% of cases, whereas during subsequent decades cardiovascular (CVD) and renal diseases become the main determinants of mortality (Secrest et al., 2010b).

Diabetes vascular complications are divided in micro- and macrovascular disease. Microvascular complications include nephropathy (DN), retinopathy (DR) and neuropathy, whereas macrovascualar complications refer to cardiovascular, cerebrovascular and peripheral vascular disease (Marshall and Flyvbjerg, 2006). As a result of vascular complications, diabetes is the leading cause of blindness in working age people, is responsible for up to 40% cases of renal failure and is a major determinant of cardiovascular morbidity and mortality (Marshall and Flyvbjerg, 2006).

2. Microvascular complications of type 1 diabetes

Diabetic microvascular complications result from damage to the microvasculature of the kidney, retina and neurons and they generally progress throughout different stages.

2.1 Diabetic nephropathy
2.1.1 Classification of diabetic nephropathy and structural kidney changes

The changing occurring in the kidney in patients with type 1 diabetes are generally classified in five stages (Mogensen, 1999). The first stage is characterized by increases in glomerular filtration rate (GFR) and kidney hypertrophy. During the second phase subtle morphological changes occur together with progressive increases in urinary albumin excretion within the normal range. The third stage, also called incipient nephropathy, is characterized by the development of microalbuminuria, defined as an albumin excretion rate (AER) between 30-300 mg/24h or 20-200 µg/min, and by more profound structural changes. During the fourth phase there is a further increase in AER leading to macroalbuminuria (AER >200 µg/min or >300 mg/24h) and a consistent fall in GFR. Without any treatment this phase leads to the final stage of end stage renal disease (ESRD).

Typical morphological changes occurring in the diabetic kidney are represented by diffuse glomerular basement membrane thickening, mesangial expansion, hyalinosis of the mesangium and arteriolar walls, broadening and effacement of podocyte foot processes, reduction in podocyte number, glomerulosclerosis and tubule-interstitial fibrosis (Osterby, 1992). These morphological changes develop years before the clinical appearance of DN and this is an alarming aspect, given that when the disease is clinically evident some of the structural damage is already irreversible.

Thickening of the basement membrane is a common bioptic finding related to DN and is associated with loss of glycosaminoglycans and associated negative charges, with consequent increased loss of anionic albumin (Fioretto and Mauer, 2007; Fioretto et al., 1994; Mauer and Najafian, 2006). A subsequent increase in the size of membrane pores leads to the development of non-selective proteinuria. An imbalance between the production and the degradation of mesangial matrix proteins, together with an increase in mesangial cells number, is responsible for mesangial expansion in DN (Fioretto and Mauer, 2007; Mauer and Najafian, 2006).

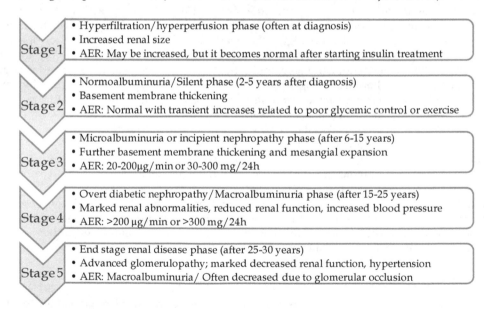

Stage 1
- Hyperfiltration/hyperperfusion phase (often at diagnosis)
- Increased renal size
- AER: May be increased, but it becomes normal after starting insulin treatment

Stage 2
- Normoalbuminuria/Silent phase (2-5 years after diagnosis)
- Basement membrane thickening
- AER: Normal with transient increases related to poor glycemic control or exercise

Stage 3
- Microalbuminuria or incipient nephropathy phase (after 6-15 years)
- Further basement membrane thickening and mesangial expansion
- AER: 20-200µg/min or 30-300 mg/24h

Stage 4
- Overt diabetic nephropathy/Macroalbuminuria phase (after 15-25 years)
- Marked renal abnormalities, reduced renal function, increased blood pressure
- AER: >200 µg/min or >300 mg/24h

Stage 5
- End stage renal disease phase (after 25-30 years)
- Advanced glomerulopathy; marked decreased renal function, hypertension
- AER: Macroalbuminuria/ Often decreased due to glomerular occlusion

Fig. 1. Stages of diabetic nephropathy

Changes in the podocyte is another key feature of DN (Mauer and Najafian, 2006). Podocytes are highly specialised epithelial cells, interconnected by foot processes, which delimit the slit diaphragm, the main size-selective barrier in the glomerulus. The first detectable alteration in podocytes in the context of DN is a broadening and effacement of their foot processes (Kriz et al., 1998), which leads to a decrease in their density and number and a detachment from the glomerular basement membrane. The last phenomena are directly correlated to levels of albumin-creatinine ratio (ACR) and to the decline in GFR (Fioretto and Mauer, 2007). Podocytes can also undergo hypertrophy, apoptosis and increased synthesis of collagen IV, whereas there is a decreased synthesis of proteins, such as nephrin (Fioretto and Mauer, 2007).

Another characteristic of DN is the hyalinosis of the afferent and efferent arterioles in the glomerulus, due to the accumulation of complement components, fibrinogen, immunoglobulins, albumin and other plasma proteins (Fioretto and Mauer, 2007). Hypertrophy and sclerosis of the iuxtaglomerular apparatus is another frequent finding in DN (Mauer and Najafian, 2006).

2.1.2 Epidemiology of diabetic nepropathy

DN affects about one third of people with type 1 diabetes after a disease duration of 20 years and represents an important determinant of mortality (Jones et al., 2005). This has been recently confirmed in patients with both childhood-onset and adult-onset type 1 diabetes (Groop et al., 2009; Orchard et al., 2010). In a large cohort of adults with type 1 diabetes the presence of microalbuminuria, macroalbuminuria and ESRD was associated with 2.8, 9.2, and 18.3 times higher standardized mortality ratio, respectively (Groop et al., 2009). Similarly, Orchard et al. reported a standardized mortality ratio of 6.4, 12.5 and 29.8 for individuals with microalbuminuria, proteinuria and ESRD, respectively, in a cohort with childhood-onset type 1 diabetes followed longitudinally for 30 years (Orchard et al., 2010).

The natural history of DN has changed over the last decades and, whereas earlier landmark studies indicated that patients with microalbuminuria had a 60-85% risk of progressing to overt proteinuria within 6-14 years (Mogensen and Christensen, 1984; Parving et al., 1982; Viberti et al., 1982), more recent studies have reported a rate of progression of 30% over 10 years, and an increasing number of cases of regression to normoalbuminuria (31 to 58%) (de Boer et al., 2011; Hovind et al., 2004; Perkins et al., 2003). Regression to normoalbuminuria has been associated with a better metabolic control, a better lipid and blood pressure profile as well as with non-modifiable risk factors, such as younger age and shorter duration of microalbuminuria (Hovind et al., 2004; Perkins et al., 2003). These data are encouraging and highlight the positive effect of improvements in treatment, particularly glycemic (1993) and blood pressure control (Lewis et al., 1993), in influencing the natural history of DN. However, this changing trend may be also related to an overestimation of the rate of progression in earlier studies.

With regards to young people with childhood onset type 1 diabetes, recent studies from Sweden (Nordwall et al., 2004) and Australia (Mohsin et al., 2005) have shown a decreasing trend in DN. However, these positive results have not been consistently reported. In fact, data from Iceland (Tryggvason et al., 2005) and the UK (Amin et al., 2009) indicated an unchanged trend in the incidence of microalbuminuria and DN over the last decades.

2.1.3 Early manifestations of diabetic nephropathy in youth with type 1 diabetes

Microalbuminuria is the most common abnormal finding in children and adolescents with type 1 diabetes, whereas overt proteinuria is found in less than 1–1.5% of them (Jones et al., 1998; Schultz et al., 1999b). Microalbuminuria often develops during puberty, whereas its prevalence during prepubertal years is rare (Janner et al., 1994; Lawson et al., 1996; Norgaard et al., 1989; Rudberg et al., 1993). The overall prevalence of microalbuminuria in youth with type 1 diabetes ranges between 4 and 26% (Bojestig et al., 1996; Cook and Daneman, 1990; Dahlquist and Rudberg, 1987; Joner et al., 1992; Jones et al., 1998; Mathiesen et al., 1986; Moore and Shield, 2000; Norgaard et al., 1989; Olsen et al., 2000; Rudberg et al., 1993; Schultz et al., 1999b). This large variation in the prevalence of microalbuminuria is due to differences in study design, duration of diabetes, age range, and glycemic control. Most studies investigating microalbuminuria have been cross-sectional and clinic based, with only a few being longitudinal, but mainly with a retrospective design. Jones *et al.* (Jones et al., 1998) reported a prevalence of 14.5% during 8.5 years of diabetes duration, whereas Rudberg *et al.* (Rudberg et al., 1993) reported a prevalence of 24% after 15 years diabetes duration. The most recent data from the Oxford Regional Prospective Study (ORPS), a population-based inception cohort of children with type 1 diabetes, has shown a cumulative prevalence of microalbuminuria of 25.7% after 10 years and of 50.7% after 19 years of diabetes duration (Amin et al., 2008).

After puberty, rates of rise in albumin excretion tend to decline and, longitudinal studies suggest that microalbuminuria is persistent in only 50% of adolescents; whereas in the other 40-50% urinary albumin excretion returns into the normal range after 3-10 years from the onset of microalbuminuria (Amin et al., 2008; Gorman et al., 1999). However, with longer follow-up cases of transient or intermittent microalbuminuria may become persistent. In addition, although urinary albumin excretion may return into the normal range, the renal morphological changes associated with microalbuminuria can persist and increase the risk of its recurrence and progression (Steinke and Mauer, 2008). Few data are available on the rate of progression of microalbuminuria to macroalbuminuria in young people with type 1 diabetes. The ORPS has shown a progression rate of around 13% after 3.2 years from the onset of microalbuminuria, a rate similar to that reported in adults (Amin et al., 2008).

Another renal abnormality often detected in youth with type 1 diabetes is increased GFR (Amin et al., 2005; Rudberg et al., 1992). Hyperfiltration, which has been associated with increased renal size often precedes the onset of microalbuminuria (Amin et al., 2005; Rudberg et al., 1992). In some, although not all studies, increased GFR has emerged as an independent predictor of microalbuminuria, and a recent meta-analysis has reported a 2.7 increased risk of developing microalbuminuria associated with hyperfiltration (Magee et al., 2009).

2.2 Diabetic retinopathy

2.2.1 Classification and structural changes

DR begins with the appearance of non-proliferative retinal abnormalities, which then progress to sight-threatening proliferative lesions (Aiello et al., 1998; Williams and Pickup, 2004) . The early stage of DR is characterised by the development of capillary microaneuryms, which consist in small blind outgrowths of retinal capillaries developing in areas where the wall is weakened (Aiello et al., 1998; D'Amico, 1994; Williams and Pickup, 2004). As the retinal damage progresses, there is the appearance of non-proliferative abnormalities, including hemorrhages, exudates and the development of vascular obstruction, intraretinal microvascular abnormalities, and infarction of the retinal nerve fibers causing cotton wool spots (Aiello et al., 1998; D'Amico, 1994; Williams and Pickup, 2004). Although this stage is not sight-threatening, it is highly predictive of progression to more advanced stages of retinopathy. Proliferative retinopathy is characterized by the development of new vessels, secondary to ischemia, on the surface of the retina and/or the optic disc (Aiello et al., 1998; D'Amico, 1994; Williams and Pickup, 2004). These new vessels can bleed into the vitroretinal space, and cause visual loss. In addition, the subsequent formation of fibrous tissue can cause tractional retinal detachment (Williams and Pickup, 2004). This stage is associated with a high risk for visual impairment related to hemorrhages and retinal detachment.

Diabetic macular oedema can complicate both non-proliferative and proliferative retinopathy and is a serious cause of vision loss in patients with diabetes (Ciulla et al., 2003). It is characterized by increased microvascular permeability and deposition of hard retinal exudates (Ciulla et al., 2003). This stage involves the breakdown of the blood-retinal barrier, with leakage of plasma from small blood vessels in the macula. Swelling of the macula is then followed by deposition of hard retinal exudates as a consequence of deposition of lipids and lipoproteins following plasma re-absorption (Ciulla et al., 2003).

Proposed disease severity level	Dilated ophthalmoscopy findings
No apparent retinopathy	No abnormalities
Mild nonproliferative DR	Microaneurysms only
Moderate nonproliferative DR	More than just microaneurysms, but less than severe nonproliferative DR
Severe nonproliferative DR	No signs of proliferative DR, with any of the following: - More than 20 intraretinal hemorrhages in each of four quadrants - Definite venous beading in two or more quadrants - Prominent intaretinal microvascular anomalies in one or more quadrants
Proliferative DR	One or more of the following: - Neovascularization - Vitreous or preretinal hemorrhage

Table 1. International clinical DR disease severity scale

Retinal damage in diabetes is mainly due to leakage of retinal blood vessels and inadequate retinal perfusion (Aiello et al., 1998; D'Amico, 1994; Williams and Pickup, 2004). It has been suggested that one of the initial alterations in the retinal hemodynamic is represented by retinal vasodilatation and hyperperfusion, due to hypoxia and increased release of nitric oxide (Joussen et al., 2004). This is followed by an impairment of the retinal vascular autoregulation with increased tension in the epithelial wall and increased vascular permeability, which, in turn, cause vascular leakage and aneurysm formation (Kohner et al., 1995; Scherrer et al., 1994).

Early structural abnormalities in the retinal microvasculature are characterised by thickening of the basement membrane, loss of endothelial cells and pericytes and increased capillary permeability (Kohner et al., 1995). An important characteristic of retinopathy is the loss of pericytes from the retinal capillaries (D'Amico, 1994; Feng et al., 2007; Frank, 2004). Pericytes are contractile cells which have an important role in the regulation of the capillary blood flow and their loss has been associated with the development of retinal microaneurysms (Feng et al., 2007; Kuwabara and Cogan, 1963). The loss of pericytes, associated with that of capillary endothelial cells, contributes to the disruption of the integrity of the blood–retinal barrier. Thickening of the capillary basement membrane and deposition of extracellular matrix components are additional mechanisms contributing to the alterations in the retinal blood flow (Feng et al., 2007).

Retinal leukostasis has been also associated with DR and, in particular, with capillary occlusion and the consequent appearance of retinal areas of non perfusion (Aiello et al., 1998; D'Amico, 1994; Williams and Pickup, 2004). These alterations contribute, in turn, to retinal ischemia, which is a potent stimulus for vascular neoformation (Miyamoto and Ogura, 1999).

2.2.2 Epidemiology of retinopathy

DR is the leading cause of blindness in people of working age in Western countries (Ciulla et al., 2003). The prevalence of DR increases with age and its was approximately 17.7 per 100 people with diabetes in the year 2005 (Deshpande et al., 2008). DR can be diagnosed already after 5 years from the onset of diabetes, and almost all patients will show variable degrees of DR after 20 years diabetes duration.

Recent data from the Wisconsin Epidemiologic Study of DR have shown that the 25-year cumulative incidence of visual impairment in adults with type 1 diabetes was 13% and that of severe visual impairment was 3%. Patients with onset of diabetes during more recent years have a lower prevalence of visual impairment when compared with those diagnosed in the past, independently of duration of diabetes (Klein et al., 2010). This is in agreement with some other recent studies reporting a declining incidence of retinopathy and other microvascular complications (Nathan et al., 2009; Nordwall et al., 2004).

2.2.3 Early manifestations of retinopathy in youth with type 1 diabetes

Early stages of DR can be detected in young people with type 1 diabetes, as shown by a population based study from Australia, where early background retinopathy was detected in 24% of the study population after 6-year diabetes duration (Donaghue et al., 2005). Similarly, in a Swedish study retinopathy was detected in 27% of young patients after 13 years of duration (Nordwall et al., 2006). Children with type 1 diabetes under the age of 10 years are at minimal risk of DR, but the prevalence rate increases after 5 years from diagnosis in post-pubertal patients (Klein et al., 1984). In an incident cohort, early retinopathy was detected in 12% of prepubertal children compared to 29% of adolescents, after 6 year type 1 diabetes duration (Donaghue et al., 2005). Interestingly, adolescents with type 1 diabetes have a higher risk of progression to sight-threatening DR when compared to adults and the progression may be particularly rapid when glycemic control is poor (Maguire et al., 2005). As for DN, cases of regression have also been reported for DR (Maguire et al., 2005).

2.3 Diabetic neuropathy

Diabetic neuropathy is the most common neuropathy in industrialized countries, and it is associated with a wide range of clinical manifestations (Tesfaye et al., 2010). Diabetic neuropathy is defined as a clinical or subclinical disorder, without any additional causes other than diabetes, and can be either somatic or autonomic (Boulton et al., 2005). Early diagnosis and treatment of diabetic neuropathy are important given that peripheral neuropathy is associated with a high risk of feet injury in patients with type 1 diabetes (Boulton et al., 2005). In addition, diabetic autonomic neuropathy can lead to a significantly increased morbidity and mortality, mainly when involves the cardiovascular system (Boulton et al., 2005).

2.3.1 Classification and epidemiological data of diabetic neuropathy

Chronic distal symmetric polyneuropathy (DPN) is the most common form of diabetic neuropathy and affects 30-50% of patients with type 1 diabetes and can be asymptomatic in up to 50% of them (Tesfaye et al., 2010). DPN implies symmetric damage of peripheral small sensory and large motor nerve fibres. It generally starts from the most distal end of the feet and then extend proximally over time and can lead to foot ulceration and amputation of lower limbs (Boulton et al., 2005). Dysfunction of peripheral small nerve fibres is characterised by parasthesiae, burning, and deep aching pain. If larger nerve fibres are affected, vibration, light touch and joint position senses are impaired, and tendon reflexes are absent (Boulton et al., 2005). Less common forms of diabetic somatic neuropathy include focal or multifocal neuropathies, which are characterized by entrapment of a peripheral nerve commonly the median, ulnar or peroneal nerve (Boulton et al., 2005).

Diabetic autonomic neuropathy is a disorder of the autonomic nervous system in the context of diabetes and can affect the cardiovascular, gastrointestinal, urogenital systems and the sudomotor function (Tesfaye et al., 2010). Autonomic neuropathy can be observed in around 20% of asymptomatic patients with diabetes (Tesfaye et al., 2010). Clinical symptoms of autonomic neuropathy do not generally occur until long after the onset of diabetes. Subclinical autonomic dysfunction can, however, occur within two years of diagnosis in patients with type 1 diabetes (Boulton et al., 2005). Dysautonomic features may reflect the involvement of different systems and manifest as postural hypotension and orthostatic lightheadedness, gastroparesis, gastric fullness, early satiety, sexual dysfunction, bladder dysfunction, gustatory sweating or anhidrosis and pupillomotor dysfunction (Boulton et al., 2005).

Peripheral neuropathies	Autonomic neuropathy
Generalized symmetric polyneuropathies	- *Cardiovascular:* Postural hypotension, resting tachicardia, exercise intolerance
- Acute sensory	- *Genitourinary:* Bladder dysfunction, Erectile dysfunction
- Chronic sensorimotor	
- Autonomic	- *Gastrointestinal:* Gastric paresis, constipation/diarrhea, fecal inconinence
Focal and multifocal neuropathies	
- Cranial	
- Truncal	- *Sudomotor:* Gustatory sweating, Anhidrosis, Heat intolerance, Dry skin
- Focal limb	
- Proximal motor	- *Metabolic:* hypoglycemia unawareness
	- *Pupillomotor dysfunction*

Table 2. Neuropathies in diabetes

Diabetic neuropathy is characterized by a reduction in the number of fibers, degeneration of the myelin sheath as well as changes affecting the endoneurial connective tissue, vessels and perineurium (Greene et al., 1992). The process of nerve demyelination may progress to Wallerian degeneration, in which the nerve axon is also injured and the distal part of the axon dies (Greene et al., 1992).

2.3.2 Early signs of diabetic neuropathy in youth with type 1 diabetes
In the most comprehensive epidemiological studies involving both adult and pediatric patients, DPN was detected in 9 to 58% of the study populations (Boulton et al., 2005). Data on autonomic neuropathy indicate a prevalence ranging from 14% to 75%, with a high number of youth with type 1 diabetes presenting suclinical signs of autonomic dysfunction, even after a short duration of T1D. This variability across different studies is mainly related to differences in the characteristics of the study cohorts as well as to the use of different testing modalities and different criteria and cut off values (Trotta et al., 2004; Verrotti et al., 2009).

3. Macrovascular complications of type 1 diabetes

Patients with type 1 diabetes have an increased risk of developing cardiovascular disease (CVD) relative to the nondiabetic population, and premature atherosclerosis represents the main cause of morbidity and mortality in type 1 diabetes populations (Laing et al., 2003).
There is extensive evidence in support of the concept that atherosclerosis begins early in life (Ross, 1993) and therefore identification of CVD risk factors and preventive strategies should be started during childhood and adolescence (Dahl-Jorgensen et al., 2005). Children and adolescents with type 1 diabetes represent a high risk population with regards to CVD, given that cardiovascular risk factors are common among them (Dahl-Jorgensen et al., 2005; Margeirsdottir et al., 2008; van Vliet et al.) and they can contribute to their poor long-term prognosis (Skrivarhaug et al., 2006). A recent study has shown that as many as 86% of youth with type 1 diabetes has at least one, 45% at least two and 15% at least three CVD risk factors, including high HbA1c, high blood pressure, dyslipidemia, smoking and family history of CVD events (Margeirsdottir et al., 2008). These data are alarming given that it is well known that CVD risk factors can persist or track over time (Berenson, 2002) and therefore contribute to the overall burden associated with type 1 diabetes.

3.1 Early signs of macrovascular disease in youth with type 1 diabetes
The early stages of the atherosclerotic process are silent, but autopsy studies have detected early structural alterations in the arteries of youth, where they have been associated with the same risk factors than in adults (Berenson et al., 1998). The earliest recognizable pathologic intimal lesions are the fatty streaks, which make their appearance in the aorta of children even before 3 years of age (McGill et al., 2000; Williams et al., 2002). Fatty streaks represent an early manifestation of lipid accumulation in the vessel wall and they have been associated with increased cholesterol levels as well as with hyperglycemia (McGill et al., 2000).
Technology progresses over the last years have made possible to look for early surrogate markers of atherosclerotic vascular disease. These markers are represented by structural alterations such as increased intima-media thickness as well as functional changes represented by decreased flow-mediated dilatation and increased arterial stiffness, as detected by pulse wave velocity (Dahl-Jorgensen et al., 2005).

Several studies have consistently shown that children and adolescents with type 1 diabetes present signs of endothelial dysfunction, as measured by flow-mediated dilation in the brachial artery (Jarvisalo et al., 2004; Singh et al., 2003). In addition, increased aortic and carotid intima-media thickness has been reported in children with type 1 diabetes (Harrington et al., 2010; Jarvisalo et al., 2001). Besides, markers of inflammation and oxidative stress are significantly increased in youth with type 1 diabetes when compared with age-matched controls and they can mediate vascular damage (Snell-Bergeon et al., 2010).

Progression of CVD in youth with type 1 diabetes can be more aggressive than in adults with diabetes, therefore highlighting the importance of early preventive strategies (Dahl-Jorgensen et al., 2005).

Early manifestations of CVD in youth with type 1 diabetes
• Increased inflammatory markers
• Increased oxidative stress
• Increased intima-media thickness
• Decreased flow-mediated dilatation
• Increased pulse wave velocity

Table 3. Early manifestations of CVD in youth with type 1 diabetes

4. Pathogenesis of micro- and macrovascular complications

Vascular complications in the context of diabetes are the result of an interplay between hemodynamic and metabolic factors and the consequent activation of common intermediate pathways, associated with increased synthesis and release of growth factors, cytokines, chemokines and oxidant species, which are all final mediators of vascular damage (Cooper, 2001).

A strong association exists between the presence of micro- and macrovascular complications in people with type 1 diabetes (Girach and Vignati, 2006). In particular, it is well known that DN is a key risk factor for cardiovascular complications and many patients with renal impairment die of CVD-related causes even before developing ESRD (Groop et al., 2009). In addition, there is growing evidence suggesting that increases in albumin excretion, even within the normal range, in the general population as well as in people with type 1 diabetes, represents a determinant of CVD (Klausen et al., 2004). The link between micro- and macrovascular disease could be represented by endothelial dysfunction, as an underlining feature of both processes, as well as by a certain degree of inflammation, which has been associated to the presence of both micro- and macrovascular complications (Schalkwijk and Stehouwer, 2005).

4.1 Glycemic control

Chronic hyperglycemia is known to activate several deleterious pathways implicated in the damage of vessels: protein glycation, increased glucose flux through alternative polyol and hexosamine pathways, increased oxidative stress, which then stimulate secondary intracellular signaling pathways leading to production of growth factors, cytokines and inflammatory factors (Brownlee, 2001).

Several epidemiological studies have shown a direct and strong association between long-term glycemic control, as expressed by HbA1c levels, and the risk of developing nephropathy, retinopathy and neuropathy (Amin et al., 2008; Danne et al., 1998; Gallego et al., 2008; Nordwall et al., 2009). In addition, HbA1c has been shown to be a key determinant also of early signs of atherosclerosis (McGill et al., 1995).

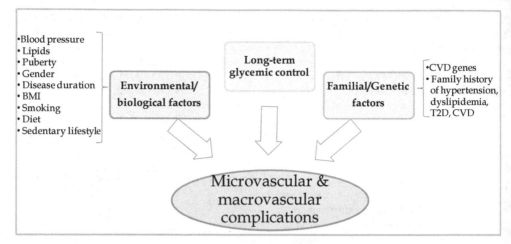

Fig. 2. Risk factors for the development of vascular complications in adolescents with type 1 diabetes

The Diabetes Control and Complications Trial (DCCT) and the Epidemiology of Diabetes Interventions and Complications (EDIC) studies have clearly shown the beneficial effect of strict glycemic control in reducing the risk of microvascular and macrovascular complications in subjects with type 1 diabetes (1993; 2003). In the adolescent cohort of the DCCT, a positive effect of improved glycemic control on complication risk was obtained. Intensive insulin therapy reduced the risk for the development and progression of DR by 76% and 54%; the occurrence of microalbuminuria and proteinuria by 39% and 54% and that of clinical neuropathy by 60% when compared to the conventional treated group (1994). Data from the DCCT/EDIC study also showed that intensive insulin therapy reduced the risk for any cardiovascular disease by 42% and of nonfatal myocardial infarction, stroke or death from CVD cause by 57% (Nathan et al., 2005). The beneficial effect of intensive insulin treatment in patients with childhood-onset type 1 diabetes also emerged from the Oslo study, where long-term glycemic control predicted coronary atherosclerosis (Larsen et al., 2002).

In addition, the EDIC study raised the important concept of 'metabolic memory'; in other words although after the end of the DCCT HbA1c levels became comparable between the intensively and conventionally treated groups, patients belonging to the first group still kept an advantage from prior better HbA1c levels (2003). Therefore, the EDIC data highlighted the need of implementing intensive management as soon as type 1 diabetes is diagnosed. This was further supported by recent data related to DR, showing that, although at year 10 of the EDIC there was still a decrease in DR progression risk in the intensively treated adult group, in the adolescent cohort retinopathy progression at year 10 of the EDIC did not differ between the previous DCCT intensively and conventionally treated groups, thus indicating loss of the metabolic memory (White et al., 2010). Interestingly, 79% of the difference in the metabolic effect between adults and adolescents after 10 years from the end of the DCCT was due to the difference in mean HbA1c levels during the DCCT between the two cohorts. This 1% difference, which did not seem to play a major role during the DCCT and early EDIC years with regards to the outcomes, seems to be a major player in the long run (White et al., 2010).

4.2 Blood pressure and plasma lipids

Elevated blood pressure and alterations in its circadian rhythm are common findings in people with type 1 diabetes and have been associated with the risk of developing vascular complications (Gallego et al., 2008; Marcovecchio et al., 2009b; Tesfaye et al., 1996). Increases in blood pressure have been found to precede or occur concomitant with the appearance of microalbuminuria in adolescents with type 1 diabetes (Marcovecchio et al., 2009b; Schultz et al., 2001). Similarly, higher than normal systolic and diastolic blood pressure independently contribute to the development of DR (Gallego et al., 2008). Blood pressure has been also associated with early markers of atherosclerosis (Dahl-Jorgensen et al., 2005).

Lipid abnormalities have also been linked to the development and progression of micro- and macrovascular complications in adolescents with diabetes (Dahl-Jorgensen et al., 2005; Kordonouri et al., 1996; Marcovecchio et al., 2009a).

4.3 Duration and age at onset of type 1 diabetes

Duration of diabetes is another major determinant of complication risk. Although vascular complications rarely appear before puberty, prepubertal duration of diabetes is an important determinant for their development (Coonrod et al., 1993; Orchard et al., 1990). Patients with type 1 diabetes from early childhood and especially those diagnosed under five years of age seem to have slightly delayed onset of persistent microalbuminuria during the first 10 to 15 years duration compared with patients diagnosed later in childhood or during puberty. However, this initial protective effect of a younger age at diagnosis disappears over time (Amin et al., 2008; Donaghue et al., 2003). After 15 years of diabetes duration the risk of developing microalbuminuria is similar between subjects diagnosed with diabetes before 5 years of age when compared with those diagnosed between 5-11 years of age or after the age of 11 years, suggesting that age at the onset of diabetes does not influence the overall risk for microalbuminuria (Amin et al., 2008). A recent study has highlighted that also for DR, although patients diagnosed at a young age have a longer time free of proliferative retinopathy, this advantage then gradually disappears and youth diagnosed before the age of 15 years have a higher risk of proliferative retinopathy when compared with those diagnosed when aged 15-40 years (Hietala et al., 2010).

4.4 Puberty

Puberty is an important factor implicated in the development and progression of vascular complications. Poor glycemic control is a common finding among adolescents with type 1 diabetes (1994; Holl et al., 2003). In addition, puberty is associated with a decrease in insulin sensitivity, and adolescents with type 1 diabetes are more insulin resistant when compared with healthy controls (Dunger, 1992). Rapid growth, hormonal and metabolic changes characterise this period of life and can influence complications risk (Dunger, 1992).

4.5 Gender

A gender dimorphism has been reported for vascular complications. In particular, during adolescence the risk for microalbuminuria is higher in female than in male subjects with comparable glycemic control (Amin et al., 2008; Jones et al., 1998), whereas among adults with type 1 diabetes the risk is higher for males (Hovind et al., 2004). These differences have been related to variations in the hormonal milieu and to a higher degree of insulin resistance in girls (Schultz et al., 1999a).

4.6 Other factors
Genetic factors represent another important contributing factor for the development of vascular complications, as suggested by their familial clustering, and by the observation that only a subset of patients with poor glycemic control develop severe long-term complications (1997). Family history of cardiovascular risk factors is associated with increased risk of microvascular complications in the offspring (Monti et al., 2007; Seaquist et al., 1989).

A high body mass index (BMI) represents another potential risk factor for microvascular complications in youth with type 1 diabetes (Stone et al., 2006). In addition, obesity is a well-known risk factor for cardiovascular disease (Dahl-Jorgensen et al., 2005).

Environmental factors, including diet and lifestyle, can also contribute to the risk of developing vascular complications. Smoking in people with type 1 diabetes has been associated with an increased risk of developing vascular complications (Chase et al., 1991; Mohamed et al., 2007).

5. Management of microvascular and macrovascular complications

5.1 Screening
Diabetic microvascular and macrovascular complications are often asymptomatic during their early stages, and once symptoms develop, they may be difficult to reverse. Therefore, longitudinal repeated screening for vascular complications initiated during early adolescence is currently recommended

The American Diabetes Association (ADA) recommends to start screening in patients with type 1 diabetes aged 10 years or older after a disease duration of 3-5 years, with yearly follow-up (Silverstein et al., 2005). The International Society for Pediatric and Adolescent Diabetes (ISPAD) recommends screening from the age of 11 years in those with 2 year diabetes duration and from 9 years in those with a 5 year duration for both nephropathy and retinopathy (Donaghue et al., 2007). Measurement of urinary albumin excretion is the basis for early detection of microalbuminuria and can be achieved with: 1) 24-hour urine collection; 2) overnight timed urine collections; 3) albumin-creatinine ratio (ACR) or albumin concentration on a early morning spot urinary sample (Donaghue et al., 2007). 24-hour or timed urine collections are often difficult to collect in children and adolescents. Assessing ACR in early morning urines is the easiest method to carry out in an office setting and it generally provides accurate information (Donaghue et al., 2007).

With regards to DR, several techniques can be used, including direct and indirect ophthalmoscopy, stereoscopic digital and color film based fundus photography, mydriatic or nonmydriatic digital color or monochromatic single-field photography. The best technique to identify and grade retinopathy is represented by retinal photography, through dilated pupils, but dilated indirect ophtalmoscopy associated with biomicroscopy is an acceptable alternative (Ciulla et al., 2003).

In contrast to well-established criteria for when starting screening for DN and DR, it is unclear when to commence screening for neuropathy. History and physical examination are generally the recommended methods of screening (Donaghue et al., 2007). Clinical examination, including history of pain, paresthesia, numbness and physical examination of ankle reflexes and vibration and light touch sensation, is a fundamental part of screening, although not being as sensitive or specific as nerve conduction studies (Donaghue et al., 2007). Autonomic neuropathy can be assessed with specific autonomic nerve tests, such as heart rate response to deep breathing, standing from a lying position, Valsalva maneuver, heart rate variations at rest, QT interval, postural changes in BP and pupil responses to light and dark adaptation (Donaghue et al., 2007). These tests need to be carefully standardized and therefore they are largely used as screening methods for complications at a population level.

Additional screening concerns risk factors for CVD, such as dyslipidemia and hypertension. Blood lipids should be checked soon after diagnosis and if normal then repeated after 5 years (Donaghue et al., 2007). Office blood pressure should be assessed annually and in case of abnormal values, hypertension needs to be confirmed by ambulatory blood pressure monitoring.

When to start
• Microvascular complications: at age 11 with 2 year duration of type 1 diabetes or from age 9 with 5 year duration (for nephropathy and retinopathy; unclear for neuropathy) • Macrovascular complications: after 12 years

Screening Method:
1) Diabetic nephropathy
  • Annual albumin-creatinine ratio in a spot urine sample or first morning albumin concentration
2) Diabetic retinopathy
  • Annual dilated fundus ophthalmoscopy or fundal photography
3) Diabetic neuropathy
  • History and physical examination
  • Nerve conduction and autonomic tests
4) Macrovascular disease
  • Annual assessments of blood pressure
  • Assessment of lipid levels every 5 years

Table 4. Screening for micro- and macrovascular complications in youth with type 1 diabetes

5.2 Interventions

Improving glycemic control is the cornerstone of treatment strategies aiming at reducing the development and progression of microvascular and macrovascular complications. The DCCT and EDIC study clearly showed the importance of a strict glycemic control both in adults and in adolescents with type 1 diabetes (1994). The importance of keeping HbA1c within targets has also been highlighted by other studies, but similarly to the DCCT, subsequent studies have confirmed the difficulties encountered when dealing with young people with type 1 diabetes (Holl et al., 2003; Petitti et al., 2009). Tight glycemic control in the DCCT and subsequent studies was associated with a higher risk of complications, such as hypoglycemia and weight gain (1994). In addition, poor compliance is an important issue to be taken into account in adolescents with type 1 diabetes. Furthermore, other factors besides insulin therapy are relevant for metabolic control, such as dietary habits, education, family interactions, cultural and psychological aspects (Holl et al., 2003), and therefore they need to be taken into account in order to define a successful treatment plan.

Treatment with angiotensin converting enzyme inhibitors (ACEIs) is recommended when hypertension is confirmed (Donaghue et al., 2007). ACEIs are treatment of choice in adults with microalbuminuria, based on evidence that their use decrease the rate of progression and even increase rates of regression of microalbuminuria (Lewis et al., 1993). A beneficial effect of anti-hypertensive treatment, and in particular of treatment with ACEIs, has also been demonstrated for DR (Chaturvedi et al., 1998). The EURODIAB Controlled Trial of Lisinopril in type 1 diabetes showed a significant effect of lisinopril in reducing by around 50% the progression of retinopathy in normotensive and normo- or microalbuminuric patients (Chaturvedi et al., 1998). However, there is no universal recommendation for the use of ACEIs in children and adolescents with microalbuminuria. The ADA recommends to start treatment with ACEIs in presence of persistent microalbuminuria (Silverstein et al., 2005). Similarly, the recent ISPAD guidelines suggest to use ACEIs or angiotensin receptor blockers in presence of persistent microalbuminuria, in order to prevent progression to proteinuria (Donaghue et al., 2007), even though the lack of evidence in this context is acknowledged.

Dyslipidemia should be managed firstly with improvements in glycemic control and dietary changes and, in case of persistence of high cholesterol levels, treatment with statins should be considered, although there is no enough evidence of their use in children apart from those with familial hypercholesterolemia (Donaghue et al., 2007). However, in adults statins have been shown to be effective in the primary and secondary prevention of major cardiovascular events (2002).

Adolescents with type 1 diabetes need to be persuaded to avoid smoking. In addition, it is of paramount importance also to avoid increases in BMI, given that adiposity is a well known risk factor for cardiovascular complications, and in some studies it has also been associated with microvascular complications of type 1 diabetes (Donaghue et al., 2007).

Targets to reduce diabetic vascular complications
• HbA1c: ≤7.5% (without severe hypoglycemia)
• LDL cholesterol: <2.6mmol/l
• HDL cholesterol: >1.1mmol/l
• Triglycerides: <1.7mmol/l
• Blood pressure: <90th percentile for age, sex and height
• BMI <95th centile
• Avoid smoking
• Physical activity: moderate: >1hr/day
• Sedentary activities: <2hr/day
• Healthy diet

Table 5. Recommendations to reduce diabetic vascular complications (ISPAD guideline 2006-2007)

New potential therapeutic possibilities for the treatment of vascular complications are emerging and they include drugs targeting specific pathways implicated in their pathogenesis. These include inhibitors of aldose reductase, inhibitors of protein kinase C, antagonists of advanced glycation end-products, glycosaminoglycans, inhibitors of growth factors and anti-oxidants (Soro-Paavonen and Forbes, 2006). Up to now, there are no definitive data to recommend the use of these new potential therapies but the overall objective of targeting specific metabolic and hemodynamic pathways implicated in the pathogenesis of diabetic vascular complications could lead to validation of these classes of drugs and discovery of novel pharmaceuticals.

6. Conclusions

The risk for micro- and macrovascular complications is high in young patients with childhood-onset type 1 diabetes and their development negatively influence their long-term prognosis.
Early identification of risk factors and prevention of diabetes complications are of paramount importance in children and adolescents. Diabetic vascular complications are often asymptomatic during their early stages, and once symptoms develop, it can be difficult to reverse them. Therefore, screening for vascular complications started during early adolescence, as currently recommended, is essential. Identification of risk factors and subclinical signs of complications is of paramount importance for the early implementation of preventive and therapeutic strategies, which could change the course of vascular complications and improve the prognosis of youth with diabetes. Efforts should be made for optimizing glycemic control, to keep blood pressure and lipid levels within target levels, to avoid smoking, promote exercise and a healthy diet. Future studies are required to test the efficacy and safety of new therapies, which could target specific metabolic or hemodynamic pathways implicated in the pathogenesis of diabetic complications.
Further advances in genomics, proteomics and in other 'omics' and the integration of the findings of these different sciences will hopefully allow a better understanding of the pathogenesis of diabetic vascular complications in the near future and will potentially lead to a personalized medicine for young patients with diabetes

7. References

(1993). The effect of intensive treatment of diabetes on the development and progression of long-term complications in insulin-dependent diabetes mellitus. The Diabetes Control and Complications Trial Research Group. N Engl J Med 329, 977-986.

(1994). Effect of intensive diabetes treatment on the development and progression of long-term complications in adolescents with insulin-dependent diabetes mellitus: Diabetes Control and Complications Trial. Diabetes Control and Complications Trial Research Group. J Pediatr 125, 177-188.

(1997). Clustering of long-term complications in families with diabetes in the diabetes control and complications trial. The Diabetes Control and Complications Trial Research Group. Diabetes 46, 1829-1839.

(2002). MRC/BHF Heart Protection Study of cholesterol lowering with simvastatin in 20,536 high-risk individuals: a randomised placebo-controlled trial. Lancet 360, 7-22.

(2003). Sustained effect of intensive treatment of type 1 diabetes mellitus on development and progression of diabetic nephropathy: the Epidemiology of Diabetes Interventions and Complications (EDIC) study. Jama 290, 2159-2167.

Aiello, L.P., Gardner, T.W., King, G.L., Blankenship, G., Cavallerano, J.D., Ferris, F.L., 3rd, and Klein, R. (1998). Diabetic retinopathy. Diabetes Care 21, 143-156.

Amin, R., Turner, C., van Aken, S., Bahu, T.K., Watts, A., Lindsell, D.R., Dalton, R.N., and Dunger, D.B. (2005). The relationship between microalbuminuria and glomerular filtration rate in young type 1 diabetic subjects: The Oxford Regional Prospective Study. Kidney Int 68, 1740-1749.

Amin, R., Widmer, B., Dalton, R.N., and Dunger, D.B. (2009). Unchanged incidence of microalbuminuria in children with type 1 diabetes since 1986: a UK based inception cohort. Arch Dis Child 94, 258-262.

Amin, R., Widmer, B., Prevost, A.T., Schwarze, P., Cooper, J., Edge, J., Marcovecchio, L., Neil, A., Dalton, R.N., and Dunger, D.B. (2008). Risk of microalbuminuria and progression to macroalbuminuria in a cohort with childhood onset type 1 diabetes: prospective observational study. Bmj 336, 697-701.

Asao, K., Sarti, C., Forsen, T., Hyttinen, V., Nishimura, R., Matsushima, M., Reunanen, A., Tuomilehto, J., and Tajima, N. (2003). Long-term mortality in nationwide cohorts of childhood-onset type 1 diabetes in Japan and Finland. Diabetes care 26, 2037-2042.

Berenson, G.S. (2002). Childhood risk factors predict adult risk associated with subclinical cardiovascular disease. The Bogalusa Heart Study. The American journal of cardiology 90, 3L-7L.

Berenson, G.S., Srinivasan, S.R., Bao, W., Newman, W.P., 3rd, Tracy, R.E., and Wattigney, W.A. (1998). Association between multiple cardiovascular risk factors and atherosclerosis in children and young adults. The Bogalusa Heart Study. N Engl J Med 338, 1650-1656.

Bojestig, M., Arnqvist, H.J., Karlberg, B.E., and Ludvigsson, J. (1996). Glycemic control and prognosis in type I diabetic patients with microalbuminuria. Diabetes Care 19, 313-317.

Boulton, A.J., Vinik, A.I., Arezzo, J.C., Bril, V., Feldman, E.L., Freeman, R., Malik, R.A., Maser, R.E., Sosenko, J.M., and Ziegler, D. (2005). Diabetic neuropathies: a statement by the American Diabetes Association. Diabetes care 28, 956-962.

Brownlee, M. (2001). Biochemistry and molecular cell biology of diabetic complications. Nature 414, 813-820.

Chase, H.P., Garg, S.K., Marshall, G., Berg, C.L., Harris, S., Jackson, W.E., and Hamman, R.E. (1991). Cigarette smoking increases the risk of albuminuria among subjects with type I diabetes. JAMA 265, 614-617.

Chaturvedi, N., Sjolie, A.K., Stephenson, J.M., Abrahamian, H., Keipes, M., Castellarin, A., Rogulja-Pepeonik, Z., and Fuller, J.H. (1998). Effect of lisinopril on progression of retinopathy in normotensive people with type 1 diabetes. The EUCLID Study Group. EURODIAB Controlled Trial of Lisinopril in Insulin-Dependent Diabetes Mellitus. Lancet 351, 28-31.

Ciulla, T.A., Amador, A.G., and Zinman, B. (2003). Diabetic retinopathy and diabetic macular edema: pathophysiology, screening, and novel therapies. Diabetes Care 26, 2653-2664.

Cook, J.J., and Daneman, D. (1990). Microalbuminuria in adolescents with insulin-dependent diabetes mellitus. Am J Dis Child 144, 234-237.

Coonrod, B.A., Ellis, D., Becker, D.J., Bunker, C.H., Kelsey, S.F., Lloyd, C.E., Drash, A.L., Kuller, L.H., and Orchard, T.J. (1993). Predictors of microalbuminuria in individuals with IDDM. Pittsburgh Epidemiology of Diabetes Complications Study. Diabetes Care 16, 1376-1383.

Cooper, M.E. (2001). Interaction of metabolic and haemodynamic factors in mediating experimental diabetic nephropathy. Diabetologia 44, 1957-1972.

Craig, M.E., Hattersley, A., and Donaghue, K.C. (2009). Definition, epidemiology and classification of diabetes in children and adolescents. Pediatr Diabetes 10 Suppl 12, 3-12.

D'Amico, D.J. (1994). Diseases of the retina. N Engl J Med 331, 95-106.

Dahl-Jorgensen, K., Larsen, J.R., and Hanssen, K.F. (2005). Atherosclerosis in childhood and adolescent type 1 diabetes: early disease, early treatment? Diabetologia 48, 1445-1453.

Dahlquist, G., and Rudberg, S. (1987). The prevalence of microalbuminuria in diabetic children and adolescents and its relation to puberty. Acta Paediatr Scand 76, 795-800.

Danne, T., Kordonouri, O., Enders, I., Hovener, G., and Weber, B. (1998). Factors modifying the effect of hyperglycemia on the development of retinopathy in adolescents with diabetes. Results of the Berlin Retinopathy Study. Hormone research 50 Suppl 1, 28-32.

de Boer, I.H., Rue, T.C., Cleary, P.A., Lachin, J.M., Molitch, M.E., Steffes, M.W., Sun, W., Zinman, B., and Brunzell, J.D. (2011). Long-term Renal Outcomes of Patients With Type 1 Diabetes Mellitus and Microalbuminuria: An Analysis of the Diabetes Control and Complications Trial/Epidemiology of Diabetes Interventions and Complications Cohort. Arch Intern Med 171, 412-420.

Deshpande, A.D., Harris-Hayes, M., and Schootman, M. (2008). Epidemiology of diabetes and diabetes-related complications. Phys Ther 88, 1254-1264.

Donaghue, K.C., Chiarelli, F., Trotta, D., Allgrove, J., and Dahl-Jorgensen, K. (2007). ISPAD clinical practice consensus guidelines 2006-2007. Microvascular and macrovascular complications. Pediatr Diabetes 8, 163-170.

Donaghue, K.C., Craig, M.E., Chan, A.K., Fairchild, J.M., Cusumano, J.M., Verge, C.F., Crock, P.A., Hing, S.J., Howard, N.J., and Silink, M. (2005). Prevalence of diabetes complications 6 years after diagnosis in an incident cohort of childhood diabetes. Diabet Med 22, 711-718.

Donaghue, K.C., Fairchild, J.M., Craig, M.E., Chan, A.K., Hing, S., Cutler, L.R., Howard, N.J., and Silink, M. (2003). Do all prepubertal years of diabetes duration contribute equally to diabetes complications? Diabetes care 26, 1224-1229.

Dunger, D.B. (1992). Diabetes in puberty. Arch Dis Child 67, 569-570.

Feng, Y., vom Hagen, F., Lin, J., and Hammes, H.P. (2007). Incipient diabetic retinopathy--insights from an experimental model. Ophthalmologica 221, 269-274.

Fioretto, P., and Mauer, M. (2007). Histopathology of diabetic nephropathy. Semin Nephrol 27, 195-207.

Fioretto, P., Steffes, M.W., and Mauer, M. (1994). Glomerular structure in nonproteinuric IDDM patients with various levels of albuminuria. Diabetes 43, 1358-1364.

Frank, R.N. (2004). Diabetic retinopathy. N Engl J Med 350, 48-58.

Gallego, P.H., Craig, M.E., Hing, S., and Donaghue, K.C. (2008). Role of blood pressure in development of early retinopathy in adolescents with type 1 diabetes: prospective cohort study. BMJ (Clinical research ed 337, a918.

Girach, A., and Vignati, L. (2006). Diabetic microvascular complications--can the presence of one predict the development of another? J Diabetes Complications 20, 228-237.

Gorman, D., Sochett, E., and Daneman, D. (1999). The natural history of microalbuminuria in adolescents with type 1 diabetes. J Pediatr 134, 333-337.

Greene, D.A., Sima, A.A., Stevens, M.J., Feldman, E.L., and Lattimer, S.A. (1992). Complications: neuropathy, pathogenetic considerations. Diabetes care 15, 1902-1925.

Groop, P.H., Thomas, M.C., Moran, J.L., Waden, J., Thorn, L.M., Makinen, V.P., Rosengard-Barlund, M., Saraheimo, M., Hietala, K., Heikkila, O., and Forsblom, C. (2009). The presence and severity of chronic kidney disease predicts all-cause mortality in type 1 diabetes. Diabetes 58, 1651-1658.

Harrington, J., Pena, A.S., Gent, R., Hirte, C., and Couper, J. 2010. Aortic intima media thickness is an early marker of atherosclerosis in children with type 1 diabetes mellitus. J Pediatr 156, 237-241.

Hietala, K., Harjutsalo, V., Forsblom, C., Summanen, P., and Groop, P.H. (2010). Age at onset and the risk of proliferative retinopathy in type 1 diabetes. Diabetes care.

Holl, R.W., Swift, P.G., Mortensen, H.B., Lynggaard, H., Hougaard, P., Aanstoot, H.J., Chiarelli, F., Daneman, D., Danne, T., Dorchy, H., Garandeau, P., Greene, S., Hoey, H.M., Kaprio, E.A., Kocova, M., Martul, P., Matsuura, N., Robertson, K.J., Schoenle, E.J., Sovik, O., Tsou, R.M., Vanelli, M., and Aman, J. (2003). Insulin injection regimens and metabolic control in an international survey of adolescents with type 1 diabetes over 3 years: results from the Hvidore study group. Eur J Pediatr 162, 22-29.

Hovind, P., Tarnow, L., Rossing, P., Jensen, B.R., Graae, M., Torp, I., Binder, C., and Parving, H.H. (2004). Predictors for the development of microalbuminuria and macroalbuminuria in patients with type 1 diabetes: inception cohort study. Bmj 328, 1105.

Janner, M., Knill, S.E., Diem, P., Zuppinger, K.A., and Mullis, P.E. (1994). Persistent microalbuminuria in adolescents with type I (insulin-dependent) diabetes mellitus is associated to early rather than late puberty. Results of a prospective longitudinal study. Eur J Pediatr 153, 403-408.

Jarvisalo, M.J., Jartti, L., Nanto-Salonen, K., Irjala, K., Ronnemaa, T., Hartiala, J.J., Celermajer, D.S., and Raitakari, O.T. (2001). Increased aortic intima-media thickness: a marker of preclinical atherosclerosis in high-risk children. Circulation 104, 2943-2947.

Jarvisalo, M.J., Raitakari, M., Toikka, J.O., Putto-Laurila, A., Rontu, R., Laine, S., Lehtimaki, T., Ronnemaa, T., Viikari, J., and Raitakari, O.T. (2004). Endothelial dysfunction and increased arterial intima-media thickness in children with type 1 diabetes. Circulation 109, 1750-1755.

Joner, G., Brinchmann-Hansen, O., Torres, C.G., and Hanssen, K.F. (1992). A nationwide cross-sectional study of retinopathy and microalbuminuria in young Norwegian type 1 (insulin-dependent) diabetic patients. Diabetologia 35, 1049-1054.

Jones, C.A., Krolewski, A.S., Rogus, J., Xue, J.L., Collins, A., and Warram, J.H. (2005). Epidemic of end-stage renal disease in people with diabetes in the United States population: do we know the cause? Kidney Int 67, 1684-1691.

Jones, C.A., Leese, G.P., Kerr, S., Bestwick, K., Isherwood, D.I., Vora, J.P., Hughes, D.A., and Smith, C. (1998). Development and progression of microalbuminuria in a clinic sample of patients with insulin dependent diabetes mellitus. Arch Dis Child 78, 518-523.

Joussen, A.M., Poulaki, V., Le, M.L., Koizumi, K., Esser, C., Janicki, H., Schraermeyer, U., Kociok, N., Fauser, S., Kirchhof, B., Kern, T.S., and Adamis, A.P. (2004). A central role for inflammation in the pathogenesis of diabetic retinopathy. FASEB J 18, 1450-1452.

Klausen, K., Borch-Johnsen, K., Feldt-Rasmussen, B., Jensen, G., Clausen, P., Scharling, H., Appleyard, M., and Jensen, J.S. (2004). Very low levels of microalbuminuria are associated with increased risk of coronary heart disease and death independently of renal function, hypertension, and diabetes. Circulation 110, 32-35.

Klein, R., Klein, B.E., Moss, S.E., Davis, M.D., and DeMets, D.L. (1984). The Wisconsin epidemiologic study of diabetic retinopathy. II. Prevalence and risk of diabetic retinopathy when age at diagnosis is less than 30 years. Arch Ophthalmol 102, 520-526.

Klein, R., Lee, K.E., Gangnon, R.E., and Klein, B.E. (2010). The 25-year incidence of visual impairment in type 1 diabetes mellitus the wisconsin epidemiologic study of diabetic retinopathy. Ophthalmology 117, 63-70.

Kohner, E.M., Patel, V., and Rassam, S.M. (1995). Role of blood flow and impaired autoregulation in the pathogenesis of diabetic retinopathy. Diabetes 44, 603-607.

Kordonouri, O., Danne, T., Hopfenmuller, W., Enders, I., Hovener, G., and Weber, B. (1996). Lipid profiles and blood pressure: are they risk factors for the development of early background retinopathy and incipient nephropathy in children with insulin-dependent diabetes mellitus? Acta Paediatr 85, 43-48.

Kriz, W., Gretz, N., and Lemley, K.V. (1998). Progression of glomerular diseases: is the podocyte the culprit? Kidney Int 54, 687-697.

Kuwabara, T., and Cogan, D.G. (1963). Retinal vascular patterns. VI. Mural cells of the retinal capillaries. Arch Ophthalmol 69, 492-502.

Laing, S.P., Swerdlow, A.J., Slater, S.D., Burden, A.C., Morris, A., Waugh, N.R., Gatling, W., Bingley, P.J., and Patterson, C.C. (2003). Mortality from heart disease in a cohort of 23,000 patients with insulin-treated diabetes. Diabetologia 46, 760-765.

Larsen, J., Brekke, M., Sandvik, L., Arnesen, H., Hanssen, K.F., and Dahl-Jorgensen, K. (2002). Silent coronary atheromatosis in type 1 diabetic patients and its relation to long-term glycemic control. Diabetes 51, 2637-2641.

Lawson, M.L., Sochett, E.B., Chait, P.G., Balfe, J.W., and Daneman, D. (1996). Effect of puberty on markers of glomerular hypertrophy and hypertension in IDDM. Diabetes 45, 51-55.

Lewis, E.J., Hunsicker, L.G., Bain, R.P., and Rohde, R.D. (1993). The effect of angiotensin-converting-enzyme inhibition on diabetic nephropathy. The Collaborative Study Group. N Engl J Med 329, 1456-1462.

Magee, G.M., Bilous, R.W., Cardwell, C.R., Hunter, S.J., Kee, F., and Fogarty, D.G. (2009). Is hyperfiltration associated with the future risk of developing diabetic nephropathy? A meta-analysis. Diabetologia 52, 691-697.

Maguire, A., Chan, A., Cusumano, J., Hing, S., Craig, M., Silink, M., Howard, N., and Donaghue, K. (2005). The case for biennial retinopathy screening in children and adolescents. Diabetes Care 28, 509-513.

Marcovecchio, M.L., Dalton, R.N., Prevost, A.T., Acerini, C.L., Barrett, T.G., Cooper, J.D., Edge, J., Neil, A., Shield, J., Widmer, B., Todd, J.A., and Dunger, D.B. (2009a). Prevalence of abnormal lipid profiles and the relationship with the development of microalbuminuria in adolescents with type 1 diabetes. Diabetes care 32, 658-663.

Marcovecchio, M.L., Dalton, R.N., Schwarze, C.P., Prevost, A.T., Neil, H.A., Acerini, C.L., Barrett, T., Cooper, J.D., Edge, J., Shield, J., Widmer, B., Todd, J.A., and Dunger, D.B. (2009b). Ambulatory blood pressure measurements are related to albumin excretion and are predictive for risk of microalbuminuria in young people with type 1 diabetes. Diabetologia 52, 1173-1181.

Margeirsdottir, H.D., Larsen, J.R., Brunborg, C., Overby, N.C., and Dahl-Jorgensen, K. (2008). High prevalence of cardiovascular risk factors in children and adolescents with type 1 diabetes: a population-based study. Diabetologia 51, 554-561.

Marshall, S.M., and Flyvbjerg, A. (2006). Prevention and early detection of vascular complications of diabetes. BMJ (Clinical research ed 333, 475-480.

Mathiesen, E.R., Saurbrey, N., Hommel, E., and Parving, H.H. (1986). Prevalence of microalbuminuria in children with type 1 (insulin-dependent) diabetes mellitus. Diabetologia 29, 640-643.

Mauer, M., and Najafian, B. (2006). The structure of human diabetic nephropathy. In The Diabetic Kidney. P. Cortes, and C.E. Mogensen, eds. (Humana Press), pp. 361-374.

McGill, H.C., Jr., McMahan, C.A., Herderick, E.E., Malcom, G.T., Tracy, R.E., and Strong, J.P. (2000). Origin of atherosclerosis in childhood and adolescence. Am J Clin Nutr 72, 1307S-1315S.

McGill, H.C., Jr., McMahan, C.A., Malcom, G.T., Oalmann, M.C., and Strong, J.P. (1995). Relation of glycohemoglobin and adiposity to atherosclerosis in youth. Pathobiological Determinants of Atherosclerosis in Youth (PDAY) Research Group. Arterioscler Thromb Vasc Biol 15, 431-440.

Miyamoto, K., and Ogura, Y. (1999). Pathogenetic potential of leukocytes in diabetic retinopathy. Semin Ophthalmol 14, 233-239.

Mogensen, C.E. (1999). Microalbuminuria, blood pressure and diabetic renal disease: origin and development of ideas. Diabetologia 42, 263-285.

Mogensen, C.E., and Christensen, C.K. (1984). Predicting diabetic nephropathy in insulin-dependent patients. N Engl J Med 311, 89-93.

Mohamed, Q., Gillies, M.C., and Wong, T.Y. (2007). Management of diabetic retinopathy: a systematic review. JAMA 298, 902-916.

Mohsin, F., Craig, M.E., Cusumano, J., Chan, A.K., Hing, S., Lee, J.W., Silink, M., Howard, N.J., and Donaghue, K.C. (2005). Discordant trends in microvascular complications in adolescents with type 1 diabetes from 1990 to 2002. Diabetes care 28, 1974-1980.

Monti, M.C., Lonsdale, J.T., Montomoli, C., Montross, R., Schlag, E., and Greenberg, D.A. (2007). Familial risk factors for microvascular complications and differential male-female risk in a large cohort of American families with type 1 diabetes. The Journal of clinical endocrinology and metabolism 92, 4650-4655.

Moore, T.H., and Shield, J.P. (2000). Prevalence of abnormal urinary albumin excretion in adolescents and children with insulin dependent diabetes: the MIDAC study. Microalbinuria in Diabetic Adolescents and Children (MIDAC) research group. Arch Dis Child 83, 239-243.

Nathan, D.M., Cleary, P.A., Backlund, J.Y., Genuth, S.M., Lachin, J.M., Orchard, T.J., Raskin, P., and Zinman, B. (2005). Intensive diabetes treatment and cardiovascular disease in patients with type 1 diabetes. N Engl J Med 353, 2643-2653.

Nathan, D.M., Zinman, B., Cleary, P.A., Backlund, J.Y., Genuth, S., Miller, R., and Orchard, T.J. (2009). Modern-day clinical course of type 1 diabetes mellitus after 30 years' duration: the diabetes control and complications trial/epidemiology of diabetes interventions and complications and pittsburgh epidemiology of diabetes complications experience (1983-2005). Arch Intern Med 169, 1307-1316.

Nordwall, M., Arnqvist, H.J., Bojestig, M., and Ludvigsson, J. (2009). Good glycemic control remains crucial in prevention of late diabetic complications--the Linkoping Diabetes Complications Study. Pediatr Diabetes 10, 168-176.

Nordwall, M., Bojestig, M., Arnqvist, H.J., and Ludvigsson, J. (2004). Declining incidence of severe retinopathy and persisting decrease of nephropathy in an unselected population of Type 1 diabetes-the Linkoping Diabetes Complications Study. Diabetologia 47, 1266-1272.

Nordwall, M., Hyllienmark, L., and Ludvigsson, J. (2006). Early diabetic complications in a population of young patients with type 1 diabetes mellitus despite intensive treatment. J Pediatr Endocrinol Metab 19, 45-54.

Norgaard, K., Storm, B., Graae, M., and Feldt-Rasmussen, B. (1989). Elevated albumin excretion and retinal changes in children with type 1 diabetes are related to long-term poor blood glucose control. Diabet Med 6, 325-328.

Olsen, B.S., Sjolie, A., Hougaard, P., Johannesen, J., Borch-Johnsen, K., Marinelli, K., Thorsteinsson, B., Pramming, S., and Mortensen, H.B. (2000). A 6-year nationwide cohort study of glycaemic control in young people with type 1 diabetes. Risk markers for the development of retinopathy, nephropathy and neuropathy. Danish Study Group of Diabetes in Childhood. J Diabetes Complications 14, 295-300.

Orchard, T.J., Dorman, J.S., Maser, R.E., Becker, D.J., Drash, A.L., Ellis, D., LaPorte, R.E., and Kuller, L.H. (1990). Prevalence of complications in IDDM by sex and duration. Pittsburgh Epidemiology of Diabetes Complications Study II. Diabetes 39, 1116-1124.

Orchard, T.J., Secrest, A.M., Miller, R.G., and Costacou, T. (2010). In the absence of renal disease, 20 year mortality risk in type 1 diabetes is comparable to that of the general population: a report from the Pittsburgh Epidemiology of Diabetes Complications Study. Diabetologia 53, 2312-2319.

Osterby, R. (1992). Glomerular structural changes in type 1 (insulin-dependent) diabetes mellitus: causes, consequences, and prevention. Diabetologia 35, 803-812.

Parving, H.H., Oxenboll, B., Svendsen, P.A., Christiansen, J.S., and Andersen, A.R. (1982). Early detection of patients at risk of developing diabetic nephropathy. A longitudinal study of urinary albumin excretion. Acta Endocrinol (Copenh) 100, 550-555.

Patterson, C.C., Dahlquist, G.G., Gyurus, E., Green, A., and Soltesz, G. (2009). Incidence trends for childhood type 1 diabetes in Europe during 1989-2003 and predicted new cases 2005-20: a multicentre prospective registration study. Lancet 373, 2027-2033.

Perkins, B.A., Ficociello, L.H., Silva, K.H., Finkelstein, D.M., Warram, J.H., and Krolewski, A.S. (2003). Regression of microalbuminuria in type 1 diabetes. N Engl J Med 348, 2285-2293.

Petitti, D.B., Klingensmith, G.J., Bell, R.A., Andrews, J.S., Dabelea, D., Imperatore, G., Marcovina, S., Pihoker, C., Standiford, D., Waitzfelder, B., and Mayer-Davis, E. (2009). Glycemic control in youth with diabetes: the SEARCH for diabetes in Youth Study. J Pediatr 155, 668-672 e661-663.

Ross, R. (1993). The pathogenesis of atherosclerosis: a perspective for the 1990s. Nature 362, 801-809.

Rudberg, S., Persson, B., and Dahlquist, G. (1992). Increased glomerular filtration rate as a predictor of diabetic nephropathy--an 8-year prospective study. Kidney Int 41, 822-828.

Rudberg, S., Ullman, E., and Dahlquist, G. (1993). Relationship between early metabolic control and the development of microalbuminuria--a longitudinal study in children with type 1 (insulin-dependent) diabetes mellitus. Diabetologia 36, 1309-1314.

Schalkwijk, C.G., and Stehouwer, C.D. (2005). Vascular complications in diabetes mellitus: the role of endothelial dysfunction. Clin Sci (Lond) 109, 143-159.

Scherrer, U., Randin, D., Vollenweider, P., Vollenweider, L., and Nicod, P. (1994). Nitric oxide release accounts for insulin's vascular effects in humans. J Clin Invest 94, 2511-2515.

Schultz, C.J., Konopelska-Bahu, T., Dalton, R.N., Carroll, T.A., Stratton, I., Gale, E.A., Neil, A., and Dunger, D.B. (1999a). Microalbuminuria prevalence varies with age, sex, and puberty in children with type 1 diabetes followed from diagnosis in a longitudinal study. Oxford Regional Prospective Study Group. Diabetes Care 22, 495-502.

Schultz, C.J., Konopelska-Bahu, T., Dalton, R.N., Carroll, T.A., Stratton, I., Gale, E.A., Neil, A., and Dunger, D.B. (1999b). Microalbuminuria prevalence varies with age, sex, and puberty in children with type 1 diabetes followed from diagnosis in a longitudinal study. Oxford Regional Prospective Study Group. Diabetes Care 22, 495-502.

Schultz, C.J., Neil, H.A., Dalton, R.N., Konopelska Bahu, T., and Dunger, D.B. (2001). Blood pressure does not rise before the onset of microalbuminuria in children followed from diagnosis of type 1 diabetes. Oxford Regional Prospective Study Group. Diabetes care 24, 555-560.

Seaquist, E.R., Goetz, F.C., Rich, S., and Barbosa, J. (1989). Familial clustering of diabetic kidney disease. Evidence for genetic susceptibility to diabetic nephropathy. N Engl J Med 320, 1161-1165.

Secrest, A.M., Becker, D.J., Kelsey, S.F., LaPorte, R.E., and Orchard, T.J. (2010a). All-cause mortality trends in a large population-based cohort with long-standing childhood-onset type 1 diabetes: the Allegheny County type 1 diabetes registry. Diabetes care 33, 2573-2579.

Secrest, A.M., Becker, D.J., Kelsey, S.F., Laporte, R.E., and Orchard, T.J. (2010b). Cause-specific mortality trends in a large population-based cohort with long-standing childhood-onset type 1 diabetes. Diabetes 59, 3216-3222.

Silverstein, J., Klingensmith, G., Copeland, K., Plotnick, L., Kaufman, F., Laffel, L., Deeb, L., Grey, M., Anderson, B., Holzmeister, L.A., and Clark, N. (2005). Care of children and adolescents with type 1 diabetes: a statement of the American Diabetes Association. Diabetes care 28, 186-212.

Singh, T.P., Groehn, H., and Kazmers, A. (2003). Vascular function and carotid intimal-medial thickness in children with insulin-dependent diabetes mellitus. J Am Coll Cardiol 41, 661-665.

Skrivarhaug, T., Bangstad, H.J., Stene, L.C., Sandvik, L., Hanssen, K.F., and Joner, G. (2006). Long-term mortality in a nationwide cohort of childhood-onset type 1 diabetic patients in Norway. Diabetologia 49, 298-305.

Snell-Bergeon, J.K., West, N.A., Mayer-Davis, E.J., Liese, A.D., Marcovina, S.M., D'Agostino, R.B., Jr., Hamman, R.F., and Dabelea, D. (2010). Inflammatory markers are increased in youth with type 1 diabetes: the SEARCH Case-Control study. J Clin Endocrinol Metab 95, 2868-2876.

Soro-Paavonen, A., and Forbes, J.M. (2006). Novel therapeutics for diabetic micro- and macrovascular complications. Curr Med Chem 13, 1777-1788.

Steinke, J.M., and Mauer, M. (2008). Lessons learned from studies of the natural history of diabetic nephropathy in young type 1 diabetic patients. Pediatr Endocrinol Rev 5 Suppl 4, 958-963.

Stone, M.L., Craig, M.E., Chan, A.K., Lee, J.W., Verge, C.F., and Donaghue, K.C. (2006). Natural history and risk factors for microalbuminuria in adolescents with type 1 diabetes: a longitudinal study. Diabetes care 29, 2072-2077.

Tesfaye, S., Boulton, A.J., Dyck, P.J., Freeman, R., Horowitz, M., Kempler, P., Lauria, G., Malik, R.A., Spallone, V., Vinik, A., Bernardi, L., and Valensi, P. (2010). Diabetic neuropathies: update on definitions, diagnostic criteria, estimation of severity, and treatments. Diabetes care 33, 2285-2293.

Tesfaye, S., Stevens, L.K., Stephenson, J.M., Fuller, J.H., Plater, M., Ionescu-Tirgoviste, C., Nuber, A., Pozza, G., and Ward, J.D. (1996). Prevalence of diabetic peripheral neuropathy and its relation to glycaemic control and potential risk factors: the EURODIAB IDDM Complications Study. Diabetologia 39, 1377-1384.

Trotta, D., Verrotti, A., Salladini, C., and Chiarelli, F. (2004). Diabetic neuropathy in children and adolescents. Pediatr Diabetes 5, 44-57.

Tryggvason, G., Indridason, O.S., Thorsson, A.V., Hreidarsson, A.B., and Palsson, R. (2005). Unchanged incidence of diabetic nephropathy in Type 1 diabetes: a nation-wide study in Iceland. Diabet Med 22, 182-187.

van Vliet, M., Van der Heyden, J.C., Diamant, M., Von Rosenstiel, I.A., Schindhelm, R.K., Aanstoot, H.J., and Veeze, H.J. 2010. Overweight is highly prevalent in children with type 1 diabetes and associates with cardiometabolic risk. J Pediatr 156, 923-929.

Verrotti, A., Loiacono, G., Mohn, A., and Chiarelli, F. (2009). New insights in diabetic autonomic neuropathy in children and adolescents. Eur J Endocrinol 161, 811-818.

Viberti, G.C., Jarrett, R.J., and Keen, H. (1982). Microalbuminuria as prediction of nephropathy in diabetics. Lancet 2, 611.

White, N.H., Sun, W., Cleary, P.A., Tamborlane, W.V., Danis, R.P., Hainsworth, D.P., and Davis, M.D. (2010). Effect of prior intensive therapy in type 1 diabetes on 10-year progression of retinopathy in the DCCT/EDIC: comparison of adults and adolescents. Diabetes 59, 1244-1253.

Williams, C.L., Hayman, L.L., Daniels, S.R., Robinson, T.N., Steinberger, J., Paridon, S., and Bazzarre, T. (2002). Cardiovascular health in childhood: A statement for health professionals from the Committee on Atherosclerosis, Hypertension, and Obesity in the Young (AHOY) of the Council on Cardiovascular Disease in the Young, American Heart Association. Circulation 106, 143-160.

Williams, G., and Pickup, J.C. (2004). Diabetic eye disease. (Blackwell Publishing).

10

Type 1 Diabetes Mellitus: Redefining the Future of Cardiovascular Complications with Novel Treatments

Anwar B. Bikhazi, Nadine S. Zwainy, Sawsan M. Al Lafi,
Shushan B. Artinian and Suzan S. Boutary
American University of Beirut,
Lebanon

1. Introduction

Diabetes Mellitus (DM) is a disease that was identified centuries ago, in around 1500 BC (King and Rubin, 2003). The word 'Diabetes' means "running through" (Holt, 2004) which is used to describe the excessive output of urine in this disease. "Mellitus" meaning "sweet" identifies the nature of the urine in patients suffering from DM (Widmaier *et al.*, 2004). Thomas Willis was the first to differentiate DM from other polyurias in 1674 (Eknoyan and Nagy, 2005). In 1776, Matthew Dobson demonstrated that the sugar present in the urine was also present in the blood and was associated with its rise (Holt, 2004). In 1848, Claude Bernard's experiments on the liver showed that glycogen stored in the liver produced sugar and he hypothesized that glycogenolysis caused the disease. Although his discovery that "sugar production is a normal function of the animal" was revolutionary, it did not quite explain the etiology of the disease. In 1889, Oskar Minkowski confirmed that the ablation of the pancreas in dogs resulted in DM (Farmer, 1952). Frederick Banting and Charles Best were the medical scientists that discovered insulin, later in 1921, the lack of which, it was made clear, caused DM (Voet and Voet, 2004). They used the extract of a dog's fresh pancreas and demonstrated that upon administration of 10mL of extract to blood, blood glucose level is decreased from 0.3% to 0.17% (Rosenfeld, 2002). Some 30 years later, in 1953, Frederick Sanger was able to determine the complete amino acid sequence of the protein for the first time in history (Boron and Boulpaep, 2009).

Today, DM is defined as a carbohydrate disorder characterized by impaired insulin secretion and/or peripheral insulin resistance leading to hyperglycemia (Beers and Berkow. 1999). It is considered to be the third leading cause of death after heart disease and cancer in the United States (Voet and Voet, 2004) and its incidence is expected to rise to 366 million people by the year 2030 (Wild *et al.*, 2004).

Diabetic patients have symptoms such as, thirst, polyuria, blurring of vision and weight loss. In extreme cases, ketoacidosis may develop leading to coma and ultimately death (Alberti and Zimmet, 1998). Diabetes Mellitus is classified according to etiology to two major types:

1.1 Type 1 diabetes mellitus

Although both type 1 Diabetes Mellitus (type 1 DM) and type 2 Diabetes Mellitus (type 2 DM) are characterized clinically by hyperglycemia, they have their differences. Type 1 DM occurs commonly during childhood or adolescence therefore also named juvenile onset DM and may develop diabetic ketoacidosis (Beers and Berkow, 1999). Of all diabetes cases, 10% are type 1 DM (Holt, 2004). It includes all autoimmune and idiopathic causes of insulin-secreting β cell destruction resulting in absolute insulin deficiency (Alberti and Zimmet, 1998). The patient is usually genetically predisposed to DM, however, an environmental insult, such as a virus is needed to trigger the pathological process of the disease (Wilson *et al.* 1991). It is evident that CD4+ and CD8+ T lymphocytes are activated in the pancreatic lymph node and later infiltrate the pancreas causing inflammation (insulitis) (Yang and Santamaria, 2003). During this time, the body develops an immune response that sees pancreatic islet cells as 'nonself' and starts destroying its β cells (Wilson *et al.*, 1991). Specific causes of β cell destruction, such as cystic fibrosis or mitochondrial defects, are excluded from this classification (Alberti and Zimmet, 1998). Recently, type 1 DM was subdivided into type 1 A and type 1 B. Type 1A diabetes mellitus is described as a disease with immune mediated, selective destruction of insulin producing β cells, with the presence of anti-islet autoantibodies. Whereas type 1B diabetes mellitus, exhibits inflammation of the pancreas, but lack of anti-islet autoantibodies (Rhoades and Bell, 2009). Patients with type 1 DM require daily subcutaneous insulin administration as a treatment (Seifter *et al.*, 2005). Administration of exogenous insulin cannot be compared to the fine control of minute to minute insulin secretion that the pancreas provides (Hakim, 2002); for that reason, human islet cell transplantation has been accepted and applied as an alternative treatment for patients with type 1 DM (George, 2009).

1.2 Type 2 diabetes mellitus

Type 2 DM is also known "Adult-onset Diabetes" (Beers *et al.*, 2006), and represents 90-95% of diabetic patients (Creager *et al.*, 2003; Seifter *et al.*, 2005). This percentage is expected to increase in the year of 2025 to reach 300 million diabetic patients (Rhoades and Bell, 2009) due to sedentary lifestyle and increase in obesity in addition to age progression (Boron and Boulpaep, 2009; King *et al.*, 2005). As the intake of glucose increases insulin secretion is elevated. After a while, insulin secretion becomes inadequate due to peripheral resistance of insulin receptors (Beers *et al.*, 2006; King *et al.*, 2005). Insulin resistance decreases glucose-mediated insulin transport and metabolism (Rhoades and Bell, 2009), resulting in a defect of the compensatory insulin secretion (Mcphee *et al.*, 2008). It is worth noting that in type 2 DM reactive oxygen species are generated resulting in endothelial dysfunction, cardiovascular complications and renal disease (Hayashi *et al.*, 2010; Seifter *et al.*, 2005).

Insulin resistance develops when insulin signaling pathway is interfered in adipose, skeletal and hepatic cells (Seifter *et al.*, 2005). As a result of insulin resistance, glucose transport inside adipocytes and skeletal muscle is reduced and the suppression of glucose output from the liver is impaired. (Rhoades and Bell, 2009)

2. Complications of diabetes mellitus

Chronic hyperglycemia causes blood vessels injury (Seifter *et al.*, 2005) which is divided into two types depending on the size of vessels injured. Small vessels injury in diabetes is a microvascular complication whereas injury of large blood vessels determines a macrovascular complication (Hayashi *et al.*, 2010, Kalani, 2008). Microvascular and macrovascular complications occur in DM both types 1 and 2 (Retenakaran and Zinman,

2008; Rhoades and Bell, 2009). These injuries cause on the long run acceleration in atherosclerotic formation (Seifter *et al.*, 2005). In type 1 diabetic patients, hyperglycemia has been correlated with a variety of events in cardiovascular pathology, initiated with endothelial dysfunction and progressed to develop arterial stiffness (Tabit *et al.*, 2010). Thus, a relation has been clearly established to link glycemia with cardiovascular events in type 1 DM, based on the fact that glycemia itself is the only factor mediating a risk factor for cardiovascular risk in the absence of other risk factors (Retenakaran and Zinman, 2008). One way of reducing cardiovascular risk and renal outcomes in type 1 DM is to initiate an early intensive therapy for its management.

2.1 Microvascular complications
Microvascular complications include nephropathy, retinopathy and neuropathy (Coccheri, 2007; Fowler, 2008; Seifter *et al.*, 2005). There is a direct clinical practice to link these complications with DM type 1 rather than type 2 (Retenakaran and Zinman, 2008). Of note, type 2 DM may manifest development of microvascular complication 7 years preceding diagnosis (King *et al.*, 2005).

2.2 Macrovascular complications
These define the pathophysiology of cardiac disease in type 1 DM which includes atherosclerosis, coronary artery diseases, stroke and peripheral arterial disease (Retenakaran and Zinman, 2008; Seifter *et al.*, 2005). These cardiovascular complications are mostly focused in clinical practice to type 2 DM (Fowler, 2008), and increased in rate as well in type 1 DM (Mcphee *et al.*, 2008); however, the mortality impact of cardiovascular diseases in both DM types 1 and 2 is similar (Juutilainen *et al.*, 2008) contributing to 80 % of the mortality and morbidity (Coccheri, 2007). More alarmingly, development of macrovascular complication might not manifest in type 1 DM until 10 years proceeding diagnosis (King *et al.*, 2005).

Endothelial and smooth muscle dysfunction has been associated with type 1 diabetic patients, which in turn might cause hypertension, a major risk factor for developing cardiovascular diseases (Retenakaran and Zinman, 2008). Also lipid abnormalities in type 1 DM, decrease in HDL and increase in LDL compositions, are being incidents of causing cardiovascular diseases (Retenakaran and Zinman, 2008). High levels of ketone bodies are produced from the body as an alternate fuel in the absence of glucose as a main source of energy in severe starving conditions, mainly hyperglycemia (Seifter *et al.*, 2005), or an acute multiplication of type 1 but not type 2 DM (Rhoades and Bell, 2009). Three types of ketones can be generated in the body these are acetone whose odor can be detected overtly *via* breath, acetacetic acid and β-hydroxybutyric acid whose levels may elevate in the blood and be excreted in urine, which is followed by cations and fluid loss ultimately leading to coma (Rhoades and Bell, 2009).

3. Renin angiotensin system
With the discovery of renin in 1898, Robert Tigerstedt and Per Bergman were able to fill a gap present in the understanding of fluid balance, hypertension and cardiovascular disease (Basso and Terragno, 2001; Phillips and Schmidt-Ott, 1999). The Renin Angiotensin System (RAS) plays an important role in maintaining normal blood volume and blood pressure. When salt and water intake is reduced, the role of RAS becomes critical (Rhoades and Bell, 2008). Upon low plasma volume, intrarenal baroreceptors found in the afferent arteriole

walls sense a decrease in stretch and neighboring granular cells increase renin synthesis and release (Boron and Boulpaep, 2009). The granular cells of the juxtaglomerular apparatus of the kidney produce renin (Widmaier *et al.*, 2004). At first, preprorenin is synthesized in the granular cells; its 23 amino acid signal peptide is then cleaved to form prorenin (Sepehrdad *et al.*, 2007). This proenzyme undergoes further modification- clipping the 43 amino acid segment from the N-terminal – to produce renin (Pool, 2007). Despite the conversion of prorenin to renin, prorenin remains the predominant form in the systemic circulation and represents 90% of the total plasma renin in humans (Pimenta and Oparil, 2009). Renin belongs to the family of aspartyl proteases, including pepsin, cathepsin D and chymosin (Verdeccia *et al.*, 2008). Unlike other aspartyl proteases however, renin is able to work at neutral pH. Moreover, renin is specific for one substrate only- angiotensinogen (Sepehrdad *et al.*, 2007). Made up of two lobes with a cleft in between renin accommodates the liver-derived angiotensinogen in its active site, where a peptide bond of angiotensinogen is hydrolyzed and the decapeptide Angiotensin I (Ang I) is released (Verdeccia *et al.*, 2008). Furthermore, this conversion is catalyzed 4-fold upon the binding of renin to its receptor (Pool, 2007). Angiotensin converting enzyme (ACE) is the principal enzyme that converts Ang I to the octapeptide Ang II (60% conversion); some other enzymes such as chymases, cathepsin G and other serine proteases account for the rest of the conversion (Weir, 2007).

3.1 Cross talk between RAS and IItus

Angiotensin II was always considered in close proximity with diseases and vascular complications. This is implied from data linking high levels of Ang II to DM and vasoconstriction (causing hypertension) (Karam *et al.*, 2005), in addition to glomerular damaging ending up with nephropathy (Coccheri, 2007). Other than its direct effect as a potent vasoconstrictor, it was denoted to alter Endothelin-1 (ET-1) production (Karam *et al.*, 2005), remodel cardiovascular structure (Parmar and Jadav, 2007), modulate heart and vessels (Nuwayri-salti *et al.*, 2007), augment transforming growth factor–beta (TGF-β) and boost proliferative and inflammatory events (Wiggins and Kelly, 2009). In conjunction; modulation of insulin significance is obtained (Karam *et al.*, 2005), either by directly halting signaling mechanism of insulin per se or damaging structure and function of β-cells *via* local pancreatic RAS (Coccheri, 2007). Angiotensin II has 2 receptors: Ang II Type 1 receptor (AT1R) and Ang II Type 2 receptor (AT2R). But until now AT1R rather than AT2R is assessed in the pathophysiology (Karam *et al.*, 2005; Rao, 2010) directing therapeutic agents either to target Ang II formation or block its binding to AT1R *via* Angiotensin converting enzyme inhibitors (ACEIs) and Ang II Receptor Blocker(ARB) respectively (Karam *et al.*, 2005). AT1R blockers improved vascular smooth muscle cell vasoconstriction and declined the hypertrophy of cardiomyocytes (CM) counteracting Ang II deleterious effect (Al Jaroudi *et al.*, 2005) once bound to the G-coupled protein receptor (AT1 R) (Parmar and Jadav, 2007; Wiggins and Kelly, 2009). Quite interestingly, ACEIs ameliorated insulin sensitivity and mitigated new onset of DM type 2 (Hadi and Suwaidi, 2007; Scheen, 2004). Pooled together, these G-coupled transmembrane proteins mimic insulin receptor action (Nuwayri-Salti *et al.*, 2007). Among several evidences, AT2R is more related to apoptotic actions thereby antagonizing insulin's growth effect, resulting in one way or another to boost cardiac hypertrophy mainly in type 1 DM (Al Jaroudi *et al.*, 2005). To complete this picture, a balance should be assured between both Ang II receptors to modulate a normal cardiac status in type 1 DM along the endothelial cells and cardiomyocytes (Al Jaroudi *et al.*, 2005).

The idea of blocking RAS at its point of origin was initiated around 50 years ago (Pool, 2007). The origin of these direct renin inhibitors (DRIs) was either analogues of the prosegment peptide of renin or of the AGT's N-terminal amino acid sequence (Gradman and Kad, 2008). Many peptidomimetic synthetic drugs used for renin inhibition have been launched including pepsatitn (the first renin inhibtor) and other oral drugs, including remikiren, enalkiren and zankiren (Pimenta and Oparil, 2009), but their low efficiency related to large molecular size, first-pass metabolism, incomplete intestinal absorption, hydrophobicity and short half-lives attributed their poor oral activity and bioavailability, besides the high production cost (Pool, 2007; Waldmeier *et al.*, 2007). The drug Tekturna® (United States) or Rasilez® (Europe) , known with the generic name of Aliskiren, ascribed to Dr. Alice Huxley (Gradman and Kad, 2008), manufactured by Novartis Pharmaceuticals, was the first of the nonpeptide DRIs to be approved by the Food and Drug Administration (FDA) (Azizi, 2008). Thereby becoming the commercially available renin blocker in markets, prescribed through United States and Canada for an effective essential hypertension treatment in March 2007 (Azizi, 2008), and approved by European Medicine Agency (EMEA) in August 2007 (Pool, 2007; Azizi, 2008).

4. Endothelin system

In 1985, Hickey *et al.* discovered a potent vasoconstricting substance from cultured endothelial cells and named it endotensin or endothelial contracting factor. Later on, Yanagisawa *et al.* isolated the same substance from cultured porcine aortic and endothelial cells and renamed it endothelin. Endothelin (ET) is a naturally occurring polypeptide (Prasad *et al.*, 2009) produced by the endothelium (Shah et al.,2009; Wikes et al., 2003; Ying wu, 2003) and consists of 21 amino acids. It is present in three isoforms ET-1, ET-2 and ET-3 (Agapitov *et al.*, 2002; Prasad *et al.*, 2009). These three isoforms are encoded by different genes but have similar structure and function (Wilkes *et al.*, 2003). They have conserved sequences of amino acids mainly at the 6 C terminus and 4 cysteine residues that form 2 disulfide bridges between residues 1 to 15 and 3 to 11 and the main difference is at the N-terminus (Prasad *et al.*, 2009). They are vasoconstrictors synthesized by vascular, right atrial and left ventricular endothelial cells, vascular smooth muscle cells and fibromyocytes. In addition, they are synthesized in extra vascular tissues such as the lungs, spleen, pancreas and nervous system (Penna *et al.*, 2006). All studies done on endothelial systems focused on ET-1, because represents the majority of the circulating endothelins (Prasad *et al.*, 2009; Schneider *et al.*, 2002) and has important role in the regulation of the cardiovascular system (Penna *et al.*, 2006; Prasad *et al.*, 2009).

4.1 Endothelin-1

Endothelin-1 is the most common isoform correlated with the cardiovascular system (Kalani, 2008). It was identified in the late 1980s by Dr. Yanagisawa and his colleagues and found to be a very potent vasoconstrictor (Prasad *et al.*, 2009; Steiner and Preston, 2008; Thorin and Webb, 2009). It has ionotropic, chemotactic and mitogenic activities. It influences salt and water retention through its effect on RAS, vasopressin release and stimulation of sympathetic nervous system. So the ultimate role of ET-1 is to increase blood pressure (Agapitov *et al.*, 2002) and to maintain vascular tone (Thorin and Webb, 2009). It is produced mostly from endothelial cells in addition to fibroblasts, cardiacmyocytes (Agapitov *et al.*,

2002; Schorlemmer *et al.*, 2008), leukocytes, macrophages (Thorin and Webb, 2009), kidney, central nervous system and posterior pituitary (Agapitov *et al.*, 2002).

Endothelin-1 exerts a paracrine/autocrine effect. In the circulation, the levels of ET-1 are in picomolars lower than that needed to cause vasoconstriction (Prasad *et al.*, 2009). Also endothelial cells secrete more ET-1 toward the vicinity of vascular smooth muscle cells than into the lumen of the blood vessels (Agapitov *et al.*, 2002).

4.2 Endothelin-1 synthesis and clearance

Endothelin-1 synthesis begins with the cleavage of a 200 amino acid peptide called pre-proendothelin-1 (preproET-1) to form preendothelin-1 (preET-1) (Agapitov *et al.*, 2002; Penna *et al.*, 2006). PreET-1 is then cleaved by furin endopeptidase to form big endothelin-1 (big ET-1) of 38-39 amino acids that is further metabolized by Endothelin Converting Enzyme-1 (ECE-1) to generate ET-1 of 21 amino acids (Agapitov *et al.*, 2002; Penna *et al.*, 2006). Moreover, chymase enzyme was found to produce ET(1-31) by breaking down big ET-1 at Tyr31-Gly32 bond (Agapitov *et al.*, 2002).

Furthermore, the regulation of ET-1 synthesis is at the gene level which means at the level of ET-1 messenger RNA (mRNA). The ET-1 mRNA is up-regulated by several factors including: interleukins, insulin, Ang II, tumor necrosis factor alpha and growth factor while it is down regulated by hypoxia, shear stress and nitric oxide (Thorin and Webb, 2009). The clearance of ET-1 from the plasma involves different mechanisms including: (1) endocytosis in the lungs, (2) enzymatic degradation in the liver and the kidney and (3) ET-1 binding to ET_B receptor thus forming ET_B Receptor-Legand complex that is broken down by endocytosis (Kalani, 2008).

4.3 Cross talk between endothelin system and renin angiotensin system

The Renin Angiotensin and the Endothelin Systems are the most potent identified vasoconstrictory systems and has been suggested to be correlated with each other (Rossi *et al.*, 1999; McEwan *et al.*, 2000). This was demonstrated by several cell culture studies in cardiac fibroblasts. These studies showed that AngII increases preproET-1 mRNA expression, ET-1 levels and thus causes cardiomyocyte hypertrophy through regulation of $ET_A R$. Also increased levels of $ET_B R$ via Ang II have also been identified in cultured CM (McEwan *et al.*, 2000).

The potential sites at which RAS increases ET-1 levels may be at the preproET-1 gene that possesses a *jun* sequence which is defined as the regulatory region of preproET-1. It is the site at which transcriptional regulation takes place by factors acting through G-protein-phospholipase and C-protein kinase C pathway. Another site for interaction of RAS and ET system is at the chymase enzyme which is abundant in the myocardium where it was found to produce ET (1-31) from big ETs, bearing in mind that the main function of chymase enzyme in the heart is to produce Ang II from Ang I (Rossi *et al.*, 1999). Therefore, elevated levels of ET-1 can be reduced by blocking the RAS system. Studies on patients suffering from hypertension or diabetes showed decrease in the level of ET-1 when ACEI was administered (Schneider *et al.*, 2002).

Therapies targeting these complications include the use of ARBs which proved their value as antihypertensive drugs. Losartan, an ARB, was found to decrease the destructive changes caused by Ang II on cardiac muscle beside its (Berk, 1999; Fiordaliso *et al.*, 2000) capacity to reduce blood pressure. Recently, Al Jaroudi *et al.* proved that losartan in diabetic normotensive rats supplemented with insulin was able to prevent nearly totally myocardial degeneration caused by diabetes (Al Jaroudi *et al.*, 2005) (Fig. 1).

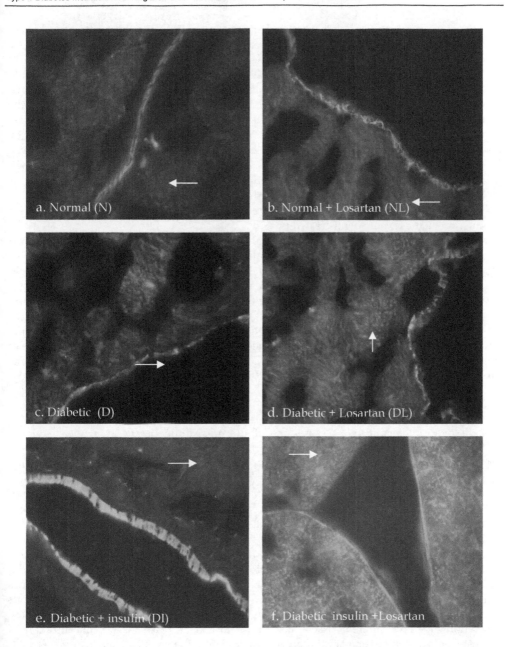

Fig. 1. Indirect immunofluorescence of CM and vascular endothelium from the different rat groups depicting insulin receptors. Noted is the increase of fluorescence in the NL group (Fig. b) when compared to the normal (N) (Fig. a) at the myocytes (arrow). There is also increase fluorescence of the myocytes of the (DL) group as compared to the (D) group, and of the (DIL) group as compared to the (DI) group (arrow).

Later, Karam *et al.* reported that the supplementation with insulin and administration of pharmacologic doses of losartan could improve cardiac contraction as well as coronary blood flow in the same normotensive rat model for type 1 DM as the one used by Jaroudi *et al.* through the modification of the affinity of ET type 1 receptor subtypes ET_AR and ET_BR to ET-1, a potent vasoconstrictor largely stimulated by Ang II (Karam *et al.*, 2005). In fact, Kakoki *et al.* have demonstrated that the ET_BRs are down-regulated by Ang II in the endothelial cells of the renal artery of diabetic rats through stimulation of increased ET-1 production (Kakoki *et al.*, 1999). On the other hand, these effects of Ang II are prevented by the ACE inhibitor Imidapril (Kakoki *et al.*, 1999). ACE inhibitors reduced also the plasma ET-1 levels in type 1 DM (Schneider *et al.*, 2002). Administration of Losartan to Ang II-treated rats restored the vasoconstrictive effect of ET-1 and decreased its tissue levels (D'Uscio *et al.*, 1997). Mc Ewan *et al.* showed that the blockade of the AT1Rs by Losartan, in the presence of a high plasma Ang II levels, is accompanied by an increase in ET-1 production by the CM of Ang II-treated rats.

In addition to this, an increase in the ET_BRs mRNA but a decrease in the ET_ARs mRNA was also noted (Mc Ewan *et al.*, 2000). On the other hand, treatment with the selective ET_AR blocker LU135252 normalized the increased ET-1 level in the aorta, femoral artery and kidney, and the ECE activity in isolated aorta and femoral artery of rats treated with Ang II (Barton *et al.*, 1997). In cultured heart endothelial cells, Ang II stimulates ppET-1 mRNA and ET-1 production via Protein Kinase C (PKC) - dependent pathway. Calphostin, a PKC inhibitor, blocks Ang II effects (Chua *et al.*, 1993). Taken together, these results show that the ET and the RA systems are related to each other. They also demonstrate the beneficial role of ARBs and ACE inhibitors in the amelioration of the blood flow which can be altered in some disease states due to the ET-1 and Ang II constrictor effects.

5. Insulin

The discovery of insulin in 1921 was one of the most dramatic events in the history of diabetes therapy. Insulin is a small globular protein comprising of two polypeptide chains A (21 amino acid residues) and B (30 amino acid residues) held together by two disulfide bonds (Docherty and Steiner. 2003; Joshi *et al.* 2007). It is produced in the β-cells of the islets of Langerhans in the form of preproinsulin which is rapidly cleaved by the action of proteolytic enzymes into proinsulin. Further catalysis of proinsulin results in insulin and a 31 amino acid connecting peptide, C-peptide, both of which are stored for secretion in secretory vesicles in β-cells (Docherty and Steiner. 2003). The biosynthesis and secretion of insulin by β-cells primarily occurs in response to increased circulating glucose levels. During feeding, elevated glucose concentrations in the blood increase the plasma insulin level, which facilitates glucose uptake through GLUT-4 into muscle tissues for utilization as a source of energy and into adipose tissues for synthesis of glycerol. Insulin also exerts its action on liver cells as well thus promoting glycogen formation. Consequently, glucose utilization by these different tissues contribute to the decrease in the concentration of glucose in blood. On top of its profound effect in carbohydrate metabolism, insulin has a fat-sparing effect. Not only does it promote the synthesis of fatty acids in the liver, it also inhibits the breakdown of fats in adipose tissue thereby inducing fat accumulation. Hence, insulin is the major determinant of carbohydrate and lipid metabolism and has significant effects on protein metabolism. Insulin acts by binding to a receptor molecule embedded in the plasma membrane of its target tissues (Docherty and Steiner. 2003).

5.1 Insulin receptor

Insulin receptor is a member of the receptor tyrosine kinase family (De Meyts and Whittaker, 2002; Kanzaki, 2006; Klarlund et al., 2003; Lawrence et al., 2007; Stern, 1995; Ward et al., 2008). It is a large cell-surface multi-domain glycoprotein that consists of two extracellular α-subunits (MW~125 kDa) and two transmembrane β-subunits (MW~95 kDa) (Kanzaki, 2006; Klarlund et al., 2003; Lawrence et al., 2007; Stern, 1995; Ward et al., 2008) linked by disulfide bonds (Kanzaki, 2006; Lawrence et al., 2007) into an $\alpha_2\beta_2$ heterotetrameric complex (Kanzaki, 2006). Extracellular α-subunits contain the insulin-binding site (Klarlund et al., 2003) while intracellularly transmembrane β-subunits contain the insulin-regulated tyrosine kinase catalytic domain (De Meyts and Whittaker, 2002; Klarlund et al., 2003; Ward et al., 2008). Two nearly identical isoforms (A and B) of the insulin receptor exist due to tissue specific alternative splicing of the receptor m-RNA at exon 11. Isoforms A and B differ by the presence or absence of a 12 amino acid sequence at the carboxyl-terminus of the α-subunit (Anderson et al. 1993; De Meyts and Whittaker. 2002; Klarlund et al., 2003; Lawrence et al., 2007). Despite the known biochemical and physiologic differences of these isoforms, changes in their expression levels have not been consistently found in patients with DM (Klarlund et al., 2003). Once insulin binds to the α-subunit of the insulin receptor, it induces a conformational change in the receptor that subsequently leads to the stimulation of the intrinsic tyrosine kinase activity in the β-subunits (Kanzaki, 2006; Klarlund et al., 2003; Stern, 1995). This results in the transfer of phosphate groups from ATP to several tyrosine residues on the insulin receptor itself as well as phosphorylation of cellular proteins such as insulin receptor substrate-1 (IRS-1) and Shc (Klarlund et al., 2003; Stern, 1995). The stimulation of the receptor tyrosine kinase allows transmission of the insulin signal to metabolic pathways such as glucose uptake upon translocation of GLUT-4 glucose transporters to the plasma membrane, glycogen synthesis, protein synthesis, and lipid metabolism within the cell. The various biological responses generated upon insulin receptor activation through insulin binding granted insulin a role in DM treatment due to its glucose lowering effects. Nevertheless, daily insulin injections continue to be a treatment for diabetic patients since 1922 despite the increasing worldwide prevalence of this disease (Sparre et al., 2005). Furthermore, insulin treatment dramatically prolongs survival, but does not cure diabetes (Myers and Zonszein, 2002). Insulin treatment does not seem to be beneficial for many patients and is associated with weight gain, hypoglycemia, and failure of their glycemic control (Halimi, 2008). Therefore, new treatment modalities are intensively studied mainly the incretins, exemplified by GLP-1.

6. Definition of incretins

The intravenous infusion of glucose at a constant rate results in a biphasic insulin secretory response, in which the first peak rises rapidly followed by a slower second peak. In contrast, an oral administration of glucose followed by its gastrointestinal absorption, triggers a hormonal pathway that eventually leads to a far greater response of insulin secretion which can last as long as glucose is administered. This phenomenon is termed as the 'Incretin Effect' (Rhoades and Bell, 2008).

Incretins are hormones that are secreted by the gut upon feeding; their release alerts the pancreatic islets that nutrients will come through the gastrointestinal tract and islets start priming by vagal stimulation (Boron and Boulpaep, 2009). Glucagon-Like Peptide-1 (GLP-1) and Glucose Dependent Insulinotropic Peptide (GIP) are the major incretin hormones produced by the L cells of the ileum and colon, and K cells of the duodenum and jejunum, respectively (Inzucchi and McGuire, 2008).

6.1 Synthesis of glucagon-like peptide-1

The proglucagon gene, located on chromosome 2 in humans, has the coding sequence of GLP-1. Pancreatic α-cells, intestinal L-cells and neural cells in the caudal brainstem and hypothalamus, express the proglucagon gene (Baggio and Drucker, 2007) and the mRNAs produced in the pancreas and intestine are identical. Its post-translational processing, however, differs in the two tissues. The post translational processing of proglucagon in pancreatic α- cells results in Glucagon, Glicentin-Related Pancreatic Polypeptide (GRPP), Intervening peptide-1 (IP-1) and the major proglucagon fragment (MPGF) (Holst, 2007). The latter codes for the production of GLP-1 (1-36 amide) and GLP-1 (1-37) and GLP-2 in the pancreas (Hui *et al.*, 2005). Whereas the intestinal L and brain cells produce GLP-1 (7-36 amide), GLP-1 (7-37), GLP-2, IP-2, and glicentin that if further cleaved produces GRPP and oxyntomodulin (Holst, 2007). The enzyme prohormone convertase (PC) 1/3 cleaves proglucagon to generate GLP-1 (Shin *et al.*, 2008). GLP-1 is an incretin hormone produced primarily by the L-cells in the mucosa of the ileum and the colon (Mannucci and Rotella, 2008). Small neurons found in the Nucleus Tractus Solitarius (NTS), caudal brainstem, also produce GLP-1 that plays the role of a neuromodulator (Berthoud, 2009). The central nucleus of the amygdala (CeA) and the paraventricular nucleus of the hypothalamus (PVN) are also sites of GLP-1 production (Kinzig *et al.*, 2002).

Recently, GLP-1 production was shown to exist in taste bud cells (Shin *et al.*, 2008; Berthoud, 2009) and in particular in α-gustducin and the sweet taste receptor subunit T1R3, that play an important role in mediating the glucose dependent secretion of GLP-1 (Shin *et al.*, 2008). GLP-1 is usually present in the circulation minutes after meal intake- far before food reaches the L-cells in the gut. Hence, its stimulation is believed to be controlled by both endocrine and neural signals (Drucker, 2007). The two active forms of GLP-1 are the 30 amino acid GLP-1 (7-36) amide and the 31 amino acid glycine extended GLP-1 (7-37) (Ban *et al.*, 2009; Mannucci and Rotella, 2008). GLP-1 (7-36) amide is far more abundant than GLP-1 (7-37) in the circulation (Manucci and Rotella, 2008), but both have short half-lives (1.5-2 minutes) (Hui *et al.*, 2002). They are rapidly degraded into their inactive forms, GLP-1(9-36) amide and GLP-1 (9-37), respectively, by the enzyme Dipeptidyl-Peptidase-IV (DPP-IV) (Mannucci and Rotella, 2008) and eliminated through renal clearance (Hui *et al.*, 2002).

6.2 Effects of GLP-1

GLP-1 has numerous effects on glucose homeostasis. Upon interaction with its receptor on β-cells, GLP-1 increases the intracellular levels of cAMP and calcium, thereby releasing insulin (Drucker, 2007). Furthermore, sustained GLP-1 receptor (GLP-1R) signaling leads to enhanced gene transcription, insulin biosynthesis and β-cell proliferation (Elahi *et al.*, 2008; Drucker, 2007). GLP-1 was shown to increase the expression of glucose transporter 2 (GLUT2) (Elahi *et al.*, 2008), a hepatic glucose transporter that facilitates glucose transport in or out of the liver regulated by insulin (Eisenberg *et al.*, 2005) and glucokinase (Elahi *et al.*, 2008) the enzyme that phosphorylates glucose to glucose-6-phosphate (G6P) (Voet and Voet, 2004). GLP-1 has also inhibitory effects on Glucagon secretion from the α-cells, gastric emptying and food ingestion (Drucker, 2007). The role of GLP-1 in relaxing the proximal stomach and increasing gastric capacity has been demonstrated (D'Alessio and Vahl, 2004).

GLP-1 also exerts effects on the central nervous system: it promotes satiety and weight loss, inhibits food and water intake and improves memory and neuronal survival (Mannucci and Rotella, 2008; Drucker, 2007).

6.3 GLP-1 receptor

The GLP-1R belongs to the Guanine Nucleotide-Binding Protein (G-protein) coupled receptor family (GPCR) (Drucker, 2007). This seven transmembrane receptor protein is 90% identical to the rat GLP-1R and shows a 95% homology in amino acid. Its gene is found on the long arm of chromosome 6p21 in humans (Doyle and Egan, 2007). GLP-1 receptor is made up of 463 amino acid residues and has a molecular weight of approximately 65 kDa (Hui *et al.*, 2005). GLP-1 receptors are expressed in many tissues including, the central and peripheral nervous systems, heart, kidney, lungs and the gastrointestinal tract (Drucker and Nauk, 2006).

However, GLP-1 receptor expression in the pancreas is controversial. Studies have confirmed the detection of GLP-1 receptors in α, β and δ cells of the islets of Langerhans, whereas other studies indicate their expression exclusively in β cells (Doyle and Egan, 2007). In the heart, GLP-1 receptor expression was shown to exist in CM, microvascular endothelium, coronary smooth muscle cells and the highest in endocardium. In cardiac fibroblasts, however, there was no evidence in GLP-1R expression (Ban *et al.*, 2009). Low detection of GLP-1 receptor gene expression proves the existence of GLP-1 receptor in liver and muscles (MacDonald *et al.*, 2002). Abundant GLP-1R specific transcripts were found in lungs and detectable amounts in the heart (Ban *et al.*, 2009). When fragments of the N-terminus are denatured, GLP-1R loses its affinity for GLP-1. This asserts that GLP-1 receptor's N-terminus plays an important role in recognizing and binding of the GLP-1 (Doyle and Egan. 2007). Upon binding of the GLP-1 to its receptor numerous signaling messengers are activated; first, GLP-1 receptor can couple to G proteins, including $G\alpha_s$, $G\alpha_q$, $G\alpha_i$ or $G\alpha_o$ (Baggio and Drucker, 2007). Adenylate cyclase uses ATP to form cAMP via the stimulatory G protein. Following the increase of cAMP is a chain of events is triggered: ATP-sensitive K^+ channels shut and L-type voltage gated Ca^{2+} channels open; together with the efflux of Ca^{2+} molecules from intracellular Ca^{2+} stores, these ion channel alterations result in a subsequent intracellular rise in Ca^{2+} ions (Gomez *et al.*, 2002) and the ultimate exocytosis of granules that contain insulin. A sustained receptor signaling results in the activation of Protein Kinase A (PKA), gene transcription, insulin biosynthesis and β-cell proliferation (Drucker and Nauk, 2006). Additionally, the binding of GLP-1 to its receptor activates protein kinase B, which is linked to glucose transporting in muscles, glycogen synthesis and lipolysis in various tissues (Peyot *et al.*, 2009).

6.4 GLP-1 in diabetes mellitus and the heart

A recent study showed that GLP-1 receptor expression is downregulated in β-cells exposed to high glucose concentrations in vitro and hyperglycemia in vivo (Xu *et al.*, 2007). Diabetic individuals' β-cells exhibit attenuated sensitivity to GLP-1. In both type 1 and type 2 DM, there is a marked reduction in the incretin effect (Knop *et al.*, 2007). On the other hand, a study reported that GLP-1 levels are not decreased in type 2 diabetic patients (Lee *et al.*, 2010). The European GLP-1 Club held a meeting recently and debated this controversial issue and came to a conclusion that more data is required to determine the exact effect of DM on GLP-1 secretion from L-cells (Burcelin, 2008). GLP-1 has been suggested to ameliorate left ventricular function, because of its antiapoptotic and insulin-like properties (Inzucchi and McGuire, 2008). In fact, one study confirmed that GLP-1 enhances the regulation of phosphatydil inositol 3 kinase (PI3K), that plays a key role in activating the antiapoptotic pathway, thus promoting cardioprotection in the ischemic rat hearts. Therefore, a direct effect of GLP-1 against apoptosis in cardiac cells is possible (Bose *et al.*, 2005).

6.5 Dipeptidyl-peptidase IV

DPP-IV grasped a great deal of the interest of the scientific, pharmaceutical, and medical community (Lambeir *et al.*, 2003). Every year, an increasing number of publications tend to elucidate the diverse compelling questions concerning the various properties of DPP-IV and its multiple functions in the different fields of Biology (Lambeir *et al.*, 2003). DPP-IV is a 766 amino acid serine protease that belongs to the prolyloligopeptidase family. It is a widely distributed cell surface peptidase expressed to different degrees in a variety of tissues such as the kidney, intestine, liver, placenta, uterus, prostate, skin, and capillary endothelium. Another soluble form of DPP-IV (sDPP-IV) also exists in the plasma and other body fluids (Drucker, 2007; Idris and Donnelly, 2007; Lambeir *et al.*, 2003). This proteolytic enzyme acts by specifically cleaving the N-terminal dipeptide of peptide hormones containing proline or alanine in the second position (Drucker, 2007; Idris and Donnelly, 2007; Lambeir *et al.*, 2003). Hence, DPP-IV truncates several biologically active peptides of medical importance. Furthermore, it has been implicated in glucose homeostasis through proteolytic degradation of the incretins (Drucker, 2007). In the case of GLP-1(7-36), proline and alanine are key determinants in incretin receptor activation therefore DPP-IV-mediated proteolysis results in the biologically inactive truncated molecules GLP-1(9-36) (Drucker, 2007; Idris and Donnelly, 2007). DPP-IV is a critical determinant of incretin inactivation (Drucker, 2007). Thus chemical inhibition of DPP-IV activity results in increased level of biologically active GLP-1 (Drucker, 2007). Therefore, extensive research studies were carried to create highly selective DPP-IV inhibitors.

6.6 DPP-IV inhibitors

DPP-IV inhibitors can be used as a potential treatment for diabetes due to their capability to potentiate the levels of active incretins (Lambeir *et al.*, 2003; Halimi, 2008; Inzucchi and McGuire, 2008) by reducing the enzymatic activity of DPP-IV by more than 80% for duration up to 24 hours (Inzucchi and McGuire, 2008). Oral inhibitors of DPP-IV reduce glycosylated hemoglobin (HbA$_{1C}$) (Drucker, 2007; Halimi, 2008; Moritoh *et al.*, 2008). Various studies reported the multiple metabolic effects of DPP-IV inhibitors including enhancement of glucose-dependent stimulation of pancreatic insulin release as well as attenuation of glucagon secretion (Drucker, 2007; Halimi, 2008; Lambeir *et al.*, 2003; Moritoh *et al.*, 2008). Furthermore, DPP-IV inhibitors demonstrated modestly effective glucose-lowering actions without being associated with hypoglycemia (Halimi, 2008; Lambeir *et al.*, 2003; Moritoh *et al.*, 2008) due to the fact that they are remarkably able to specifically end the insulin-secreting effect and glucagon inhibition once glycemic levels are normalized (Halimi, 2008). Moreover, loss of DPP-IV activity is associated with improved glucose tolerance, reduced glycemic excursion following oral glucose challenge, and increased pancreatic insulin content (Drucker, 2007). A cardinal role of DPP-IV inhibitors is their potential to significantly augment β-cell mass in streptozotocin (STZ)-injected diabetic rats (Moritoh *et al.*, 2008) and enhance pancreatic islet cell function in animal models of type 2 diabetes and in diabetic patients (Lambeir *et al.*, 2003). In contrast to GLP-1 mimetics, there are no data indicating inhibition of gastric emptying or appetite or weight reduction due to a treatment with DPP-IV inhibitors (Inzucchi and McGuire, 2008). Thus, chronic treatment with orally administered DPP-IV inhibitors has neutral effects on body weight and food consumption (Halimi, 2008).

6.7 GLP-1 receptor agonists and GLP-1 analogues

In April 2005, the FDA approved the subcutaneous injectable exenatide with the brand name Byetta® to be launched as a GLP-1 analogue (Inzucchi and McGuire, 2008; Rhoades and Bell, 2009) with longer half life to maintain its glycemic control as diabetic medication (Behme *et al.*, 2003). Exenatide exhibits a half-life of 60-90 minutes and a single injection of exenatide makes its concentration in the blood last for 4-6 hours (Drucker and Nauk, 2006). Exenatide exhibits antidiabetic effects similar to those of GLP-1 and is shown to improve β cell functioning (Baggio and Drucker, 2007). It also reduces the glycated Hemoglobin-HbA1c- levels that reflect mean blood glucose levels of the last 6-8 weeks. In addition, exenatide affects gastric emptying, appetite and consequently causes weight loss (Inzucchi and McGuire, 2008). GLP-1 agonists have exhibited vasodilating and diuretic effects. Recently, Laugero *et al.* showed that Exenatide may display antihypertensive effects mediated by pathways independent from glucose control, but possibly by altering steroid hormones (Laugero *et al.*, 2009).

6.7.1 GLP-1 analogue, exendin-4

The short half-life of GLP-1 limits itself from performing as a good therapeutic agent, as it is rapidly degraded by the serine protease DPP-IV (Hirata *et al.*, 2009). The search for biologically active peptides in lizard venom, led to the discovery of Exendin-4, a naturally occurring GLP-1 analogue (Drucker and Nauk, 2006). Exendin-4 is a peptide naturally found in the saliva of heloderma suspectum - the Gila monster (Laugero *et al.*, 2009; Zhou *et al.*, 2008). Exendin-4 is a peptide made up of 39 amino acid residues that shares a 53% structural homology to GLP-1 (Zhou *et al.*, 2008).This long acting GLP-1 receptor agonist has an N-terminus almost identical to that of the GLP-1, except that the second amino acid residue is glycine in exendin-4 while alanine in GLP-1 (Hui *et al.*, 2005). This one amino acid difference makes it resistant to degradation by the enzyme DPP-IV, hence explaining its long half-life in vivo (Lovshin and Drucker, 2009). Studies have shown that GLP-1 receptor agonists like exendin-4, exhibit cardioprotective effects such as modifications in contractility, cardiac output and blood pressure (Ban *et al.*, 2009).

6.7.2 Mode of action of exendin-4

Endogenous GLP-1 action is inhibited upon degradation by DPP-IV (De Koning *et al.*, 2008; Mann *et al.*, 2007), an enzyme expressed in many organs mainly kidney, small intestine, liver, and lung (Inzucchi and McGuire, 2008). More apt, exendin-4 is synthetic, thus not recognized by DPP-IV enzyme, thereby not degraded (Rhoades and Bell, 2009). This resistance allows it to stay in the circulation longer mimicking GLP-1 role in bolstering insulin secretion but with 5 to 10 times more powerful insulinotrpic effect (Hantouche *et al.*, 2010; Xu *et al.*, 1999). Moreover, it binds to GLP-1R with high affinity even after truncation of the first 8 amino acids at the N-terminal of the peptide unlike the endogenous GLP-1 (Mann *et al.*, 2007). GLP-1R is a G-coupled transmembrane receptor (GPCR) that is found in many organs, most importantly the pancreatic β-cells and ducts, heart, lung, kidneys (Ban *et al.*, 2008), brain and stomach (Hantouche *et al.*, 2010). Conceptual understanding of this receptor delineates its advantages in cardiac management (Ban *et al.*, 2008). On the initiation of treatment, slight adverse effects might arise as nausea and vomiting (Inzucchi and McGuire, 2008), which are dose-dependent and will vanish with time (Mcphee *et al.*, 2008). It can be used efficiently in type 1 DM (Behme *et al.*, 2003) in conjunction with insulin irrespective of hypoglycemic effects attributed to its glucose-dependent action; in spite of insulin low efficiency with type 2 DM (Inzucchi and McGuire, 2008).

6.8 Exendin-4 in the treatment of diabetes mellitus correlated with cardiovascular risk

In conjunction to insulinotropic action of GLP-1 role, exendin-4 also mimics the action of insulin itself, through reinforcing the heart to uptake glucose irrespective of insulin level in both diabetic and non-diabetic cases (Hantouche *et al.*, 2010) STZ-induced diabetic rats acquire cardiomyopathic damage on day 1 starting with apoptosis and ending with hypertrophied hearts (Al Jaroudi *et al.*, 2005), particularly myocardial atrophy (Poornima *et al.*, 2006). Thereby, associated with its glucose lowering effect, certain data emphasized a potential benefit of exendin-4 in recovery of heart failure and function of left ventricle (Inzucchi and McGuire, 2008). Just similar to that of GLP-1 in improving ventricular contractions (Hantouche *et al.*, 2010) upon activation of pancreatic GLP-1R to boost insulin synthesis and secretion (De Koning *et al.*, 2008). Treatment with exendin-4 was concomitant with no cardiovascular complications, inexorable renal progression, or escalating plasma lipid (De Fronzo *et al.*, 2005). In type 2 DM exendin-4 has completed a novel fruition in the arena of organ rejuvenation especially at the level of both α and β cells mass, implementing a new born anti-hyperglycemic drug for solving the diabetes conundrum (Xu *et al.*, 1999). This increase in pancreatic mass happens as a post hoc to β-cells neogenesis from either existing duct cells and/or replication of the already present β-cells (hyperplasia) and not from hypertrophy (escalating cell size) (De Koning *et al.*, 2008). Pooled together, this regimen was found to be concomitant with cardioprotection, judicious vascular and cardiac actions based on the fact that endogenous GLP-1 has the same sequence in humans, rats and mice (Ban *et al.*, 2008). Recently, it was found that exendin-4 ameliorates the sensitivity of insulin receptors towards insulin at both the CM and coronary endothelium (CE) level (Hantouche *et al.*, 2010). This effect is achieved by either enhancing the sensitivity of insulin towards insulin or augmenting β-cells to release more of the hypoglycemic hormone (De Koning *et al.*, 2008). Valuable efficacy of treatment with both exendin-4 and insulin alleviates cardiomypathic regressions associated in type 1 DM at the level of receptor affinity enhancement and insulin secretion bolstering (Hantouche *et al.*, 2010) (Fig. 1 and 2).

Insulin affinity (τ) to its receptor was shown to be decreased in the diabetic state at the level of the CE as compared to normal. Exendin-4 treatment increases insulin receptor affinity at the CE in both diabetic and normal rat groups; whereas insulin tends to normalize the affinity irrespective of exendin-4 absence or presence (Table 1). Exendin-4 treatment probably augments insulin receptor affinity both in normal and diabetic state through exerting its insulinotropic actions (Nikolaidis *et al.*, 2005) and/or by improving insulin sensitivity (Ebinger *et al.*, 2000). The dramatic increase in the affinity of insulin to its receptor in the normal group treated with exendin-4 might be attributed to both of the previously mentioned causes. Yet the rise in insulin receptor affinity in exendin-4-treated diabetic group is not as remarkable as in NE which may be due to the lack of β-cells in diabetic type 1 state thus abolishing the insulinotropic effect of exendin-4.

Rat Group	τ (min) ± SEM
Normal (N)	0.279 ± 0.004 [a']
Normal + Exendin-4 (NE)	0.370 ± 0.007 [b']
Normal + DPP-IV inhibitor (N-Dp)	0.311 ± 0.005 [c']
Diabetic (D)	0.252 ± 0.003 [d']
Diabetic + Insulin (DI)	0.292 ± 0.004 [e']
Diabetic + Exendin-4 (DE)	0.327 ± 0.005 [f]
Diabetic + Insulin + Exendin-4 (DIE)	0.295 ± 0.004 [g']
Diabetic + DPP-IV inhibitor (D-Dp)	0.255 ± 0.003 [h']
Diabetic + Insulin + DPP-IV inhibitor (DI-Dp)	0.321 ± 0.005 [i']

Table 1. The calculated affinity constant (τ) of insulin to its receptor at CE (CHAPS-untreated) in normal and diabetic rats

Rat Group	τ (min) ± SEM
Normal (N)	0.337 ± 0.006 [a']
Normal + Exendin-4 (NE)	0.424 ± 0.009 [b']
Normal + DPP-IV inhibitor (N-Dp)	0.234 ± 0.003 [c']
Diabetic (D)	0.368 ± 0.007 [d']
Diabetic + Insulin (DI)	0.331± 0.006 [e']
Diabetic + Exendin-4 (DE)	0.328 ± 0.005 [f]
Diabetic + Insulin + Exendin-4 (DIE)	0.331 ± 0.006 [g']
Diabetic + DPP-IV inhibitor (D-Dp)	0.376 ± 0.007 [h']
Diabetic + Insulin + DPP-IV inhibitor (DI-Dp)	0.382 ± 0.007 [i']

Table 2. The calculated affinity constant (τ) of insulin to its receptor at CM (CHAPS-treated) in normal and diabetic rats.

Therefore, in diabetes type 1, exendin-4 increases the insulin receptor affinity only by improving insulin sensitivity. As a conclusion, exendin-4 seems to have supplementary effects which might explain the increase in τ value at the level of the CE. First, it augments insulin release from pancreatic β-cells when present in the normal state. This is its insulinotropic effect. Second, it improves insulin sensitivity possibly by inducing a conformational change in the insulin receptor (Ebinger et al., 2000). On the other hand, DPP-IV inhibitor (KR-62436, Sigma Chemical Company) treatment solely does not seem to be implicated in modulating insulin receptor affinity at the endothelial site in diabetic rats treated with DPP-IV inhibitor as compared to diabetics. Yet the effect of DPP-IV inhibitor at the CE becomes obvious in the presence of insulin, as seen in the diabetic group co-treated with insulin and DPP-IV inhibitor (DI-Dp) compared to diabetics (D) and in the normal group treated with DPP-IV inhibitor (N-Dp) with respect to normal. This could be due to some kind of a cross-talk between insulin and DPP-IV inhibitor which results in an increase of τ value in both N-Dp and DI-Dp. Moreover, insulin receptor affinity is not altered at the level of the CM in diabetics treated with DPP-IV inhibitor (D-Dp) and/or insulin (DI-Dp) when compared to diabetic rats (D) (Table 2). The major difference between the CE and CM upon DPP-IV inhibitor treatment could be attributed to the fact that the already limited increase of GLP-1 by DPP-IV inhibitor is primarily imposed on endothelial cells which are the first site of encounter with systemic GLP-1. The difference in affinities observed between DPP-IV inhibitor and exendin-4 treatment might be due to the fact that DPP-IV inhibitor increases the systemically available GLP-1 levels; whereas exendin-4, besides its quantitative systemic effect, has a higher physiologic quality in term of being 5- to 10- fold more potent than GLP-1 (Saraceni and Broderick, 2007).

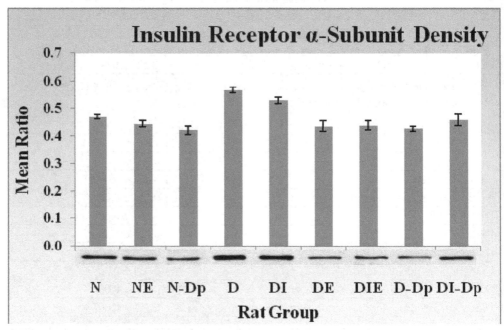

Fig. 2. Insulin receptor α-subunit (MW~125 kDa) density in the heart of the different rat groups.

Western blotting was performed on protein extracts from rat heart homogenates in order to assess the variation in the insulin receptor subunits density among the different treated and untreated normal and diabetic rat groups. Both insulin receptor α-subunit (IR-α) (Fig. 2) and insulin receptor β-subunit (IR-β) (Fig. 3) levels are augmented in diabetic state indicating that there is an increase in the level of cardiac insulin receptor protein in diabetics (D) compared with normal controls (N). These results indicate that cardiac insulin receptors are up-regulated in the heart of diabetic rats as a feedback mechanism probably due to the lack of insulin. This is consistent with the results demonstrated by Al Jaroudi et al. 2005 in the study done on insulin receptor regulation in the diabetic heart. Our results indicate that insulin administration to diabetic rats reduces the number of IR-α and IR-β to near normal values. Interestingly, exendin-4 treatment normalizes insulin receptor subunits density in diabetic rat hearts (Fig. 2 and 3). The regression in insulin receptor density with exendin-4 treatment is suggested to be attributable to the insulinomimetic effects of exendin-4 (Sokos et al., 2006) which result in a cross-talk between GLP-1 and insulin signaling pathways (Ebinger et al., 2000).

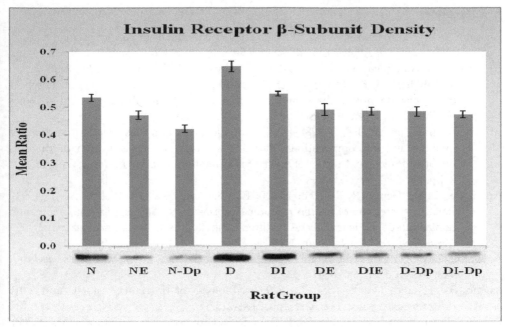

Fig. 3. Insulin receptor β-subunit (MW~95 kDa) density in the heart of the different rat groups.

There is no further attenuation in the level of insulin receptor upon insulin administration in combination with exendin-4 in diabetic rat groups. Thus, it is conceivable that GLP-1 is a key player in insulin receptor regulation in the diabetic state. GLP-1 also induces its insulinomimetic effects in the normal state thereby resulting in a slight decrease of insulin receptor density in NE. DPP-IV inhibitor induces similar effects as exendin-4 on IR-α and IR-β levels and this could be attributed as well to the insulinomimetic effects of GLP-1 (Fig. 2 and 3). There is a similar attenuation in receptor density in non-diabetic DPP-IV inhibitor treated rats (N-Dp). This reflects the actions of DPP-IV inhibitor treatment on the modulation of insulin receptor density not only in the diabetic but also in the normal state.

7. Conclusion

In conclusion, insulin, Losartan, exendin-4 and DPP-IV inhibitor have demonstrated their ability as promising candidates for treating type 1 diabetic patients. Moreover, exendin-4 and DPP-IV inhibitor appear to be promising in their efficacy and prolonged antidiabetic properties. Their actions on cardiovascular function, in both the preclinical and clinical realms, warrant future investigation.

8. Acknowledgement

The authors would like to acknowledge funding from the University Research Board and Medical Practice Plan of the American University of Beirut.

9. References

Agapitov, A. V. and Haynes, W. G., .(2002). Role of endothelin in cardiovascular disease. *Journal of Renin-Angiotensin-Aldosterone System,* Vol. 3, No. 1, pp. 1

Al Jaroudi, W. A., Nuwayri-Salti, N., Usta, J. A., Zwainy, D. S., Karam, C. N., Bitar, K. M. and Bikhazi, A. B., .(2005). Effect of insulin and angiotensin II receptor subtype-1 antagonist on myocardial remodelling in rats with insulin-dependent diabetes mellitus. *Journal of hypertension,* Vol. 23, No. 2, pp. 381

Alberti, K. and Zimmet, PZ, .(1998). Definition, diagnosis and classification of diabetes mellitus and its complications. Part 1: diagnosis and classification of diabetes mellitus. Provisional report of a WHO consultation. *Diabetic Medicine,* Vol. 15, No. 7, pp. 539-553

Anderson, C. M., Henry, R. R., Knudson, P. E., Olefsky, J. M. and Webster, NJ, .(1993). Relative expression of insulin receptor isoforms does not differ in lean, obese, and noninsulin-dependent diabetes mellitus subjects. *Journal of Clinical Endocrinology & Metabolism,* Vol. 76, No. 5, pp. 1380

Azizi, M. .(2008). Direct renin inhibition: clinical pharmacology. *Journal of molecular medicine,* Vol. 86, No. 6, pp. 647-654

Baggio, L. L. and Drucker, D. J., .(2007). Biology of incretins: GLP-1 and GIP. *Gastroenterology,* Vol. 132, No. 6, pp. 2131-2157

Ban, K., Noyan-Ashraf, M. H., Hoefer, J., Bolz, S. S., Drucker, D. J. and Husain, M., .(2008). Cardioprotective and vasodilatory actions of glucagon-like peptide 1 receptor are mediated through both glucagon-like peptide 1 receptor-dependent and - independent pathways. *Circulation,* Vol. 117, No. 18, pp. 2340-2350, 1524-4539; 0009-7322

Barton, M. and Yanagisawa, M., .(2008). Endothelin: 20 years from discovery to therapy. *Canadian journal of physiology and pharmacology,* Vol. 86, No. 8, pp. 485-498, 0008-4212; 0008-4212

Basso, N. and Terragno, N. A., .(2001). History about the discovery of the renin-angiotensin system. *Hypertension,* Vol. 38, No. 6, pp. 1246

Beers, M. H. and Berkow, R., .(1999). The Merck manual of diagnosis and therapy. *Merck Research Laboratories* Vol. 2833

Beers M. H. and Berkow R. (2006) In: Disorders of Carbohydrate Metabolism. *The Merck Manual of diagnosis and therapy.* 18:1274-1276

Behme, M. T., Dupre, J. and McDonald, T. J., .(2003). Glucagon-like peptide 1 improved glycemic control in type 1 diabetes. *BMC endocrine disorders* Vol. 3, No. 1, pp. 3, 1472-6823; 1472-6823

Berk, B. C. .(1999). Angiotensin II signal transduction in vascular smooth muscle: pathways activated by specific tyrosine kinases. *Journal of the American Society of Nephrology : JASN,* Vol. 10 Suppl 11, pp. S62-8, 1046-6673; 1046-6673

Berthoud, H. R. .(2008). Paying the Price for Eating Ice Cream: Is Excessive GLP-1 Signaling in the Brain the Culprit? *Endocrinology,* Vol. 149, No. 10, pp. 4765

Bikhazi, A. B., Khalifeh, A. M., Jaroudi, W. A., Saadeddine, R. E., Jurjus, A. R., El-Sabban, M. E. and Bitar, K. M., .(2003). Endothelin-1 receptor subtypes expression and binding in a perfused rat model of myocardial infarction. *Comparative biochemistry and physiology.Toxicology & pharmacology : CBP*, Vol. 134, No. 1, pp. 35-43, 1532-0456; 1532-0456

Boron WF and Boulpaep EL. (2009). The Endocrine Pancreas. In: *Medical Physiology*. Elsevier Saunders. pp.1074-1093

Boron WF and Boulpaep EL. (2009) The Adrenal Gland. In: *Medical Physiology*. Elsevier Saunders. pp.1057-1073

Boron WF and Boulpaep EL. (2009) Organization of Urinary System. In: *Medical Physiology*. Elsevier Saunders. pp. 749-766

Bose, A. K., Mocanu, M. M., Carr, R. D., Brand, C. L. and Yellon, D. M., .(2005). Glucagon-like peptide 1 can directly protect the heart against ischemia/reperfusion injury. *Diabetes*, Vol. 54, No. 1, pp. 146

Braga, M. F. B. and Leiter, L. A., .(2009). Role of renin-angiotensin system blockade in patients with diabetes mellitus. *The American Journal of Cardiology*, Vol. 104, pp. 835-839

Burcelin, R. (2008). What is known, new and controversial about GLP-1? Minutes of the 1st European GLP-1 Club Meeting, Marseille, 28–29 May 2008. *Diabetes and Metabolism*, Vol. 34, No. 6, pp. 627-630

Chua, B. H. L., Chua, C. C., Diglio, C. A. and Siu, B. B., .(1993). Regulation of endothelin-1 mRNA by angiotensin II in rat heart endothelial cells. *Biochimica et Biophysica Acta (BBA)-Molecular Cell Research*, Vol. 1178, No. 2, pp. 201-206

Coccheri, S. .(2007). Approaches to prevention of cardiovascular complications and events in diabetes mellitus. *Drugs*, Vol. 67, No. 7, pp. 997-1026

Creager, M. A., Luscher, T. F., Cosentino, F. and Beckman, J. A., .(2003). Diabetes and vascular disease: pathophysiology, clinical consequences, and medical therapy: Part I. *Circulation*, Vol. 108, No. 12, pp. 1527-1532, 1524-4539; 0009-7322

D'Alessio, D. A. and Vahl, T. P., .(2004). Glucagon-like peptide 1: evolution of an incretin into a treatment for diabetes. *American Journal of Physiology-Endocrinology And Metabolism*, Vol. 286, No. 6, pp. E882

de Koning, E. J. P., Bonner-Weir, S. and Rabelink, T. J., .(2008). Preservation of β-cell function by targeting β-cell mass. *Trends in pharmacological sciences*, Vol. 29, No. 4, pp. 218-227

De Meyts, P. and Whittaker, J., .(2002). Structural biology of insulin and IGF1 receptors: implications for drug design. *Nature Reviews Drug Discovery*, Vol. 1, No. 10, pp. 769-783

DeFronzo, R. A., Ratner, R. E., Han, J., Kim, D. D., Fineman, M. S. and Baron, A. D., .(2005). Effects of exenatide (exendin-4) on glycemic control and weight over 30 weeks in metformin-treated patients with type 2 diabetes. *Diabetes care*, Vol. 28, No. 5, pp. 1092

Docherty K and Steiner DF. (2003). The Molecular and Cell Biology of the Beta Cell. In: *Ellenberg & Rifkin's Diabetes Mellitus*, San Francisco: McGraw-Hill pp.23-41

Doyle, M. E. and Egan, J. M., .(2007). Mechanisms of action of glucagon-like peptide 1 in the pancreas. *Pharmacology & therapeutics*, Vol. 113, No. 3, pp. 546-593,

Drucker, D. J. .(2007). Dipeptidyl peptidase-4 inhibition and the treatment of type 2 diabetes. *Diabetes care*, Vol. 30, No. 6, pp. 1335

Drucker, D. J. and Nauck, M. A., .(2006). The incretin system: glucagon-like peptide-1 receptor agonists and dipeptidyl peptidase-4 inhibitors in type 2 diabetes. *The Lancet*, Vol. 368, No. 9548, pp. 1696-1705

d'Uscio, L. V., Moreau, P., Shaw, S., Takase, H., Barton, M. and Luscher, T. F., .(1997). Effects of chronic ETA-receptor blockade in angiotensin II-induced hypertension. *Hypertension*, Vol. 29, No. 1, pp. 435

Ebinger, M., Jehle, D. R., Fussgaenger, R. D., Fehmann, H. C. and Jehle, P. M., .(2000). Glucagon-like peptide-1 improves insulin and proinsulin binding on RINm5F cells and human monocytes. *American Journal of Physiology-Endocrinology and Metabolism*, Vol. 279, No. 1, pp. E88

Eisenberg, M. L., Maker, A. V., Slezak, L. A., Nathan, J. D., Sritharan, K. C., Jena, B. P., Geibel, J. P. and Andersen, D. K., .(2009). Insulin receptor (IR) and glucose transporter 2 (GLUT2) proteins form a complex on the rat hepatocyte membrane. *Cellular Physiology and Biochemistry*, Vol. 15, No. 1-4, pp. 051-058

Eknoyan, G. and Nagy, J., .(2005). A history of diabetes mellitus or how a disease of the kidneys evolved into a kidney disease. *Advances in chronic kidney disease*, Vol. 12, No. 2, pp. 223-229

Elahi, D., Egan, J. M., Shannon, R. P., Meneilly, G. S., Khatri, A., Habener, J. F. and Andersen, D. K., .(2008). GLP-1 (9–36) amide, cleavage product of GLP-1 (7–36) amide, is a glucoregulatory peptide. *Obesity* Vol. 16, No. 7, pp. 1501-1509

Fiordaliso, F., Li, B., Latini, R., Sonnenblick, E. H., Anversa, P., Leri, A. and Kajstura, J., (2000). Myocyte death in streptozotocin-induced diabetes in rats is angiotensin II-dependent. *Laboratory investigation*, Vol. 80, No. 4, pp. 513-527

Fowler, M. J. (2008). Microvascular and macrovascular complications of diabetes. *Clinical Diabetes*, Vol. 26, No. 2, pp. 77

George, C. M. (2009). Future trends in diabetes management. *Nephrology nursing journal : journal of the American Nephrology Nurses' Association*, Vol. 36, No. 5, pp. 477-483, 1526-744X; 1526-744X

Gomez, E., Pritchard, C. and Herbert, T. P. (2002). cAMP-dependent protein kinase and Ca2 influx through L-type voltage-gated calcium channels mediate Raf-independent activation of extracellular regulated kinase in response to glucagon-like peptide-1 in pancreatic β-cells. *Journal of Biological Chemistry*, Vol. 277, No. 50, pp. 48146-48151

Gradman, A. H. and Kad, R., .(2008). Renin inhibition in hypertension. *Journal of the American College of Cardiology*, Vol. 51, No. 5, pp. 519

Hadi, H. A. and Suwaidi, J. A., .(2007). Endothelial dysfunction in diabetes mellitus. *Vascular health and risk management*, Vol. 3, No. 6, pp. 853-876, 1176-6344

Hakim, NS. .(2003). Pancreatic transplantation for patients with type 1 diabetes. Vol. 35, No. 7, pp. 2801-2802

Halimi, S. .(2008). DPP-4 inhibitors and GLP-1 analogues: for whom? Which place for incretins in the management of type 2 diabetic patients? *Diabetes & metabolism*, Vol. 34, pp. S91-S95

Hantouche, C. M., Bitar, K. M., Nemer, G. M., Obeid, M. Y., Kadi, L. N., Der-Boghossian, A. H. and Bikhazi, A. B., .(2010). Role of glucagon-like peptide-1 analogues on insulin receptor regulation in diabetic rat hearts. *Canadian journal of physiology and pharmacology*, Vol. 88, No. 1, pp. 54-63, 1205-7541; 0008-4212

Hayashi, T., Takai, S. and Yamashita, C., .(2010). Impact of the renin-angiotensin-aldosterone-system on cardiovascular and renal complications in diabetes mellitus. *Current vascular pharmacology*, Vol. 8, No. 2, pp. 189-197, 1875-6212; 1570-1611

Hirata, K., Kume, S., Araki, S., Sakaguchi, M., Chin-Kanasaki, M., Isshiki, K., Sugimoto, T., Nishiyama, A., Koya, D. and Haneda, M., .(2009). Exendin-4 has an anti-hypertensive effect in salt-sensitive mice model. *Biochemical and biophysical research communications*, Vol. 380, No. 1, pp. 44-49

Holst, J. J. .(2006). Glucagon-like peptide-1: from extract to agent. The Claude Bernard Lecture, 2005. *Diabetologia*, Vol. 49, No. 2, pp. 253-260, 0012-186X; 0012-186X

Holt, R. I. G. .(2004). Diagnosis, epidemiology and pathogenesis of diabetes mellitus: an update for psychiatrists. *The British Journal of Psychiatry*, Vol. 184, No. 47, pp. s55

Hui, H., Zhao, X. and Perfetti, R., .(2005). Structure and function studies of glucagon-like peptide-1 (GLP-1): the designing of a novel pharmacological agent for the treatment of diabetes. *Diabetes/metabolism research and reviews*, Vol. 21, No. 4, pp. 313-331

Ichihara, A., Sakoda, M., Kurauchi-Mito, A., Kaneshiro, Y. and Itoh, H., . Renin, prorenin and the kidney: a new chapter in an old saga. *Journal of nephrology*, Vol. 22, No. 3, pp. 306

Idris, I. and Donnelly, R., .(2007). Dipeptidyl peptidase-IV inhibitors: a major new class of oral antidiabetic drug. *Diabetes, Obesity and Metabolism*, Vol. 9, No. 2, pp. 153-165,

Inzucchi, S. E. and McGuire, D. K., .(2008). New drugs for the treatment of diabetes: part II: Incretin-based therapy and beyond. *Circulation*, Vol. 117, No. 4, pp. 574,

Joshi, S. R., Parikh, R. M. and Das, A. K., .(2007). Insulin-History, Biochemistry, Physiology and Pharmacology. *JOURNAL-ASSOCIATION OF PHYSICIANS OF INDIA*, Vol. 55, No. L, pp. 19

Juutilainen, A., Lehto, S., Rönnemaa, T., Pyörälä, K. and Laakso, M., .(2008). Similarity of the impact of type 1 and type 2 diabetes on cardiovascular mortality in middle-aged subjects. *Diabetes care*, Vol. 31, No. 4, pp. 714

Kakoki, M., Hirata, Y., Hayakawa, H., Tojo, A., Nagata, D., Suzuki, E., Kimura, K., Goto, A., Kikuchi, K. and Nagano, T., .(1999). Effects of Hypertension, Diabetes Mellitus, and Hypercholesterolemia on Endothelin Type B Receptor–Mediated Nitric Oxide Release From Rat Kidney. *Circulation*, Vol. 99, No. 9, pp. 1242

Kalani, M. .(2008). The importance of endothelin-1 for microvascular dysfunction in diabetes. *Vascular health and risk management*, Vol. 4, No. 5, pp. 1061-1068, 1176-6344

Kanzaki, M. .(2006). Insulin receptor signals regulating GLUT4 translocation and actin dynamics. *Endocrine journal*, Vol. 53, No. 3, pp. 267-293, 0918-8959; 0918-8959

Karam, C. N., Nuwayri-Salti, N., Usta, J. A., Zwainy, D. S., Abrahamian, R. E., Al Jaroudi, W. A., Baasisri, M. J., Abdallah, S. M., Bitar, K. M. and Bikhazi, A. B., .(2005). Effect of systemic insulin and angiotensin II receptor subtype-1 antagonist on endothelin-1 receptor subtype(s) regulation and binding in diabetic rat heart. *Endothelium : journal of endothelial cell research*, Vol. 12, No. 5-6, pp. 225-231, 1062-3329; 1026-793X

KING, K. M. and Rubin, G., .(2003). A history of diabetes: from antiquity to discovering insulin. *British journal of nursing,* Vol. 12, No. 18, pp. 1091-1095

King, KD, Jones, JD and Warthen, J., .(2005). Microvascular and macrovascular complications of diabetes mellitus. *Am J Pharm Educ,* Vol. 69, pp. 87

Kinzig, K. P., D'Alessio, D. A. and Seeley, R. J., .(2002). The diverse roles of specific GLP-1 receptors in the control of food intake and the response to visceral illness. *The Journal of neuroscience,* Vol. 22, No. 23, pp. 10470

Klarlund JK, Cherniack AD, Conway BR, VanRenterghem B and Czech MP. (2003). Mechanisms of Insulin Action. In: *Ellenberg & Rifkin's Diabetes Mellitus*Anonymous McGraw-Hill, pp. 67-83

Knop, F. K., Vilsbøll, T., Højberg, P. V., Larsen, S., Madsbad, S., Vølund, A., Holst, J. J. and Krarup, T. (2007). Reduced Incretin Effect in Type 2 Diabetes. *Diabetes,* Vol. 56, No. 8, pp. 1951

Lambeir, A. M., Durinx, C., Scharpé, S. and De Meester, I., .(2003). Dipeptidyl-peptidase IV from bench to bedside: an update on structural properties, functions, and clinical aspects of the enzyme DPP IV. *Critical reviews in clinical laboratory sciences,* Vol. 40, No. 3, pp. 209-294

Laugero, K. D., Stonehouse, A. H., Guss, S., Landry, J., Vu, C. and Parkes, D. G., .(2009). Exenatide improves hypertension in a rat model of the metabolic syndrome. *Metabolic Syndrome and Related Disorders,* Vol. 7, No. 4, pp. 327-334

Lawrence, M. C., McKern, N. M. and Ward, C. W., .(2007). Insulin receptor structure and its implications for the IGF-1 receptor. *Current opinion in structural biology,* Vol. 17, No. 6, pp. 699-705

Lee, S., Yabe, D., Nohtomi, K., Takada, M., Morita, R., Seino, Y. and Hirano, T., .(2010). Intact glucagon-like peptide-1 levels are not decreased in Japanese patients with type 2 diabetes. *Endocrine journal,* Vol. 57, No. 2, pp. 119

Lovshin, J. A. and Drucker, D. J., .(2009). Incretin-based therapies for type 2 diabetes mellitus. *Nature Reviews Endocrinology,* Vol. 5, No. 5, pp. 262-269

MacDonald, P. E., El-kholy, W., Riedel, M. J., Salapatek, A. M. F., Light, P. E. and Wheeler, M. B., .(2002). The multiple actions of GLP-1 on the process of glucose-stimulated insulin secretion. *Diabetes,* Vol. 51, No. suppl 3, pp. S434,

Mann, R., Nasr, N., Hadden, D., Sinfield, J., Abidi, F., Al-Sabah, S., de Maturana, R. L., Treece-Birch, J., Willshaw, A. and Donnelly, D., .(2007). Peptide binding at the GLP-1 receptor. *Biochemical Society transactions,* Vol. 35, No. Pt 4, pp. 713-716, 0300-5127; 0300-5127

Mannucci, E. and Rotella, C. M., .(2008). Future perspectives on glucagon-like peptide-1, diabetes and cardiovascular risk. *Nutrition, Metabolism and Cardiovascular Diseases,* Vol. 18, No. 9, pp. 639-645

McEwan, P. E., Sherry, L., Kenyon, C. J., Webb, D. J. and Gray, G. A., .(2000). Regulation of the myocardial endothelin system by angiotensin-II and losartan. *Journal of cardiovascular pharmacology,* Vol. 36, No. 5 Suppl 1, pp. S144-7, 0160-2446; 0160-2446

McPhee SJ, Tierney LM and Papadakis MA. (2008). Masharani U. Diabetes Mellitus & Hypoglycemia. In: *Current medical diagnosis and treatment.* Appleton & Lange, *Mc Graw Hill LANGE.* 47(Middle East Edition): 1032-1073

Moritoh, Y., Takeuchi, K., Asakawa, T., Kataoka, O. and Odaka, H., .(2008). Chronic administration of alogliptin, a novel, potent, and highly selective dipeptidyl peptidase-4 inhibitor, improves glycemic control and beta-cell function in obese diabetic ob/ob mice. *European journal of pharmacology*, Vol. 588, No. 2-3, pp. 325-332

Myers J and Zonszein J. (2002). Diagnostic Criteria and Classification of Diabetes. In: *Principles of Diabetes Mellitus*, edited by Portesky L. London: Kluwer Academic Publishers, pp. 95-106

Nikolaidis, L. A., Elahi, D., Shen, Y. T. and Shannon, R. P. (2005). Active metabolite of GLP-1 mediates myocardial glucose uptake and improves left ventricular performance in conscious dogs with dilated cardiomyopathy. *American Journal of Physiology-Heart and Circulatory Physiology*, Vol. 289, No. 6, pp. H2401

Nuwayri-Salti, N., Karam, C. N., Al Jaroudi, W. A., Usta, J. A., Maharsy, W. M., Bitar, K. M. and Bikhazi, A. B. (2007). Effect of type-1 diabetes mellitus on the regulation of insulin and endothelin-1 receptors in rat hearts. *Canadian journal of physiology and pharmacology*, Vol. 85, No. 2, pp. 215-224

Parmar, D. M. and Jadav, S. P., .(2007). Aliskiren: a novel renin inhibitor for hypertension. *Indian journal of physiology and pharmacology*, Vol. 51, No. 1, pp. 99-101, 0019-5499; 0019-5499

Penna, C., Rastaldo, R., Mancardi, D., Cappello, S., Pagliaro, P., Westerhof, N. and Losano, G., .(2006). Effect of endothelins on the cardiovascular system. *Journal of Cardiovascular Medicine*, Vol. 7, No. 9, pp. 645

Peyot, M. L., Gray, J. P., Lamontagne, J., Smith, P. J. S., Holz, G. G., Madiraju, SR, Prentki, M., Heart, E. and Maedler, K., .(2009). Glucagon-like peptide-1 induced signaling and insulin secretion do not drive fuel and energy metabolism in primary rodent pancreatic beta-cells. *PLoS One*, Vol. 4, No. 7, pp. e6221

Phillips, M. I. and Schmidt-Ott, K. M., .(1999). The Discovery of Renin 100 Years Ago. *News in physiological sciences : an international journal of physiology produced jointly by the International Union of Physiological Sciences and the American Physiological Society*, Vol. 14, pp. 271-274, 0886-1714; 0886-1714

Pimenta, E. and Oparil, S., .(2009). Role of aliskiren in cardio-renal protection and use in hypertensives with multiple risk factors. *Vascular Health and Risk Management*, Vol. 5, pp. 453

Pool, J. L. (2007). Direct renin inhibition: focus on aliskiren. *Journal of Managed Care Pharmacy*, Vol. 13, No. 8, pp. 21

Poornima, I. G., Parikh, P. and Shannon, R. P., .(2006). Diabetic cardiomyopathy: the search for a unifying hypothesis. *Circulation research*, Vol. 98, No. 5, pp. 596

Prasad, V. S., Palaniswamy, C. and Frishman, W. H., .(2009). Endothelin as a clinical target in the treatment of systemic hypertension. *Cardiology in review*, Vol. 17, No. 4, pp. 181

Rao, M. S. .(2010). Inhibition of the Renin Angiotensin Aldosterone System: Focus on Aliskiren. *Journal of Association of Physicians of India*, Vol. 58, No. FEV, pp. 102-108

Retnakaran, R. and Zinman, B., .(2008). Type 1 diabetes, hyperglycaemia, and the heart. *The Lancet*, Vol. 371, No. 9626, pp. 1790-1799

Rhoades RA and Bell DR. (2009). The Control Mechanisms in Circulatory function. In: *Principles for Clinical Medicine*. Lippincott Williams and Wilkins. 3rd Edition: 312-317

Rhoades RA and Bell DR. (2009). Physiology and Body Fluids Medical Physiology. In: *Principles for Clinical Medicine*. Lippincott Williams and Wilkins. 3rd Edition: 419-441

Rhoades RA and Bell DR. (2009). The Endocrine Pancreas. In: *Principles for Clinical Medicine*. Lippincott Williams and Wilkins. 3rd Edition: 641-655,

Rosenfeld, L. .(2002). Insulin: discovery and controversy. *Clinical chemistry*, Vol. 48, No. 12, pp. 2270

Rossi, G. P., Sacchetto, A., Cesari, M. and Pessina, A. C., .(1999). Interactions between endothelin-1 and the renin–angiotensin–aldosterone system. *Cardiovascular research*, Vol. 43, No. 2, pp. 300,

Saraceni, C. and Broderick, T. L., .(2007). Effects of glucagon-like peptide-1 and long-acting analogues on cardiovascular and metabolic function. *Drugs in R&# 38; D* Vol. 8, No. 3, pp. 145-153

Scheen, AJ. .(2004). Renin-angiotensin system inhibition prevents type 2 diabetes mellitus:: Part 2. Overview of physiological and biochemical mechanisms. *Diabetes & metabolism*, Vol. 30, No. 6, pp. 498-505

Schneider, J. G., Tilly, N., Hierl, T., Sommer, U., Hamann, A., Dugi, K., Leidig-Bruckner, G. and Kasperk, C., .(2002). Elevated plasma endothelin-1 levels in diabetes mellitus&ast.

Schorlemmer, A., Matter, M. L. and Shohet, R. V., .(2008). Cardioprotective signaling by endothelin. *Trends in cardiovascular medicine*, Vol. 18, No. 7, pp. 233-239

Seifter J, Sloane D and Ratner A. (2005). The Endothelial Function and Homeostasis. In: *Concepts in medical physiology*. Lippincott Williams & Wilkins. 142-156

Seifter J, Sloane D and Ratner A. (2005). the Endocrine Pancreas: Fed and Fasted Metabolic States. In: *Concepts in medical physiology*. Lippincott Williams & Wilkins. 498-507

Sepehrdad, R., Frishman, W. H., Stier Jr, C. T. and Sica, D. A., .(2007). Direct inhibition of renin as a cardiovascular pharmacotherapy: focus on aliskiren. *Cardiology in review*, Vol. 15, No. 5, pp. 242

Shah, A. P., Niemann, J. T., Youngquist, S., Heyming, T. and Rosborough, J. P., .(2009). Plasma endothelin-1 level at the onset of ischemic ventricular fibrillation predicts resuscitation outcome. *Resuscitation*, Vol. 80, No. 5, pp. 580-583

Shin, Y. K., Martin, B., Golden, E., Dotson, C. D., Maudsley, S., Kim, W., Jang, H. J., Mattson, M. P., Drucker, D. J. and Egan, J. M. (2008). Modulation of taste sensitivity by GLP-1 signaling. *Journal of neurochemistry*, Vol. 106, No. 1, pp. 455-463

Sokos, G. G., Nikolaidis, L. A., Mankad, S., Elahi, D. and Shannon, R. P., .(2006). Glucagon-like peptide-1 infusion improves left ventricular ejection fraction and functional status in patients with chronic heart failure. *Journal of cardiac failure*, Vol. 12, No. 9, pp. 694-699

Sparre, T., Larsen, M. R., Heding, P. E., Karlsen, A. E., Jensen, O. N. and Pociot, F., .(2005). Unraveling the pathogenesis of type 1 diabetes with proteomics: present and future directions. *Molecular & Cellular Proteomics*, Vol. 4, No. 4, pp. 441

Steiner, M. K. and Preston, I. R., .(2008). Optimizing endothelin receptor antagonist use in the management of pulmonary arterial hypertension. *Vascular health and risk management,* Vol. 4, No. 5, pp. 943

Tabit, C. E., Chung, W. B., Hamburg, N. M. and Vita, J. A., .(2010). Endothelial dysfunction in diabetes mellitus: Molecular mechanisms and clinical implications. *Reviews in endocrine & metabolic disorders,* 1573-2606; 1389-9155

Thorin, E. and Webb, D. J., . Endothelium-derived endothelin-1. *Pflügers Archiv European Journal of Physiology,* pp. 1-8

Verdecchia, P., Angeli, F., Mazzotta, G., Gentile, G. and Reboldi, G., .(2008). The renin angiotensin system in the development of cardiovascular disease: role of aliskiren in risk reduction. *Vascular Health and Risk Management,* Vol. 4, No. 5, pp. 971

Voet, D. and Voet, J.D. (2004). Energy Metabolism: Integration and Organ Specialization, In: *Biochemistry,* pp. 1054-1068, John Wiley & Sons Inc., 0-471-39223-5, United States of America

Waldmeier, F., Glaenzel, U., Wirz, B., Oberer, L., Schmid, D., Seiberling, M., Valencia, J., Riviere, G. J., End, P. and Vaidyanathan, S., .(2007). Absorption, distribution, metabolism, and elimination of the direct renin inhibitor aliskiren in healthy volunteers. *Drug metabolism and disposition: the biological fate of chemicals,* Vol. 35, No. 8, pp. 1418-1428, 0090-9556; 0090-9556

Ward, C., Lawrence, M., Streltsov, V., Garrett, T., McKern, N., Lou, M. Z., Lovrecz, G. and Adams, T., .(2008). Structural insights into ligand-induced activation of the insulin receptor. *Acta Physiologica,* Vol. 192, No. 1, pp. 3-9

Widmaier EP, Raff H and Strang KT. (2004). The Mechanisms of the Body Function. In: *Vander, Sherman, and Luciano's Human Physiology.* The McGraw-Hill Companies. p: 534-621.

Wiggins, K. J. and Kelly, D. J., .(2009). Aliskiren: a novel renoprotective agent or simply an alternative to ACE inhibitors&quest. *Kidney international,* Vol. 76, No. 1, pp. 23-31

Wiggins, K. J. and Kelly, D. J., .(2009). Aliskiren: a novel renoprotective agent or simply an alternative to ACE inhibitors&quest. *Kidney international,* Vol. 76, No. 1, pp. 23-31

Wild, S. H., Roglic, G., Green, A., Sicree, R. and King, H., .(2004). Global prevalence of diabetes: estimates for the year 2000 and projections for 2030. *Diabetes care,* Vol. 27, No. 10, pp. 2569

Wilson JD, Braunwald E, Isselbacher KJ, Peterdorf RG, Martin JB, Fauci AS, Root RK, (1991). In: *Harrison's Principles of Internal Medicine,* 12th edition, vol. 2, McGraw-Hill, Inc. pp.1739-1742

Xu, G., Kaneto, H., Laybutt, D. R., Duvivier-Kali, V. F., Trivedi, N., Suzuma, K., King, G. L., Weir, G. C. and Bonner-Weir, S., .(2007). Downregulation of GLP-1 and GIP receptor expression by hyperglycemia. *Diabetes,* Vol. 56, No. 6, pp. 1551

Xu, G., Stoffers, D. A., Habener, J. F. and Bonner-Weir, S., .(1999). Exendin-4 stimulates both beta-cell replication and neogenesis, resulting in increased beta-cell mass and improved glucose tolerance in diabetic rats. *Diabetes,* Vol. 48, No. 12, pp. 2270-2276, 0012-1797; 0012-1797

Yang, Y. and Santamaria, P., (2003). Dissecting autoimmune diabetes through genetic manipulation of non-obese diabetic mice. *Diabetologia*, Vol. 46, No. 11, pp. 1447-1464.

Zhou, J., Chu, J., Wang, Y. H., Wang, H., Zhuang, Y. P. and Zhang, S. L., .(2008). Purification and bioactivity of exendin-4, a peptide analogue of GLP-1, expressed in Pichia pastoris. *Biotechnology Letters*, Vol. 30, No. 4, pp. 651-656

11

Understanding Pancreatic Secretion in Type 1 Diabetes

Mirella Hansen De Almeida[1], Alessandra Saldanha De Mattos Matheus[2]
and Giovanna A. Balarini Lima[3]
[1]*Federal University of Rio de Janeiro (UFRJ),*
[2]*State University of Rio de Janeiro (UERJ)*
[3]*Fluminense Federal University of Rio de Janeiro (UFF)*
Brazil

1. Introduction

Type 1 Diabetes Mellitus (T1DM) is a chronic disease characterized by the immune-mediated destruction of β cells of pancreatic islets. Despite the increase of its incidence observed in last decades, it has not been fully elucidated the immunogenetic and environmental factors associated with the initiation and perpetuation of the pancreatic injury(1,2).

The pathogenic process in T1DM begins with insulitis, which progresses and expands so as to be accompanied by cell necrosis. The rate of progression of the lesion is variable and may be related to age at onset of the disease, being faster in cases diagnosed in children (3). When approximately 80-90% of insulin-secreting cells have been destroyed, T1DM is clinically overt (4).

T1DM patients may have some residual insulin secretion at diagnosis (5-8). Several studies indicate that the loss of functional capacity usually occurs within three to five years. Most patients with long duration of disease do not present clinical evidence of preservation of β cells (9-11). However, the conservation of some residual secretion, even insufficient to cure or prevent T1DM from using insulin, has been associated with a better prognosis regarding glycemic control, lower rates of hypoglycemia, diabetic retinopathy and nephropathy (12).

One of the most frequently used method to assess β cell function in patients with T1DM is the determination of C-peptide (CP), a molecule secreted by β cells in equimolar concentrations with insulin and without significant liver metabolism (13-15). Taking into consideration the potential benefits of preserving a residual insulin secretion in patients with T1DM, experimental treatments have been proposed in order to maintain detectable levels of CP in these individuals.

Developments in research aiming for the prevention and cure of T1DM, increased the need to elucidate the contributing factors for the maintenance of residual insulin secretion in patients affected by the disease. This is because individuals who still exhibit residual insulin secretion could be ideal candidates for new curative treatments. Furthermore, most studies of pancreatic function in T1DM have been performed in Caucasians and Asians. We do not know whether the results obtained so far can be extrapolated to other ethnic populations (16).

2. Type 1 diabetes mellitus (T1DM)

2.1 Definition

T1DM is a chronic disease characterized by the destruction of pancreatic β cells, which leads to absolute deficiency in insulin production.

There are two subgroups of T1DM: type 1A, mediated by autoimmune destruction of β cells and type 1B, without an identifiable cause and more common among Asian and Afro-American people (17).

2.2 Epidemiology

The incidence of T1DM is rising in recent decades (18-20). This has been observed mainly in developed countries, mainly among children younger than four years-old (18,20-22). It is estimated that 15 to 30 million people in the world population have the disease with a growth rate of approximately 3-5% per year (19,20,23,24).

Epidemiological data suggest that 30 to 50% of T1DM cases may occur after the age of 20 and 50-60% of these patients were younger than 16-18 years at diagnosis. The incidence declines throughout the adult life (25-28).

The incidence among men and women is equal. However, there is a predominance of females in populations at low risk for T1DM, while the opposite occurs in high-risk populations (29).

There is also variation in relation to different countries. There is a high incidence in Finland and Sardinia, Italy (36.5 and 36.8 individuals per 100,000, respectively) and low in Germany and Pakistan. In countries like Brazil and Portugal, the incidence of T1DM is intermediate, as shown in Table 1. In Brazil, there is about 8.0 new cases per 100,000 inhabitants (30).

Regarding ethnicity, individuals of Caucasian origin have a higher incidence of T1DM than Hispanic, African, Asian or Indian descendents (31).

Country	Term	Incidence per 100,000 people Total
Germany	1990 – 1994	1.0
Brazil	1990 – 1992	8.0
Canada	1990 – 1994	24.0
Denmark	1990 – 1994	15.5
Spain	1990 – 1994	12.5
USA	1990 – 1994	
White		16.4
Non-white		13.3
Finland	1987 – 1989	36.5
Italy	1990 – 1994	
Sardinia		36.8
Sicily		11.7
Lombardy		7.2
Mexico	1990 – 1993	1.5
Norway	1990 – 1994	21.2
Pakistan	1990	0.7
Portugal	1990 – 1994	13.2
Sweden	1978 – 1987	24.2

Adapted from The WHO Diamond Project Group, 2000 (30).

Table 1. Incidence of T1DM in population under 15 years-old, in different countries.

2.3 Etiopathogenesis

In the pathogenesis of T1DM, the activation of the immune system mediated by T cells plays a central role. This process leads to an inflammatory reaction (insulitis) characterized by infiltration of pancreatic islets by mononuclear cells such as dendritic cells, macrophages, B lymphocytes and CD4 and CD8 (3,17,32). With the progression of inflammatory injury, there is a development of cellular necrosis and cellular immunity seems to be primarily responsible for this process (33).

The pathogenic process that culminates with the onset of T1DM begins with the loss of self-tolerance of T lymphocytes. Self-tolerance is defined as the process in which T cells or autoreactive B are eliminated from the body. This can be divided into central and peripheral. The central tolerance is the deletion of autoreactive T cells in the thymus and requires the presence of autoantigens in thymic environment. Peripheral tolerance mechanisms are responsible for destroying or inhibiting the function of self-reactive cells that crossed the thymic deletion process, through mechanisms such as immunological ignorance, deletion, anergy or immune inhibition (34).

Some of the risk genes for the development of T1DM are responsible for the concentration of insulin within the thymus. Thus, these genes are linked to the process of central tolerance. Moreover, changes in peripheral tolerance may also be related to the etiopathogenesis and the release of super-antigens after viral infections. Typically, the peripheral tolerance would be responsible for the sequestration of these super-antigens mediated by the immune system, which would not lead to lymphocyte activation (34,35). Another mechanism of pancreatic injury is associated with infection as a possible molecular mimicry between viral antigens and autoantigens aggravating the process of insulitis. This molecular similarity could activate autoreactive T lymphocytes and direct them to attack pancreatic cells (34).

Overt T1DM occurs when approximately 80 to 90% of the β cells have been destroyed (4). The rate of progression to classical T1DM symptoms may be related to age of onset of symptoms, being faster in cases diagnosed at young age (3).

The presence of one or more autoantibodies associated with T1DM may precede the onset of clinical disease by months or even years (28,36,37).

T1DM diagnosed in childhood may have autoantibodies to the major antigens of the pancreatic islets detectable in the first two years of life (38). This seems to be a reflection of cellular injury and its cause is not specific (33). The role of B lymphocyte cells in the pathogenesis of T1DM must also be emphasized. Several diseases mediated by T lymphocytes present B lymphocytes in the process of antigen presentation (39). A recent study revealed that patients with newly diagnosed T1DM treated with Rituximab (monoclonal anti-CD20) showed improvement in clinical and metabolic parameters after selective depletion of B lymphocytes. The explanation for this fact lies on the reduction of antigen presentation mediated by B lymphocytes, or even the reduction of cytokine production in pancreatic or peri-pancreatic lymph nodes. This suggests that B lymphocytes may have a greater role in the pathogenesis of T1DM than previously thought (40).

Although there are many hypotheses about the onset and progression to autoimmunity of T1DM, the definitive mechanism is not fully understood.

2.4 Autoantibodies

Production of pancreatic autoantibodies does not appear to be the primary mechanism of destruction of pancreatic islets (41,42). The release of antigen caused by β cell destruction leads to its detection by the immune system and immune activation, subsequently causing the production of antibodies against pancreatic components. Thus, antibodies appear to be predominantly markers of immune activation and β cell destruction, and not the cause itself (31,33).

The first autoantibody isolated was the antibody against the cytoplasm of the pancreatic islet *(islet cell cytoplasmic antibody* - ICA) and three major autoantibodies contribute to their positivity: the antiglutamic acid decarboxylase (GADA65), antibody against tyrosine phosphatase (anti-IA2, also known as ICA512) and antibodies against glycolipids (43)

The glutamic acid decarboxylase (GADA) is an enzyme involved in the synthesis of γ-amino-butiric acid (GABA) in the central nervous system (CNS) and in pancreatic islets. GADA is expressed in all cell types of pancreatic islets, not only in β cells. Two isoforms of GADA (GADA64 and GADA67) synthesized in other tissues have also been identified. GADA, used in current assays, detects pancreatic isoform of this enzyme of 65 kd and is found in 70-80% of newly diagnosed Caucasian. A lower incidence is observed in children younger than 10 years of age (43,44).

After GADA discovery, anti-IA-2 (40 kd) or ICA512, and anti-IA-2β (37 kd), known as *phorin* (45,46), were identified. Most patients with anti-IA 2β also exhibit anti-IA-2. However, about 10% of T1DM with anti-IA-2 autoantibodies are not the type-2 anti-IA. Until now, anti-IA-2 appears to be the most specific immunological marker of T1DM and is present in 32 to 75% of the new cases (47,48). Once detected, most individuals concomitantly present positive GADA and anti-insulin (IAA) (28). Another antibody has been identified as IAA. In children diagnosed under 10 years of age, sensitivity of IAA is of 50 to 60%, while in patients between 10 and 30 years   sensitivity is of 10% (47,48). There is cross-reactivity between antibodies produced against endogenous and exogenous insulin and most patients develop IAA after initiation of insulin therapy, even with the use of recombinant analogues. Thus, the measurement of this antibody in the blood is recommended only before or within 5 to 7 days after initiation of insulin therapy (32).

It has been recently described another auto-antigen associated with T1DM - the zinc transporter 8 *(zinc transporter* 8 - Znt8). Present in β cells, the Znt8 is involved in regulating the insulin secretion pathway. It regulates the entry of zinc in the lumen of the granules, where this cation binds to hexamers of insulin. Nearly 60 to 80% of individuals with newly diagnosed T1DM have antibodies against this antigen (49,50).

Most pancreatic autoantibody titers decline after the diagnosis of the disease, but GADA may remain positive for many years after diagnosis (51). This feature makes it ideal for antibody studies in patients with T1DM of long duration.

Some patients may not have pancreatic autoantibodies detectable at diagnosis. This can be explained by some reasons (5):

1.   These patients may have detectable titers in the pre clinical and became negative before diagnosis.
2.   Tests available for determination of these autoantibodies were not sensitive enough to detect low titers.
3.   There may be yet unidentified antibodies in research conducted so far.
4.   This is possibly a case of idiopathic T1DM (type 1B) without autoimmune etiology.

At diagnosis, traditionally it has been estimated that 90% of children had one or more pancreatic antibody positive. However, with the availability of anti-Znt8, measuring the combination of the four main pancreatic autoantibodies (GADA, IAA, anti-IA2 and anti-Znt8) in patients with newly diagnosed T1DM, showed a detection rate of autoimmunity against β cells of 98% (49,50).

2.5 Genetic factors associated with T1DM

Genes from the histocompatibility system HLA *(Human Leukocyte Antigen Complex)*, IDDM 1 - chromosome 6q21.31, are polymorphic and have different amino acid sequences between individuals. They are divided into HLA class I (HLA-A, B and C) and HLA class II (DP, DQ and DR) and both are related to immune response (52).

HLA class II polymorphisms are associated with an increased risk of T1DM. The main risk alleles are HLA DQB1 * 2002 / * 0302 and HLA DR03/04. The DQB1 * 0602 allele is considered protective (5).

Other genes have been associated with the pathogenesis of T1DM, as shown in Table 2, among which are the insulin gene PTPN22 and CTL4 (17,27,53-55).

* IDDM - insulin dependent diabetes mellitus	Genetic Product	Cromossomic location
IDDM1	HLA	6p21.31
IDDM2	Insulin	11p15.5
IDDM3	-	15q.26
IDDM4	-	11q13
IDDM5	-	6q25
IDDM6	-	18q21
IDDM7	-	2q31-31
IDDM8	-	6q27
IDDM9	-	3q21
IDDM10	-	10p11-q11
IDDM11	-	14q4.3-14q31
IDDM12	CTLA-4	2q33
IDDM13	-	2q34
IDDM14	-	6q21
IDDM15	-	10q25.1
IDDM17	-	CR10
PTPN22	-	

Adapted from Kelly et al. 2003 (3) and Eisenbarth, 2005 (32).

Table 2. Genes involved in the Pathogenesis of T1DM

2.6 Environmental factors associated with T1DM

Besides genetic susceptibility, exposure to environmental factors is also important for the development of T1DM. Studies suggest that these factors would be responsible for triggering the immune process that leads to β cell destruction. Specific viral infectious diseases have been included among the causes (56,57). Some of the viruses suggested as associated with T1DM are Enteroviruses, Coxsackie virus, congenital Rubella. Toxins such as nitrosamines and protein foods such as cow's milk, cereals and gluten are also considered as potential immunological triggers (58-60). Moreover, the presence of multiple infections in early life is associated with a reduced risk for the disease (1).

Recently, there has been a significant increase in diagnosed cases aged younger than four years (61,62). This shift may be explained by increased exposure to environmental factors or the increased prevalence of obesity (63,64).

One of the hypotheses to explain the development of T1DM is the controversial theory of acceleration suggested by Wilkin. It argues that T1DM and type 2 diabetes (T2DM) constitute a single disease and not two distinct comorbidities. The rate of loss of β cell mass, associated with three main factors accelerators, would define the disease. The first factor would be the intrinsic potential for high speed apoptosis of β cells, essential, but insufficient for the development of DM. The second accelerator would be insulin resistance, a result of obesity and physical inactivity, central link between the two entities. Insulin resistance overtaxes the β cell mass already at risk for accelerated apoptosis, contributing to the clinical expression of DM. The third accelerator was present only in individuals with genetic susceptibility to autoimmunity. Individuals with metabolically more active β cells, insulin resistance and genetic susceptibility would be more prone to rapid deterioration of functional and clinical expression of T1DM. In the absence of autoimmune accelerator, apoptosis rate would be slower and thus there would be progression to T2DM (65).

3. Assessment of pancreatic β cell function

A major limitation of studies of T1DM in humans is the inability to measure the mass of β cells *in vivo*, since pancreatic biopsies are associated with high morbidity and mortality. Therefore, indirect methods have been developed. The assessment of pancreatic function was shown to have a rough correlation with the mass of β cells used in islet transplantation in patients with DM (25).

Methods of imaging and nuclear medicine are being studied to assist the measurement of the mass of pancreatic islets and its correlation with insulin production, but with conflicting results (66-68).

The measurement of β cell mass does not always correlate with functional capacity. In pre-diabetes, there can be no proliferation or maintenance of cell mass (69,70). Marchetti et al suggested that patients with T1DM can have β cell secretory dysfunction and not just cell destruction (71).

In an attempt to understand the β cell function *in vivo*, it was initially developed a radioimmunoassay for measurement of serum insulin. For years, this was the gold standard for assessing the secretory activity. However, there are several factors limiting the use of serum insulin for the evaluation of pancreatic β cell function. The first is that 50 to 60% of the insulin produced by the pancreas undergoes hepatic metabolism and does not reach the systemic circulation. In addition, the peripheral *clearance* of insulin is variable and the tests available for their determination do not differentiate insulin, proinsulin, its intermediates and the use of exogenous insulin. Another limiting factor is the presence of anti-insulin antibodies (IAA) to interfere in the measurement of serum insulin (12,72,73).

Thus, other means to measure β cell function have been developed, and among them the measurement of baseline and/or stimulated CP.

3.1 C-peptide

Pancreatic β cells secrete, in addition to insulin, proinsulin, conversion intermediates of insulin (proinsulin *split*) and the connecting peptide (CP) (15).

The pro-insulin is cleaved in the Golgi apparatus of islet cells. This reaction leads to the formation of insulin, CP and two pairs of basic amino acids. Insulin and the CP are released into circulation at a ratio of 1:1, as well as small amounts of proinsulin and intermediates. The proinsulin sum 20% of molecules with insulin-immunoreactivity *simile*, seems to have no metabolic effect, undergoes extra-hepatic metabolism and is excreted exclusively by the kidneys.

The CP is a connection between the peptide chains A and B of proinsulin and facilitates the processing of biologically active insulin in secretory granules of pancreatic islets. After the cleavage of proinsulin, the intact CP is stored with insulin in these granules and is co-secreted with insulin. For this reason, the CP can be considered an independent marker of insulin secretion (16). However, in some situations, such as renal failure, the serum concentration of CP is not proportional to the rate of insulin secretion. About 85% of CP is metabolized by the kidneys and the remainder excreted intact in urine. A decrease in renal function leads to reduced metabolism of CP and elevated serum levels (74)

The CP plasma half-life is of thirty minutes, greater than that of insulin, which is only of four minutes (13-15,75). The normal value of the CP varies from 1.1 to 5.0 ng / mL.

Under standard conditions of measurement, the CP has been widely accepted as a rough measure of insulin secretion, since it is secreted into the portal circulation in equimolar, concentrations, does not undergo hepatic metabolism, its half-life is longer (30 minutes) and has low cross reactivity with proinsulin and insulin antibodies (12, 76,77).

In adverse conditions, such as hyper- or hypoglycemia, CP concentrations are not proportional to the rate of insulin secretion, and its *clearance* may vary between different individuals (78,79).

Therefore, at the moment, the most appropriate, accepted and clinically validated method to measure the ability of β cell secretion under ideal conditions is the measurement of baseline and/or stimulated CP (76). This stimulation can be done with glucose or insulin secretagogues such as glucagon, standard mixed meal or oral glucose tolerance test with 75g of anhydrous glucose (OGTT) (12,80-82).

The standard mixed meal test consists of oral administration of a liquid diet (Sustacal ® / Boost) of approximately 500 kcal containing 50% carbohydrate, 30% fat and 20% protein. Blood samples for measurement of blood glucose and CP are collected in fasting and 30, 60 and/or 90 minutes after the meal (76,80). This test shows the typical postprandial response of the cell β and its interaction with the various hormones secreted during oral feeding. It is the most physiological test among the above cited (76,83).

Oral glucose tolerance test (OGTT) is the determination of glucose, insulin and CP after 10 hours of fasting and 30, 60, 90, 120 minutes after ingestion of 75g anhydrous glucose orally administered. It is used to measure glucose tolerance and the residual function of the β cell in patients at risk, but has not yet been validated for use in T1DM patients. It is useful to predict early changes in glucose metabolism in relatives of T1DM or individuals with positive autoantibodies (76).

The glucagon stimulation test is done by measurement of CP at baseline, after 8 hours fasting, and 6 minutes after intravenous administration of 1 mg of glucagon, while its maximum concentration is observed (76,79). The most commonly observed side effects are facial flushing and nausea due to decreased gastrointestinal motility (76). The advantages of the glucagon test in relation to the standard meal test are:

1. Faster action, since glucagon is a potent supra-physiological stimulus for insulin secretion, directly and indirectly, also influenced by hyperglycemia (76).
2. Minor influence of glucotoxicity in patients with high glycated hemoglobin (HbA1C) (76,80).
3. Simple technical achievement (76).
4. Good reproducibility between individuals (76).

To avoid inaccuracy in CP measurement, caution is necessary during blood collection and processing. As the CP is a small molecule, linear and prone to degradation by proteolytic enzymes blood samples should be cleared by centrifugation for a short period of time (not more than a few hours). Palmer et al suggest that this is done within one month after collection because immunoreactivity falls with prolonged blood storage generating falsely lower results (84). This time, however, it is not well defined (12). Until the proper measurement, the serum should be stored -80 ° C.

Changes in blood glucose are factors that acutely interfere with the measurement of serum CP and can underestimate the ability of secretion. The Immunology of Diabetes Society has established that the glucagon test must be conducted during fasting and with glucose levels between 70 and 200mg/dL. The optimal level of blood glucose in these patients is around 126mg/dL. Hypoglycemia (<70 mg / dL) inhibits the insulin response while acute hyperglycemia (> 200mg/dL) may potentiate the secretory response or inhibit it. On the other hand, chronic hyperglycemia can reduce β cell function due to the phenomenon of glucotoxicity (85-86). Moreover, high glucose concentrations have been shown to damage β cells *in vitro* and *in vivo*, compromising insulin secretion (87).

The characteristics of the methods used to quantitate the CP must be well defined. The presence of cross-reactivity with proinsulin and its intermediate results in falsely elevated CP concentrations. In general, it is expected that the rate of cross-reactivity of a method is less than 10% (12).

3.2 Role of the pancreatic β cell in T1DM

In T1DM, there is a progressive loss of the ability of insulin secretion. During the process of destruction of pancreatic β cells, the first abnormality observed in the preclinical phase is the loss of first phase insulin secretion - *FPIR, First phase insulin release* (31,88). The FPIR is the sum of the plasma insulin at 1 and 3 minutes after the glucose load during an intravenous glucose tolerance test (76). Moreover, impairment in glucose tolerance test has been correlated with an increased risk of progressing from preclinical to clinical diabetes (4).

One of the first authors who studied β cell function in diabetic patients and healthy controls was OK Faber et al in 1977. He compared measurements of the CP after the standard meal and after glucagon (1 mg intravenous) and noticed that the CP, at baseline and after fasting and stimulation with glucagon, was higher in healthy controls when compared to patients with T1DM (79). Subsequently, it was identified that individuals with T1DM may have some residual insulin secretion at diagnosis especially in cases diagnosed in adulthood (5-8, 89).

The loss of this residual secretion usually occurs within three to five years after the diagnosis (86). Patients with long duration of illness tend not to have CP secretory reserves, demonstrating the exhaustion of pancreatic secretion (9-11). However, Meier et al demonstrated the preservation of β cells secreting insulin in most patients with T1DM evaluated in histopathological studies (90). In addition, Keenan and colleagues demonstrated detectable levels of CP in 18% of individuals with T1DM for over 50 years and absence of chronic complications of the disease (91).

The reason why some β cells are maintained for years after diagnosis of T1DM remains unclear. It is possible that some cells are not equally susceptible to destruction or even that the destructive process is attenuated over the years. Another possibility to explain this persistence would be a recovery in β cell by replication, which seems unlikely. Another explanation is that some cells could be inactive and not destroyed and recover their function over time (92).

3.2.1 Factors influencing the residual insulin secretion and CP

The rate of decline of pancreatic function in T1DM is heterogeneous, ranging from 13 to 58% in the first year after diagnosis (84). Some factors such as age at diagnosis and sex seem to influence this fall. Association between residual pancreatic function and female sex has also been found (93). Karjalainen et al reported that T1DM that begins in adulthood (20 to 55.8 years old) is characterized by a longer asymptomatic period before diagnosis and better preservation of residual β cell function than T1DM beginning in childhood (5,16,94).

Some studies have shown that baseline serum CP levels in patients diagnosed in adulthood and post-pubertal period are higher than in those diagnosed in the pre-puberty (7,8,12). This fact indicates a greater destruction of β cells in younger people. However, there could be a change in CP levels according to age. According to Palmer JP et al, the serum CP levels in adulthood are around 0.6 to 1.3 nmol / L during puberty between 0.3 and 0.9 nmol / L and in pre-pubertal <0.2 nmol / L (12).

In the *Diabetes Control and Complications Trial* (DCCT), patients with short disease duration (≤ 5 years) had a CP after the stimulus with mixed meal detectable (greater than 0.2 nmol / L) in 33% of those with <18 years of age and 48% in adults (10). Stimulated CP > 0.2 pmol / mL was found in 3% of children and 8% of adults with long duration of illness (> 5 years). Basal and stimulated CP were negatively correlated with disease duration (80).

The presence of antibodies is another predictor of reduction in β cell function. High levels of ICA were associated with a faster decrease in the secretion of CP (81). Aimed to modulate the immune system and prevent the destruction of β cells, studies using vaccination against GADA showed some preservation of the CP, although it did not change the needs of insulin (95,96).

There is evidence that intensive glucose control can reduce, at least temporarily, the failure of insulin secretion in T1DM. However, it is possible that the maintenance of some residual secretion facilitates the achievement of adequate metabolic control (20). The mechanisms by which intensive insulin prolongs the β-cell function in T1DM can be due to reduced glucotoxicity or by direct action in the autoimmune destruction (97).

3.2.2 Impact of maintenance of residual insulin secretion and PC

The persistence of detectable CP serum levels, especially in patients with long duration of disease, may have clinical importance. Some studies have shown that this is a prognostic factor for improved glycemic control, lower frequency of hypoglycemia, retinopathy and diabetic nephropathy (8,80,98). So far, the main information about the importance of preservation of some residual secretion in the development of chronic complications, glycemic control and incidence of hypoglycemia T1DM were obtained from the DCCT (8).

In the DCCT, the intensive glucose control significantly reduced the loss of β cell function in relation to conventional treatment. Furthermore, patients with CP ≥ 0.2 nmol / L in the intensive treatment group had lower HbA1C at baseline and through the four year follow-up period (8).

The presence of a residual capacity for insulin secretion has also been associated with a reduced risk of hypoglycemia. Data from the DCCT showed that patients with stimulated CP≥ 0.2 nmol / L for at least one year had the prevalence of hypoglycemia reduced in 30%. Among patients in intensive control group, the risk of hypoglycemia was three times lower in those who remained detectable CP than in others. In the conventional group, this difference was not observed (8).

In relation to chronic complications, the DCCT showed that patients with T1DM and undetectable levels of CP (<0.04 nmol / L) had 4.6 times greater chance of progression to diabetic retinopathy and 4.4 times greater chance of developing microalbuminuria in relation to others (8).

Some authors found no association between the frequency of chronic complications and residual β cell function. Klein and colleagues studied the relationship between serum levels of CP and severity of diabetic retinopathy in different types of diabetes in the *Wisconsin Epidemiologic Study of Diabetic Retinopathy*. Young subjects with T1DM using insulin did not present any association between CP levels and the frequency or severity of diabetic retinopathy (99). Winocour et al, on the other hand, found an association between the presence of residual secretion of CP and reduced risk of proliferative diabetic retinopathy in T1DM but no correlation to peripheral neuropathy or autonomic, hypertension, nephropathy or coronary heart disease (100).

Other studies also found no influence of CP stimulated with the development of retinopathy, neuropathy and/or microalbuminuria in T1DM. However, these studies included a small number of patients, with short time for monitoring and/or few chronic complications (100-102).

In the pathological study of Meier et al, the number of β cells found in patients with T1DM was not associated with the disease duration, but rather with glycemic control, being higher at lower blood glucose levels (90).

Today, the role of the CP only as a marker of insulin secretion is questionable. Some suggests that it may also have a direct action on target organs of chronic complications of T1DM (84). Potential actions of the CP include: improvement in nerve conduction velocity, improving the sensory and autonomic nerve function, improvement in cardiac function, decreased microalbuminuria; stimulation of the activity of nitric oxide synthase *(eNOS)* inhibition of smooth muscle cells proliferation; and decreased signal transduction of NF-kβ *(nuclear factor kappa-light-chain-enhancer of activated B cells)* with reduced inflammation. These findings have been observed *in vitro* and in clinical studies in animals and humans with T1DM (84).

3.2.3 Methods of preserving pancreatic function

The need for insulin and/or progression of pancreatic β cell damage can be avoided by preserving the ability of insulin secretion. The maintenance of some residual function, even if insufficient to avoid insulin therapy may have important advantages in better metabolic control and lower risk of chronic complications as previously described (8,84).

The DCCT showed that intensive insulin therapy can reduce the progression of β cell damage, with positive effects for up to 6 years after diagnosis (8). Brown et al in their study also confirmed this benefit (103). Intensive insulin therapy may promote survival of β cells, reducing the metabolic demand and glucotoxicity.

Immunosuppressive therapy, such as cyclosporine, azathioprine, prednisone, and anti-thymocyte globulin, aiming for depletion and inactivation of β cells, were used in newly diagnosed patients, but with limited efficacy and temporary effects due to its toxicity (104).

Immunomodulators, such as anti-CD3 monoclonal antibodies, used in newly diagnosed T1DM also allowed the maintenance of the secretion of CP for one to two years with low toxicity, and benefits in glycemic control (105-107). After 48 months of follow up, patients who received the monoclonal antibodies anti-CD3 had lower daily insulin requirements, with improved A1C and glycemic variations smaller than the control. The best results have been found in individuals under the age of 27 years and with higher CP at baseline (108).

The induction of immunological tolerance to self antigens such as GAD, insulin and oral *heat shock protein* 60 (HSP60) has been tried with controversial results in preservation of islet function (104,109,110).

Another measure that has been tested for secondary prevention of T1DM is the autologous non-myeloablative hematopoietic stem cell transplant. Voltarelli and colleagues conducted this transplant in 15 newly diagnosed patients with T1DM. Five patients have remained insulin free for up to 21 months and seven remained for more than six months without use of exogenous insulin (111). Despite the low rate of complications reported, there is a potential risk for more serious effects related to immunosuppression. (107,110). Mesenchymal stem cell therapies and combination of multiple immunomodulatory drugs are currently under study.

Several studies aiming at the preservation of β cell mass are being conducted, with a main goal: search for the cure of T1DM. The attempt to preserve β cell function even if insufficient to cure the disease, can be useful in the prevention of microvascular complications, improves glycemic control and reduced the frequency of hypoglycemic events (7,8,12,98).

In summary, we tried to emphasize some aspects of the natural history of T1DM. At first, a large mass of beta cell function is lost between the period from the surveillance diagnosis to the period of overt T1DM. Then, residual beta cell function results in better glycemic control and less microvascular complications. The rate of progression of beta cell failure may be due to several factors such as underlying genetic predisposition, age of the patient and metabolic control. Finally, CP has its role on diagnosis reserve of beta cell mass and higher levels are associated to a better glycemic control and preservation of pancreatic function. Moreover, interventions that are being held nowadays are clinically important to quality of life, mortality and morbidity of patients with T1DM.

4. References

[1] Atkinson MA et al. Type 1 Diabetes: New Perspectives On Disease Pathogenesis And Treatment. Lancet 2001; 358: 221-229.

[2] Libman IM, Laporte RE. Changing Trends In Epidemiology Of Type 1 Diabetes Mellitus Throughout The World: How Far Have We Come And Where Do We Go From Here. Pediatr Diabetes 2005; 6(3): 119-121.

[3] Kelly MA, Rayner ML, Mijovic CH et al. Molecular Aspects Of Type 1 Diabetes. Mol Pathol 2003; 56 (1): 1–10.

[4] Knip M, Kukko M, Kulmala P et al. Humoral Beta – Cell Autoimmunity In Relation To HLA-Defined Disease Susceptibility In Preclinical And Clinical Type 1 Diabetes. Am J Med Genetics 2002; 115: 48–54.

[5] Sabbah E, Savola K, Ebeling T et al. Genetic, Autoimmune And Clinical Characteristics Of Childhood And Adult Onset Type 1 diabetes. Diabetes Care 2000; 23 (9):1326-1332.

[6] Effects Of Age, Duration And Treatment Of Insulin-Dependent Diabetes Mellitus On Residual Beta-Cell Function: Observations During Eligibility Testing For The Diabetes Control And Complications Trial (DCCT). The DCCT Research Group. J Clin Endocrinol Metab 1987; 65: 30-36.

[7] The Diabetes Control And Complications Trial Research Group: The Effect Of Intensive Treatment In Diabetes On The Development And Progression Of Long-Term Complications On Insulin-Dependent Diabetes Mellitus. N Engl J Med 1993; 329: 977-986.

[8] The Diabetes Control And Complications Trial Research Group: The Effect Of Intensive Therapy On Residual Beta-Cell Function In Patients With Type 1 Diabetes In The Diabetes Control And Complications Trial. Ann Intern Med 1998; 128: 517-523.

[9] Cravarezza P, Radaeli E, Toffoli C et al. Discrimination Of Type 1 From Insulin-Treated Type II Diabetic Patients By C Peptide Measurement. Acta Diabetol Lat 1986; 23 (4): 345-350.

[10] Gottsater A, Landin-Olsson M, Fernlund P et al. Beta-Cell Function In Relation To Islet Cell Antibodies During The First 3 Years After Clinical Diagnosis Of Diabetes In Type II Diabetic Patients. Diabetes Care 1993; 16(6): 902-910.

[11] Ahn CW, Kim HS, Nam JH et al. Clinical Characteristics, GAD Antibody (GADA) And Change Of C-Peptide In Korean Young Age Of Onset Diabetic Patients. Diabet Med 2002; 19(3): 227-233.

[12] Palmer JP, Fleming GA, Greenbaum CJ et al. C-Peptide Is The Appropriate Outcome Measure For Type1 Diabetes Clinical Trials To Preserve Beta Cell Function – ADA Workshop Report. Diabetes 2004; 53: 250-264.

[13] Polonsky KS, Jaspan J, Pugh W, Cohen D, Schneider M, Schartz T, Moossa AR, Tager H, Rubenstein AH. Metabolism Of C-Peptide In The Dog; In Vivo Demonstration Of The Absence Of Hepatic Extraction. J Clin Invest 1983; 72: 1114-1123.

[14] Polonsky KS, Pugh W, Jaspan JB, Cohen DM, Karrisson T, Tager HS, Rubenstein AH. C-Peptide And Insulin Secretion: Relationship Between Peripheral Concentrations Of C-Peptide And Their Secretion Rates In The Dog. J Clin Invest 1984; 74:1821-1829.

[15] Bratusch-Marrain PR, Waldhausl WK, Gasic S, Hofer A. Hepatic Disposal Of Biosynthetic Human Insulin And Porcine Proinsulin In Humans. Metabolism 1984; 33: 151-157.

[16] Rodacki M, Zajdenverg L, Tortora RP et al. Characteristics Of Childhood And Adult-Onset Type 1 Diabetes In A Multi-Ethnic Population. Diab Res Clin Pract 2005; 69: 22-28.

[17] Daneman D. Type 1 Diabetes. Lancet 2006; 367: 847-858.

[18] Gale EA. The Rise Of Childhood Type1 Diabetes In The 20th Century. Diabetes 2002; 51(12): 3353-3361.

[19] Secular Trends In Incidence Of Childhood IDDM In 10 Countries. Diabetes Epidemiology Research International Group. Diabetes 1990; 39(7): 858-864.

[20] Variation And Trends In Incidence Of Childhood Diabetes In Europe. EURODIAB ACE Study Group. Lancet 2000; 355(9207): 873-876.

[21] Rewers M, Norris JM, Eisenbarth GS et al. Beta-Cell Autoantibodies In Infants And Toddlers Without IDDM Relatives: Diabetes Autoimmunity Study In The Young (DAISY). J Autoimmun 1996; 9(3): 405-410.

[22] Onkamo P, Vaananen S, Karvonen M et al. Worldwide Increase In Incidence Of Type I Diabetes - The Analysis Of The Data On Published Incidence Trends. Diabetologia 1999; 42(12): 1395-1403.

[23] Rosenbauer J, Herzig P, Von KR et al. Temporal, Seasonal, And Geographical Incidence Patterns Of Type 1 Diabetes Mellitus In Children Under 5 Years Of Age In Germany. Diabetologia 1999; 42(9): 1055-1059.

[24] Karvonen M, Pitkaniemi J, Tuomilehto J. The Onset Age Of Type 1 Diabetes In Finnish Children Has Become Younger. The Finnish Childhood Diabetes Registry Group. Diabetes Care 1999; 22(7): 1066-1070.

[25] Laakso M, Pyorala K. Age Of Onset And Type Of Diabetes. Diabetes Care 1985; 8: 114-117.

[26] Molbak AG, Christau B, Marner B et al. Incidence Of Insulin-Dependent Diabetes Mellitus In Age Groups Over 30 Years In Denmark. Diabetic Med 1994; 11: 650-655.

[27] Devendra D, Liu E, Eisenbarth GS. Type 1 Diabetes: Recent Developments. BMJ 2004; 328: 750–754.

[28] Barker JM, Barriga KJ, Yu L, et al. Prediction Of Autoantibody Positivity And Progression To Type 1 Diabetes: Diabetes Autoimmunity Study In The Young (DAISY). J Clin Endocrinol Metab 2004; 89: 3896–3902.

[29] Karvonen M, Pitkaniemi M, Pitkaniemi J et al. Sex Difference In The Incidence Of Insulin-Dependent Diabetes Mellitus: An Analysis Of The Recent Epidemiological Data. World Health Organization DIAMOND Project Group. Diabetes Metab Rev 1997; 13(4): 275-291.

[30] Karvonen M, Viik-Kajander M, Moltchanova E et al. Incidence Of Childhood Type 1 Diabetes Worldwide. Diabetes Mondiale DIAMOND Project Group. Diabetes Care 2000; 23(10): 1516-1526.

[31] Diagnosis And Classification/ Pathogenesis. In: Bode BW. Medical Management Of Type I Diabetes. 4a Ed. Alexandria (Virginia): American Diabetes Association; 2004. P. 4-18.

[32] Eisenbarth GS. Type 1 Diabetes Mellitus. In: Kahn CR, Weir GC, King GL, Moses AC, Smith RJ, Jacobson AM. Joslin's Diabetes Mellitus. 14a Ed. Boston, MA: Lippincott Williams & Wilkins; 2005. Cap. 23, P.399-424.

[33] Baekkeskov S, et al. Auto-Antibodies In Newly Diagnosed Diabetic Children Immunoprecipitate Human Pancreatic Islet Cell Proteins. Nature 1982; 298: 167 – 169.

[34] Kamradt,T.; Mitchison, N.A. Tolerance And Autoimmunity. N.Engl.J.Med 2001; 344(9): 655-664.

[35] Vafiadis, P. et al. Insulin Expression In Human Thymus Is Modulated By Ins Vntr Alleles At The Iddm2 Locus. Nat.Genet 1997; 15(3): 289-292.

[36] Krischer JP, Cuthbertson DD, Yu L, et al. Screening Strategies For The Identification Of Multiple Antibody-Positive Relatives Of Individuals With Type 1 Diabetes. J Clin Endocrinol Metab 2003; 88: 103–108.

[37] Maclaren N, Lan M, Coutant R, et al. Only Multiple Autoantibodies To Islet Cells (ICA), Insulin, GAD65, IA-2 And IA-2beta Predict Immune-Mediated (Type 1) Diabetes In Relatives. J Autoimmun 1999; 12: 279–287.

[38] Lohmann T, Sessler J, Verlohren HJ et al. Distinct Genetic And Immunological Features In Patients With Insulin-Dependent Diabetes Below And Above Age 40 At Onset. Diabetes Care 1997; 20: 524-529.

[39] Rivera A et al. Role Of B Cells As Antigen-Presenting Cells In Vivo Revisited: Antigen-Specific B Cells Are Essential For T Cell Expansion In Lymph Nodes And For Systemic T Cell Responses To Low Antigen Concentrations. Int Immunol; 13(12): 1583-1593.

[40] Pescovitz MD et al. Rituximab, B-Lymphocyte Depletion, And Preservation Of Beta-Cell Function. N Engl J Med 2009; 361(22): 2143-2152.

[41] Acherbach P, Bonifacio E, Koczwara K, Ziegler AG. Natural History Of Type 1 Diabetes. Diabetes 2005; 54(2): S25-S31.

[42] Pihoker C, Gilliam LK, Hampe CS et al. Autoantibodies In Diabetes. Diabetes 2005; 54(2): S52-S61.

[43] Yu L, Eisenbarth GS. Humoral Autoimmunity - Chapter 10, 2008. Em: <Http://Www.Uchsc.Edu/Misc/Diabetes/Books/Type1/Type1_Ch10.Html>. Acesso Em: Jun 2010.

[44] Winter WE, Harris N, Schatz D. Type 1 Diabetes Islet Autoantibody Markers. Diabetes Technol Ther 2002; 4(6): 817-39.

[45] Payton MA, Hawkes CJ, Christie MR. Relationship Of The 37,000- And 40,000-M(R) Tryptic Fragments Of Islet Antigens In Insulin-Dependent Diabetes To The Protein Tyrosine Phosphatase-Like Molecule IA-2 (ICA512). J Clin Invest 1995; 96(3): 1506-1511.

[46] Lu J, Li Q, Xie H et al. Identification Of A Second Transmembrane Protein Tyrosine Phosphatase, IA-2beta, As An Autoantigen In Insulin-Dependent Diabetes Mellitus: Precursor Of The 37-Kda Tryptic Fragment. Proc Natl Acad Sci USA 1996; 93(6): 2307-2311.

[47] Graham J, Hagopian WA, Kockum I et al. Genetic Effects On Age-Dependent Onset And Islet Cell Autoantibody Markers In Type 1 Diabetes. Diabetes 2002; 51(5): 1346-1355.

[48] Kawasaki E, Takino H, Yano M et al. Autoantibodies To Glutamic Acid Decarboxylase In Patients With IDDM And Autoimmune Thyroid Disease. Diabetes 1994; 43(1): 80-86.

[49] Eisenbarth GS, Jeffrey J. The Natural History Of Type 1A Diabetes. Arq Bras Endrocrinol Metab 2008;52(2): 146-155.

[50] Wenzlau JM et al. The Cation Efflux Transporter Znt8 (Slc30A8) Is A Major Autoantigen In Human Type 1 Diabetes. Proc Natl Acad Sci 2007; 104(43): 17040-17045.

[51] Zimmet PZ. The Pathogenesis And Prevention Of Diabetes In Adults. Diabetes Care 1995; 18(7): 1050-1064.

[52] Reijonen H, Concannom. Genetics Of Type 1 Diabetes. In: Kahn CR, Weir GC, King GL, Moses AC, Smith RJ, Jacobson AM. Joslin's Diabetes Mellitus. 14ª Ed. Boston, MA: Lippincott Williams & Wilkins; 2005. Cap. 21, P.355-370.

[53] Redondo MJ, Fain PR, Eisenbarth GS. Genetics Of Type 1A Diabetes. Recent Prog Horm Res 2001; 56: 69–89.

[54] Lambert AP, Gillespie KM, Thomson G, et al. Absolute Risk Of Childhood-Onset Type 1 Diabetes Defined By Human Leukocyte Antigen Class II Genotype: A Population-Based Study In The United Kingdom. J Clin Endocrinol Metab 2004; 89: 4037–4043.

[55] Anjos S, Polychronakos C. Mechanisms Of Genetic Susceptibility To Type 1 Diabetes: Beyond HLA. Mol Genet Metab 2004; 81: 187–195.

[56] Akerblom HK, Vaarala O, Hyooty H et al. Environmental Factors In The Etiology Of Type 1 Diabetes. Am J Med Genet 2002; 115: 18-29.

[57] Hyoty H, Hiltunen M, Knip M et al. The Childhood Diabetes In Finland (Dime) Study Group. A Prospective Study Of The Role Of Coxsackie B And Other Enterovirus Infections In The Pathogenesis Of IDDM. Diabetes 1995; 44: 652-657.

[58] Lammi N, Karvonen M, Tuomilehto J. Do Microbes Have A Causal Role In Type 1 Diabetes? Med Sci Monit 2005; 11: 63–69.

[59] Robles DT, Eisenbarth GS. Type 1A Diabetes Induced By Infection And Immunization. J Autoimmun 2001; 16: 355–362.

[60] Helgason T, Jonasson MR. Evidence For A Food Additive As A Cause Of Ketosis-Prone Diabetes. Lancet 1981; 318: 716–720.

[61] Dahlquist G, Mustonen L. Analysis Of 20 Years Of Prospective Registration Of Childhood Onset Diabetes Time Trends And Birth Cohort Effects. Swedish Childhood Study Group. Acta Paediatr 2000; 89: 1231–1237.

[62] Weets I, De Leeuw IH, Du Caju MV, et al. The Incidence Type1 Diabetes In The Age Group 0–39 Years Has Not Increased In Antwerp (Belgium) Between 1989 And 2000. Diabetes Care 2002; 25: 840–846.

[63] Tremblay MS, Willms JD. Secular Trends In The Body Mass Index Of Canadian Children. CMAJ 2000; 163: 1429–1433.

[64] Chinn S, Hughes JM, Rona RJ. Trends In Growth And Obesity In Ethnic Groups In Britain. Arch Dis Child 1998; 19: 162–166.

[65] Wilkin TJ. The Accelerator Hypothesis: Weight Gain As The Missing Link Between Type 1 And Type II Diabetes. Diabetologia 2001; 44: 914-922

[66] Alanentalo T, Rnblad AH, Mayans S et al. Quantification And Three-Dimensional Imaging Of The Insulitis-Induced Destruction Of _-Cells In Murine Type 1 Diabetes. Diabetes 2010; 59: 1756-1764.

[67] Meier JJ, Menge BA, Breuer T et al. Functional Assessment Of Pancreatic Cell Area In Humans. Diabetes 2009; 58: 1595-1603.

[68] Ueberberg S, Meier JJ, Waengler C et al. Generation Of Novel Single-Chain Antibodies By Phage-Display Technology To Direct Imaging Agents Highly Selective To Pancreatic - Or -Cells In Vivo. Diabetes 2009; 58: 2324-2334

[69] Screenan S, Pick AJ, Levisetti M et al. Increased Beta-Cell Proliferation And Reduced Mass Before Diabetes Onset In The Non obese Diabetic Mouse. Diabetes 1999; 48: 989-996.

[70] Shimada A, Charlton B, Taylor-Edwards C, Fathman CG: Beta-Cell Destruction May Be A Late Consequence Of Autoimmune Process In Non Obese Diabetic Mice. Diabetes 1996; 45: 1063-1067.

[71] Marchetti P, Dotta F, Zhiong L, et al. The Function Of Pancreatic Islets Isolated From Type 1 Diabetic Patient. Diabetes Care 2000; 23: 701-703.

[72] Lucinio-Paixao J, Polonsky KS, Given BD et al. Ingestion Of A Mixed Meal Does Not Affect The Metabolic Clearance Rate Of Biosynthetic Human C-Peptide. J Clin Endocrinol Metab 1983; 63: 401-403.

[73] Gumbiner B, Polonsky KS, Beltz WF et al. Effects Of Weight Loss And Reduces Hyperglycemia On The Kinetics Of Insulin Secretion In Obese Non-Insulin Dependent Diabetes Mellitus. J Clin Endocrinol Metab 1990; 70: 1594-1602.

[74] Covic AM, Schelling JR, Constantiner M et al. Serum C-Peptide Concentrations Poorly Phenotype Type 2 Diabetic End-Stage Renal Disease Patients. Kidney Intern 2000;58(4):1742-50.

[75] Cavaghan MK, Polonsky KS. Insulin Secretion In Vivo. In: Kahn CR, Weir GC, King GL, Moses AC, Smith RJ, Jacobson AM. Joslin's Diabetes Mellitus. 14ª Ed. Boston, MA: Lippincott Williams & Wilkins; 2005. Cap. 7, P.109-124.

[76] Vendrame F, Zappaterreno A, Dotta F. Markers Of Beta Cell Function In Type 1 Diabetes Mellitus. Minerva Med 2004; 95:1-6.

[77] Tsai EB, Sherry NA, Palmer JP, Herold KC. For The DPT-1 Study Group.The Rise And Fall Of Insulin Secretion In Type 1 Diabetes Mellitus. Diabetologia 2006;49:261-70.

[78] Fujisawa T, Ikegami H, Kawaguchi Y et al. Class I HLA Is Associated With Age-At-Onset Of IDDM, While Class II HLA Confers Susceptibility To IDDM. Diabetologia 1995; 38(12): 1493-1495.

[79] Faber OK, Binder C. C-Peptide Response To Glucagon. Diabetes 1977; 26: 605-610.

[80] Steele C, Hagopian WA, Gitelman S et al. Insulin Secretion In Type 1 Diabetes. Diabetes 2004; 53: 426-433.

[81] Sherry NA, Tsai EB, Palmer JP, Herold KC. Natural History Of Beta Cell Function In Type 1 Diabetes. Diabetes 2005; 54(Suppl 2): 32-39.

[82] Koskinem PJ, Viikari JS, Irjala KMA. Glucagon-Stimulated And Posprandial Plasma C-Peptide Values As Measures Of Insulin Secretory Capacity. Diabetes Care 1988; 11(4): 318- 322.

[83] Cernea S, Raz I, Kevan C et al. Challenges In Developing Endpoints For Type 1 Diabetes Intervention Studies. Diabetes Metab Res Rev 2009; 25: 694-704.

[84] Palmer J.P et al. C-Peptide In The Natural History Of Type 1 Diabetes. Diabetes Metab Res Rev 2009; 25(4): 325-328.

[85] Scheen AJ, Castillo MJ, Lefebvre PJ. Assessment Of Residual Insulin Secretion In Diabetic Patients Using The Intravenous Glucagon Stimulatory Test: Methodological Aspects And Clinical Implications. Diabetes Metab 1996; 22: 397-446.

[86] Greenbaum C, Harison IC. Guidelines For Intervention Trials In Subjects With Newly Diagnosed Type 1 Diabetes. Diabetes 2003; 52: 1059-1065.

[87] Palatnik, M et al. Ethnicity And Type 2 Diabetes In Rio De Janeiro, Brazil, With A Review Of The Prevalence Of The Disease In Amerindians. Hum Biol 2002; 74 (4): 533-544.

[88] Chase HP, Cuthbertson DD, Dolan LM et al. First-Phase Insulin Release During The Intravenous Glucose Tolerance Test As A Risk Factor For Type 1 Diabetes. J Pediatr 2001; 138(2): 244-249.

[89] Keskinen P, Korhonen S, Kupila A et al. First - Phase Insulin Response In Young Healthy Children At Genetic And Immunological Risk For Type 1 Diabetes. Diabetologia 2002; 45(12): 1639-1648.

[90] Meier JJ, Bhushan A, Butler AE et al. Sustained Beta Cell Apoptosis In Patients With Long-Standing Type 1 Diabetes: Indirect Evidence For Islet Regeneration? Diabetologia 2005; 48(11): 2221-8.

[91] Keenan HA, Berger A, Sun JK et al. Demonstration Of Islet Cell Function In Patients With 50 Years Or Longer Of Diabetes. Diabetes 2007;56(S1): 386.

[92] Rodacki M, Milech A, Oliveira JEP. A Secreção Residual Do Peptídeo C Faz Diferença No Tratamento Do Diabetes Melito Tipo 1? Arq Bras Endocrinol Metab 2008; 52(2): 322-333.

[93] Snorgaard O, Larsen LH, Binder C. Homogeneity In Patter Of Decline Of B-Cell Function In IDDM. Diabetes Care 1992; 15: 1009-1015.

[94] Karjalainen J, Salmela P, Ilonen J et al. A Comparison Of Childhood And Adult Type 1 Diabetes. N Engl J Med 1989; 320: 881-886.

[95] Ludvigsson J. The Role Of Immunomodulation Therapy In Autoimmune Diabetes. J Diabetes Sci Technol 2009; 3(2): 320-330.

[96] Ludvigsson J, Faresjö M, Hjorth M et al. GAD Treatment And Insulin Secretion In Recent-Onset Type 1 Diabetes. N Engl J Med 2008; 359(18): 1909-20.

[97] Kolb H, Gale EA. Does Partial Preservation Of Residual Beta-Cell Function Justify Immune Intervention In Recent Onset Type I Diabetes? Diabetologia 2001; 44(10): 1349-53.

[98] Sjöberg S, Gunnarsson R. Residual Insulin Production, Glycaemic Control And Prevalence Of Microvascular Lesions And Polyneuropathy In Long-Term Type 1 (Insulin-Dependent) Diabetes Mellitus. Diabetologia 1987; 30: 208-213.

[99] Klein R, Moss SE, Klein BE et al. Wisconsin Epidemiologic Study Of Diabetic Retinopathy. XII. Relationship Of C-Peptide And Diabetic Retinopathy. Diabetes 1990; 39(11): 1445-50.

[100] Winocour PH, Jeacock J, Kalsi P et al. The Relevance Of Persistent C-Peptide Secretion In Type 1 (Insulindependent) Diabetes Mellitus To Glycaemic Control And Diabetic Complications. Diabetes Res Clin Pract 1990; 9(1): 23-35.

[101] Gomes MB, Goncalves MF, Neves R et al. Residual Beta-Cell Function And Microvascular Complications In Type 1 Diabetic Patients. Braz J Med Biol Res 2000; 33(2): 211-6.

[102] S Berna P, Valentini U, Cimino A, Sabatti MC, Rotondi A, Crisetig M, Et Al. Residual B-Cell Function In Insulin-Dependent (Typei) Diabetics With And Without Retinopathy. Acta Diabetol Lat 1986; 23(4): 339-44.

[103] Brown RJ, Rother KI. Effects Of Beta-Cell Rest On Beta-Cell Function: A Review Of Clinical And Preclinical Data. Pediatric Diabetes 2008; 9(3): 14–22.

[104] Cernea S, Herold K. Drug Insight: New Immunomodulatory Therapies In Type 1 Diabetes. Nat Clin Pract Endocrinol Metab 2006; 2(2): 89-98.

[105] Herold KC, Hagopian W, Auger JA et al. Anti-CD3 Monoclonal Antibody In New-Onset Type 1 Diabetes Mellitus. N Engl J Med 2002; 346: 1692-98.

[106] Herold KC, Gitelman SE, Masharani U, et al. A Single Course Of Anti-CD3 Monoclonal Antibody Hokt3gamma1(Ala-Ala) Results In Improvement In C-Peptide Responses And Clinical Parameters For At Least 2 Years After Onset Of Type 1 Diabetes. Diabetes 2005; 54(6): 1763-9.

[107] Chéramy M, Skoglund C, Johansson I, Ludvigsson J. GAD-alum treatment in patients with type 1 diabetes and the subsequent effect on GADA IgG subclass distribution, GAD65 enzyme activity and humoral response. Clin Immunol. 2010;137 (1): 31-40.

[108] Ziegler AG, Walter M. Loss And Preservation Of B-Cell Function: Two Treatment Regimes Targeting T Or B Lymphocytes. Diabetologia 2010; 10(5): 323-325.

[109] Lazar L, Ofan R, Weintrob N, et al. Heat-Shock Protein Peptide Dia-pep277 Treatment In Children With Newly Diagnosed Type 1 Diabetes: A Randomised, Double-Blind Phase II Study. Diabetes Metab Res Rev 2007;23(4):286-91.

[110] Raz I, Avron A, Tamir M, et al. Treatment Of New-Onset Type 1 Diabetes With Peptide Dia-Pep277 Is Safe And Associated With Preserved Beta-Cell Function: Extension Of A Randomized, Double-Blind, Phase II Trial. Diabetes Metab Res Rev 2007; 23(4): 292-8.

[111] Voltarelli JC, Couri CE, Stracieri AB, et al. Autologous Nonmyeloablative Hematopoietic Stem Cell Transplantation In Newly Diagnosed Type 1 Diabetes Mellitus. JAMA 2007; 297(14): 1568-76.

12

Diabetic Nephrophaty in Children

Snezana Markovic-Jovanovic[1],
Aleksandar N. Jovanovic[2] and Radojica V. Stolic[2]
[1]*Pediatric clinic, Medical Faculty Prishtina, Kosovska Mitrovica*
[2]*Internal clinic, Medical Faculty Prishtina, Kosovska Mitrovica*
Serbia

1. Introduction

Diabetic nephropathy (DN) is one of the consequences of a long-term diabetes, typically defined by macroalbuminuria — that is, a urinary albumin excretion of more than 300 mg in a 24-hour collection — or macroalbuminuria and abnormal renal function as represented by an abnormality in serum creatinine, calculated creatinine clearance, or glomerular filtration rate (GFR). [1]

2. Prevalence

Long-term microvascular and neurologic complications cause major morbidity and mortality in patients with insulin-dependent diabetes mellitus (IDDM) [2]. The incidence of overt nephropathy rapidly grows 10-15 years after the onset of type 1 diabetes mellitus; the incidence of nephropathy declines after that period and the occurence of nephropathy after 35 years of duration of type 1 diabetes is uncommon. Diabetic nephropathy rarely develops before 10 years' duration of IDDM. The peak incidence (3% per year) is usually found in persons who have had diabetes for 10-20 years. The increased mortality risk in long-term T1DM may be due to nephropathy, which may account for about 50% of deaths.

Epidemiologic data derived from one of the studies – EDC – showed that in group of patients aged <18 and with the duration of diabetes over 5 years the prevalence of microalbuminia reached as much as 14%. Long-term diabetes further increased the prevalence of albuminiria, thus 80% of male and 50% of female patients having diabetes up to 30 years of duration had proteinuria in micro- or macroalbuminuric range. ([3-4])

3. What is microalbuminuria

Microalbuminuria is a marker for more serious proteinuria followed by azotemia in type 1 diabetic nephropathy[5] . Microalbuminuria develops in 40-60% type 1 diabetic patients and over 50% of patients with microalbuminuria evolve to macroalbuminuric stage e.g. advanced phase of overt diabetic nephropathy.

4. Risk factor for diabetes nephropathy

Reported risk factors for the development of diabetic renal disease include a longer duration of IDDM, an earlier age at the time of diagnosis, onset of puberty, poorer glycemic control during the first five years of diabetes, smoking, and a family history of diabetic nephropathy.[6-7]

Some of the factors leading to occurrence of diabetic nephropathy are hereditary predisposition (ACE genotype), poor glycemic control, diabetes - induced hyperfiltration, tissue hypoxia owing to reduction in capillary permeability, and increased postcapillary resistance . The capillary changes are caused by accumulation of glycated proteins and interaction of these proteins with cellular elements in the capillary walls, that effectuate the decrement in capillary ability for dilatation and ultimately, lead to capillary obstruction. In diabetes, morphological changes in type 4 collagen, heparin – sulphat proteoglycane, fibronectin and enectin molecules leads to structural and functional changes in basal membrane of the renal capillary bed . [8]

The theory of a reduction in nephron number at birth indicates that individuals born with a reduced number of glomeruli may be predisposed to subsequent renal injury and progressive nephropathy. This has been shown in animal studies in which the mother was exposed to hyperglycemia at the time of pregnancy. If this linkage is true in humans, that would have important implications concerning the role of maternal factors in the eventual development of kidney disease. [1]

Certain ethnic groups, particularly African Americans, persons of Hispanic origin, and American Indians, may be particularly disposed to renal disease as a complication of diabetes.

5. Pathology and patohistologic changes in diabetic nephropathy

The earliest morphologic abnormality in diabetic nephropathy is the thickening of the glomerular basement membrane (GBM) and expansion of the mesangium due to accumulation of extracellular matrix. Light microscopy findings in diffuse diabetic nephropathy show an increase in the solid spaces of the tuft, most frequently observed (by the positive periodic-acid Schiff reaction) as coarse branching of solid material. Large acellular accumulations also may be observed within these areas. These are circular on section and are known as the Kimmelstiel-Wilson lesions/nodules. Three major histologic changes occur in the glomeruli of persons with diabetic nephropathy. First, mesangial expansion which may be directly induced by hyperglycemia, perhaps via increased matrix production or glycation of matrix proteins. Second, a glomerulal basement membrane thickening may occur. Third, glomerular sclerosis being caused by intraglomerular hypertension (induced by renal vasodilatation or from ischemic injury induced by hyaline narrowing of the vessels supplying the glomeruli). These different histological patterns appear to have similar prognostic significance.

Hyperglycemia induces diverse metabolic changes which may give birth to variety of microvascular lesions. The glycation (also called non-enzymatic glycosilation) of proteins is a process induced by the incubation of soluble proteins in the solution with a high glucose concentrations. Glucation lead to three-dimensional structural and/or functional alterations of the proteins involved: thus, the glycation of the erythrocyte membrane proteins leads to its increased adherence ability; likewise, the glycation of heparin – sulphate proteoglycans leads to proliferation of mesangial cells.

High glucose level induces activation of polyol metabolic pathway resulting in increased sobritol production. Sorbitol, in turn, reduces intracellular myoinositol levels leading to increased capillary permeability and structural basal membrane changes. [9]

Hyperglycemia increases the expression of transforming growth factor-beta (TGF-beta) in the glomeruli and of matrix proteins specifically stimulated by this cytokine. TGF-beta may contribute to the cellular hypertrophy and enhanced collagen synthesis observed in persons with diabetic nephropathy. [10] High glucosae levels may also may activate protein kinase C, which further contribute to renal disease and other vascular complications of diabetes.

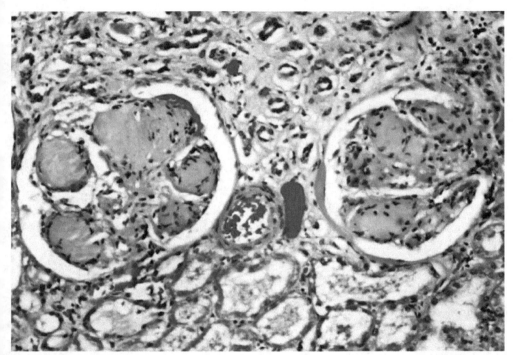

Fig. 1. Nodular glomerularsclerosis – *Nodular glomerulosclerosis in the kidney of a patient with diabetic nephropathy. US Federal Government public domain image. Source: CDC. (This image was copied from wikipediaen)*

Tissue hypoxia, augmented capillary permeability and capillary blood flow are the factors which cause increased production of angiotensin II in 45% of diabetics. Angiotensin II might generate precapillary and capillary hypertension. The presence of risk factors for hypertension is particularlly important in patients with relatively poor glucose control (hemoglobin A1 concentration above 12 percent). These patients are at increased risk of developing overt nephropathy within 20 years. [11]. Furthermore, the risk for developing diabetic nephropathy in adolescents with type 1 diabetes whose parents suffered hypertension is threefold increased. [12] The effects of prostaglandin PGI2 produced by hyperertrophic mesangial cells and atrial natriuretic polypeptide may be important in development of microvascular complications including diabetic nepropathy.

In our previous study[13], performed among the 55 pediatric patients with type 1 diabetes, who had urinary albumin excretion in the range of microalbuminuria was found in almost half (17 of 35 e.g. 48.6%) of children with diabetic ketoacidosis. Furthermore, among the 20 patients with normoalbuminuric UAE only 3 (15.0%) had ketoacidosis.

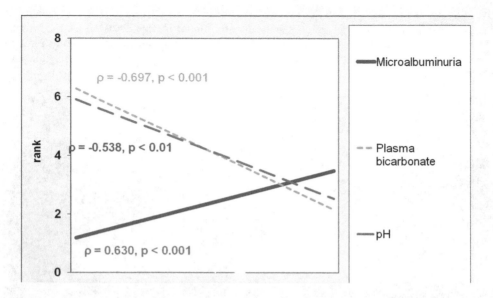

Fig. 2. Showing the correlations between the level of UAE and main parameters of acid-base staus.

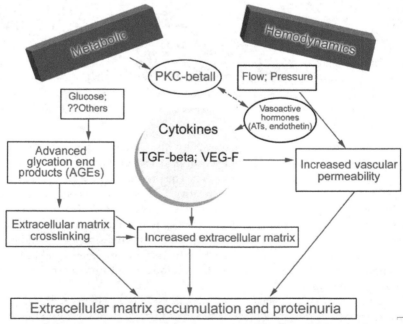

Fig. 3. The pathogenesis of diabetic nephropathy, Soman SS, Soman AS>Diabetic Nephropathy eMedicine Specialities, Endocrinology, Diabetes Mellitus, 2009.

The results of the study[13] revealed a quite significant correlation between microalbuminuria and plasma pH and bicarbonates; moreover, the level of plasma bicarbonate was a very good predictor of UAE values, depicting the aggravation of urinary albumin excretion in a response to the development of diabetic ketoacidosis

6. Alterations in renal function in diabetic nephropathy

There are 5 clinical stages of diabetic nephropathy. In the first stage, there is the substantial increase of glomerular filtration rate. Hyperglycemia and the lack of insulin along with several other hormones and factors undoubtedly contribute to development of hyperfiltration. The increase in glomerular filtration rate correlates with the enlargement of total filtration surface owing to glomerular hypertrophy; the latter reaches as much as 80% of the values existing prior to diabetes.

In the second ("silent") phase hypefunctional periods alternate the periods of normal function, and vice-versa. The periodicity of these alterations depend on quality of metabolic control. Glomerular filtration rate is, therefore, variable, arterial blood pressure is mainly within the normal range, although a mild hypertension might be present; UAE excretion rate is normal.

The third stage (the incipient nephropathy) is characterized by UAE within microalbuminuric range (30-3oo mg/24 h), there is progressive increment of arterial blood pressure, usually 5-15mmHg above the normal values, while the glomerular filtration rate may be normal, increased or reduced.

In our previous study, the total of 40% microalbuminuric children had systolic prehypertension and systolic hypertension (17.1% and 22.9%, respectively) and even 60% had diastolic blood pressure disorders: diastolic prehypertension was found in 35% and diastolic hypertension in 25% patients with microalbuminuria. While the microalbuminuric patients had significantly higher blood pressure comparing to normoalbuminuric group, its noteworthy that the percentage (15% with systolic and 20% with diastolic disturbances) of prehypertensive and hypertensive patients among the type 1 diabetic children with normal UAE was also relatively high (Fig.1 and 2). The level of blood pressure correlated significantly with UAE, but was not proved to be a predictor of microalbuminuria in children with type 1 diabetes.

The fourth stage, also known as manifest nephropathy, a clinically manifest proteinuria ensues, with UAE excretion rate exceeding 3oo mg/24h; albuminuria tends to be progressive, possibly leading to the clinical manifestations of nephritic syndrome. As nephropathy evolves to early overt stage with proteinuria (UAE >300 mg/24 hr, or >200 µg/min), it is accompanied by hypertension. The arterial blood pressure is generally raised by 7% per year, followed by the variable reduction in glomerular filtration rate. In the majority of patients, in the midst of this phase a manifest renal insufficiency characterized by overt azotemia occurs. The fourth and fifth stages almost never occur in children and are quite rare in adolescents, mostly being related to the adult population.

The fifth phase (renal insufficiency) is characterized by the general glomerular collapse, followed by overt azotemia, manifest proteinuria and grave hypertension.

Microalbuminuria is also a well-established marker of increased CVD risk [15-16]

At the beginning, proteinuria is mild and intermittent and may remain that way during 5-10 years following the first discovery. However, an increase of the amount of excreted protein and of frequency of proteinuric episodes might be expected afterwards. The beginning of retinopathy may precede or follow the occurrence of nephropathy, but in the later stages these two diabetic complications usually have roughly parallel course.

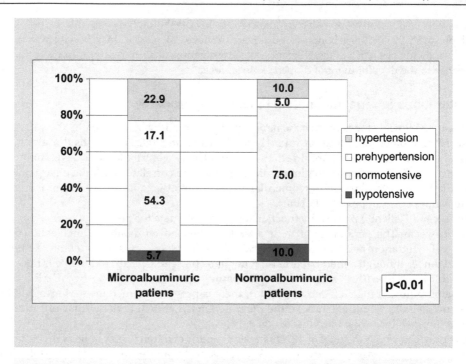

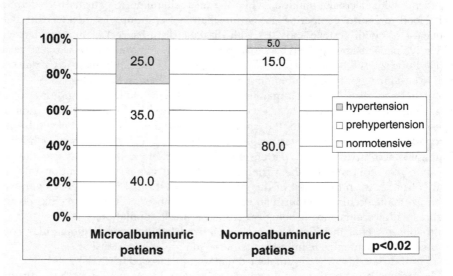

Fig. 4 and 5. Showing the percentage of blood pressure disturbances in microalbuminuric and normoalbuminuric group of children with type 1 diabetes .

Phase of constant and massive proteinuria may follow the stage of intermittent proteinuria. During the period, serum creatinine remains normal or slightly increased. The duration of this stage may be variable. Its course may accelerate leading to terminal renal insufficiency. The first sign of this acceleration is the rise in serum creatinine level.

Advanced stage nephropathy is defined by a progressive decline in renal function (declining glomerular filtration rate and elevation of serum blood urea and creatinine), progressive proteinuria, and hypertension. Progression to end-stage renal disease (ESRD) is recognized by the appearance of uremia, the nephritic syndrome.

Natural History of Diabetic Nephropathy

	Designation	Characteristics	GFR (minimum)	Albumin Excretion	Blood Pressure	Chronology
Stage 1	Hyperfunction and hypertrophy	Glomerular hyperfiltration	Increased in type 1 and type 2	May Be Increased	Type 1 normal Type 2 normal hypertension	Present at time of diagnosis
Stage 2	Silent stage	Thickend BM Expanded mesangium	Normal	Type 1 normal Type 2 may be <30-300 mg/d	Type 1 normal Type 2 normal hypertension	First 5 years
Stage 3	Incipient stage	Microalbuminuria	GFR begins to fall	30-300 mg/d	Type 1 increased Type 2 normal hypertension	6-15 years
Stage 4	Overt diabetic nephropathy	Macroalbuminuria	GFR below N	>380 mg/d	Hypertension	15-25 years
Stage 5	Uremic	ESRD	0-10	Decreasing	Hypertension	25-30 years

Fig. 6. Soman SS, Soman AS: Diabetic Nephropathy eMedicine Specialities, Endocrinology, Diabetes Mellitus, 2009.

7. The clinical features and laboratory findings in diabetic nephropathy

The first system manifestation of diabetic nephropathy is the occurrence of **peripheral oedema** usually on ankles. Contrary to the widely accepted conviction that only hypoalbuminemia gives rise to ankle oedema, the direct cause of this symptom is usually not found. It seems that the pathogenesis of this symptom is quite complex. In most of the patients, the frail capillary walls are detected very often and, thus, the oedema might be due to increased capillary permeability.

Regardless of cause, the peripheral oedema always indicate advanced stage of diabetic nephropathy and the occurrence and extent of the swelling is dependent on the duration of clinically manifest proteinuria. Also, the complaints related to lower leg muscle cramps are not unusual.

Hypertension: Incipient to mild structural glomerular lesions do not correlate with the raise in arterial blood pressure. However, in the advanced stage of diabetic nephropathy the arterial hypertension is almost always present and relates with the duration of clinically manifest proteinuria.

Some of our previous results[13] showed a very good correlation between the level of urinary albumin excretion and the values of systolic and diastolic arterial blood pressure. Still, the arterial blood pressure level was not predictive for microalbuminuria, judging by the multiple regression analysis, as already stated above.

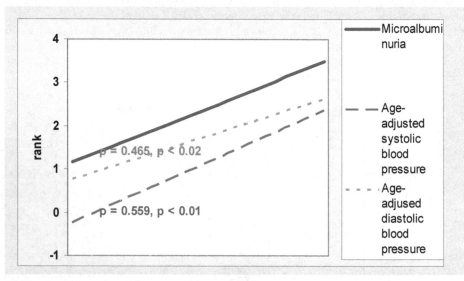

Fig. 7. Showing the relation between the arterial blood pressure level and UAE values

Paradoxally, however, there is no good correlation between the reduction in glomerular filtration rate and the rise in arterial blood pressure [17-18]. Yet, most certainly, the therapy aimed at lowering high blood pressure leads to slowing down in reduction of glomerular filtration.

Macroproteinuria: The amount of proteins daily excreted in patients with diabetic nephropathy ranges from the minimal concentrations of 30 mg/day to more than 20g/day. The average excretion is about 2,5g/24h. In about 20% of patients with nephropathy the amount is less than 1g/day and in 15% it exceeds 5g/day (nephritic syndrome). Therefore, although proteinuria is considered a marker of of chronic diabetic nephropathy, yet it relatively rarely reach the nephritic range.

Other symptoms of kidney disease include loss of sleep, poor appetite, upset stomach, weakness, and difficulty concentrating. Characteristic signs are:
- Going to the bathroom more often at night
- Less need for insulin or antidiabetic medications
- Morning sickness, nausea, and vomiting
- Weakness, paleness, and anemia
- Itching

8. Differential diagnosis

Other pathological states of potential significance in differential diagnosis are:
- Cholesterol embolization
- Chronic obstruction
- Interstitial nephritis
- Amyloidosis

Disease	Differentiating Signs/Symptoms	Differentiating Tests
Non diabetic kidney disease	• Since both diabetes mellitus and chronic kidney disease (CKD) are common disorders, patients with both conditions may or may not have DN. A diagnosis other than DN should be considered if: there is a rapid progression of renal failure, evidence of another systemic disease, or short duration of diabetes (although onset is insidious in type 2, and DN may occasionally be the presenting manifestation of type 2 DM).	• Minimal proteinuria may indicate nondiabetic kidney disease. • Other specific diagnostic tests for other systemic disorders associated with nondiabetic kidney disease may be positive.
Multiple myeloma (MM)	• Multiple myeloma (MM) patients also may present with renal failure and proteinuria. • Symptoms of bone pain and anemia are the most common presenting features, affecting 80% of patients with MM.	• The characteristic test results that differ from DN are: the presence of paraproteinemia/paraproteinuria; hypercalcemia; impaired production of normal immunoglobulin; and lytic bone lesions. Bataille R, Harousseau JL. Multiple myeloma. N Engl J Med. 1997;336:1657-1664 • Urinalysis with sulfosalicylic acid (SSA) was classically utilized to evaluate for discrepancy between albumin and total protein, as standard urinalysis dipstick detects albumin only. SSA causes precipitation of all of the urinary proteins, including paraproteins (Bence Jones proteins). • Serum protein electrophoresis (SPEP), urine protein electrophoresis (UPEP): paraprotein spike. • Serum and urine free light chains: increased concentrations of free light chain in serum. • Skull x-rays, CT or MRI bone: lytic lesions. • Bone marrow biopsy: plasma cell Proliferation
Renal tract obstruction	• Can be caused by stones, cancer, fibrosis, prostate hypertrophy/cancer, neurogenic bladder, or pelviureteric junction obstruction. • Obstruction to urine flow can result in postrenal failure. Symptoms	• Passage of Foley catheter will result in flow of urine and relief of obstruction. • Kidney ultrasound: hydronephrosis, stones. • Prostate ultrasound: hypertrophy, cancer.

Disease	Differentiating Signs/Symptoms	Differentiating Tests
	include trouble passing urine, anuria, oliguria, hematuria, pain (with kidney stones), and urinary leakage/incontinence. Physical examination findings include enlarged prostate on rectal examination, costovertebral angle tenderness, suprapubic tenderness, and bladder fullness.	• CT abdomen: hydronephrosis, stones, mass, congenital abnormalities, fibrosis. • PSA: elevated in BPH, prostate cancer. • MRI: not routine but may show hydronephrosis, stones, mass, congenital abnormalities, fibrosis
Glomerulonep hritis	Glomerulonephritis, such as lupus nephritis and cryoglobulinemia, is in the differential for DN. Patient presentation and physical examination may be similar to that of DN. However, there may be symptoms and signs of other systemic disease, such as rashes or joint involvement.	Urinalysis: hematuria, proteinuria, RBC casts, dysmorphic red cells. Albuminuria. Positive serology (e.g., ANA, ANCA, hepatitis serology). Complement: decreased in immune glomerulonephritis (e.g., lupus). Kidney biopsy: glomerulonephritis.
Renal artery stenosis	Renal artery stenosis presents either as hypertension refractory to multiple maximized antihypertensives or as renal failure shortly after the initiation of an ACE inhibitor. Physical examination is significant for an abdominal bruit. Safian RD, Textor SC. Renal-artery stenosis. N Engl J Med. 2001;344:431-442	Ultrasound, CT scan, MRI: shrunken kidney, decreased flow through the renal artery. Magnetic resonance angiography (MRA): renal artery stenosis. Renal angiogram: renal artery stenosis.

Table 1. BMJ Group: Diabetic nephropathy, diferential diagnosis , epocrates online, 2010

8.1 The diagnosis of diabetic nephropathy [19]

Patients with diabetes should be screened annually for DKD. Initial screening should commence:

• 5 years after the diagnosis of type 1 diabetes; or
• From diagnosis of type 2 diabetes.

Screening should include:

• Measurements of urinary ACR in a spot urine sample;
• Measurement of serum creatinine and estimation of GFR.

An elevated ACR should be confirmed in the absence of urinary tract infection with 2 additional first-void specimens collected during the next 3 to 6 months.

• Microalbuminuria is defined as an ACR between 30-300 mg/g.
• Macroalbuminuria is defined as an ACR > 300 mg/g.
• 2 of 3 samples should fall within the microalbuminuric or macroalbuminuric range to confirm classification.

Using the CKD staging likelihood of DN can be determined as follows:

- Normoalbuminuria in CKD stages 3 to 5 (GFR <60) is unlikely to be DN.
- Microalbuminuria in CKD stages 1 to 3 (GFR >30) is possible DN.
- Microalbuminuria in CKD stages 4 to 5 (GFR <30) is unlikely to be DN.
- Macroalbuminuria at all stages of CKD is highly likely to be DN.

Urinanalysis	proteinuria
Urinary albumin for creatinine ratio	microalbuminuria: between 30 and 300 mg/g; macroalbuminuria: >300 mg/g
Blood biochemistry	elevated creatinine
Serum creatinine with GFR estimation	Glomerular filtration rate (GFR) may be raised in CKD stage 1, normal in CKD stage 2, and reduced in CKD stages 3 to 5
Kidney ultrasound	normal-to-large kidneys with increased echogenicity; may show hydronephrosis if vesiculopathy and/or obstruction is superimposed

Table 2. Clinical tests in diagnosis of diabetic nephropathyClinical tests in diagnostics of diabetic nephropathy:

Test	Results
24 hour urine to collection	microalbuminuria: albumin 30 to 300 mg/24 hours; macroalbuminuria: albumin >300 mg/24 hours
CT-abdomen	hydronephrosis; wedge-shaped areas of low attenuation; loss of the ability to distinguish the corticomedullary border; perinephric stranding; cysts; masses; stones
Magnet resonance angiography	renal artery stenosis
Doppler ultrasound	may show renal artery stenosis
Kidney biopsy	mesangial expansion, fibrosis, Kimmelstiel-Wilson nodules

The source: epocrates online com, 2010

Table 3. Other tests to consider

High blood pressure often goes along with diabetic nephropathy. You may have high blood pressure that develops rapidly or is difficult to control.

9. Treatment and therapy

Annual screening for microalbuminuria, with a random spot urine sample for microalbumin-to-creatinine ratio, should be initiated once the child is 10 years of age and has had diabetes for 5 years.

Confirmed, persistently elevated microalbumin levels on two additional urine specimens should be treated with an ACE inhibitor titrated to normalization of microalbumin excretion if possible

Once albuminuria is diagnosed, a number of factors attenuate the effect of hyperfiltration on kidneys:

1. Control of hyperglycemia- The Diabetes Control and Complications Trial (DCCT) [21] and the United Kingdom Prospective Diabetes Study (UKPDS) [21] have definitively shown that intensive diabetes therapy can significantly reduce the risk of the development of microalbuminuria and overt nephropathy in people with diabetes.

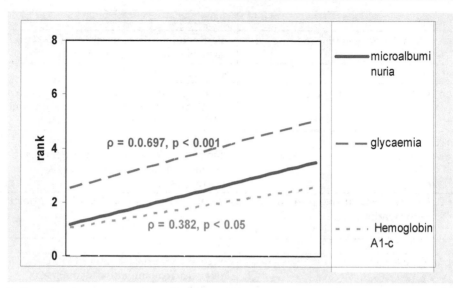

Fig. 8. Showing the relation of the parameters of metabolic regulation and the UAE level in children with type 1 diabetes

Accordingly the earlier study[13] revealed that hemoglobin A1/c and, particularly, blood glucose level were significantly related to urinary albumin excretion rate. Furthermore, blood glucose was the major predictor of microalbuminuria in children with type 1 diabetes. Lowering A1C to an average of ~7% has been shown to reduce microvascular and neuropathic complications of diabetes and, possibly, macrovascular disease. Preliminary results of the multicenter A1C-Derived Average Glucose (ADAG) Trial, presented at the European Association for the Study of Diabetes meeting in September 2007, confirmed a close correlation of A1C with mean glucose in patients with type 1, type 2, or no diabetes. Final results of this study, not available at the time this statement was completed, should allow more accurate reporting of the estimated average glucose (eAG) and improve patients' understanding of this measure of glycemia[22]

Target HbA1c for people with diabetes should be < 7.0%, irrespective of the presence or absence of CKD. [23]

Considering the high incidence of overnight hypoglycemias, in children and adolescents during the optimal regulation of blood glucosae levels, the A1C level achieved in the "intensive" adolescent cohort of the DCCT group was >1% higher than that achieved by adult DCCT subjects and above current ADA recommendations for patients in general. Standards of Medical Care in Diabetes – 2008 American Diabetes Association Tight glycemic control will delay the progression of microalbuminuria and slow the progression of diabetic nephropathy.

2. Aggressive control of systemic blood pressure- In patients with type 1 diabetes, hypertension is usually caused by underlying diabetic nephropathy and typically becomes manifest about the time that patients develop microalbuminuria . Hypertension in childhood is defined as an average systolic or diastolic blood pressure ≥95th percentile for age, sex, and height percentile measured on at least three separate days. "High-normal" blood pressure is defined as an average systolic or diastolic blood pressure ≥90th but <95th percentile for age, sex, and height percentile measured on at least three separate days.

Treatment of hi gh-normal blood pressure (systolic or diastolic blood pressure consistently above the 90th percentile for age, sex, and height) should include dietary intervention and exercise aimed at weight control and increased physical activity, if appropriate. If target blood pressure is not reached with 3–6 months of lifestyle intervention, pharmacologic treatment should be initiated.

Pharmacologic treatment of hypertension (systolic or diastolic blood pressure consistently above the 95th percentile for age, sex, and height or consistently >130/80 mmHg, if 95% exceeds that value) should be initiated as soon as the diagnosis is confirmed.

The principal agents for lowering high blood pressure are angiotensin convertase inhibitors (ACE). The beneficial effect of ACE inhibition on preventing progression from microalbuminuria to overt diabetic nephropathy is long-lasting (8 y) and is associated with the preservation of a normal GFR. ACE-I reduces the risk of progression of overt type 1 diabetic nephropathy to ESRD and in type 1 patients with microalbuminuria to overt nephropathy. [25] The results of multicentric studies showed that blood pressure in patients with chronic renal insufficiency should be lowered below normal range (as recommended by WHO) in order to achieve beneficial effect on progression of the disease.

A meta-analysis of several small studies has shown that protein restriction may be of benefit in some patients whose nephropathy seems to be progressing despite optimal glucose and blood pressure control [26]

Hypertensive people with diabetes and CKD stages 1-4 should be treated with an ACE inhibitor or an ARB (Angiotensin Receptor Blocer), usually in combination with a diuretic[27]

If needed to achieve blood pressure targets, a thiazide diuretic should be added to those with an estimated glomerular filtration rate (GFR) (see below) ≥50 ml/min per 1.73 m2 and a loop diuretic for those with an estimated GFR <50 ml/min per 1.73 m2. (E)

Normotensive people with diabetes and macroalbuminuria should be treated with an ACE inhibitor or an ARB.In type 1 diabetes with macroalbuminuria, ACE inhibitors decrease albuminuria and reduce the risk of clinical outcomes regardless of the presence or absence of hypertension. A randomized controlled trial in people with type 1 diabetes and macroalbuminuria found that ACE inhibitors reduced the risk of the combined outcome of doubling of serum creatinine level, CKD stage 5, and death. [28] A quarter of the participants were normotensive. There was no significant difference in the treatment effect between the normotensive and hypertensive individuals.

Future agents: Wenzel et al. [29] . have examined the role of avosentan (endothelin antagonist) on progression of microalbuminuria. Avosentan have demonstrated antifibrotic, anti-inflammatory, and antiproteinuric effects in experimental studies. Wenzel et al conducted a randomized, placebo-controlled, double-blind, parallel-design, dosage-range study on the effect of the endothelin-A antagonist avosentan (SPP301) on urinary albumin excretion rate in 286 patients with diabetic nephropathy, macroalbuminuria, and a blood pressure of <180/110 mm Hg. All dosages of avosentan, administered in addition to standard ACE inhibitor/ARB treatment, were found to reduce the mean relative urinary albumin excretion rate (-16.3% to -29.9%, relative to baseline) in the study's patients.

3. Selective control of arteriolar dilation by use of angiotensin-converting enzyme (ACE) inhibitors (thus decreasing transglomerular capillary pressure) This is particularly significant when lowering of systemic blood pressure is accompanied with concomitant lessening of glomerular capillary pressure. however the optimal lower limit for systolic blood pressure is unclear. [30]

4.   Dietary protein restriction (because high protein intake increases renal perfusion rate).
A meta-analysis examining the effects of dietary protein restriction (0.5-0.85 g/kg/d) in diabetic patients suggested a beneficial effect on the GFR, creatinine clearance, and albuminuria. However, a large, long-term prospective study is needed to establish the safety, efficacy, and compliance with protein restriction in diabetic patients with nephropathy. Considering the importance and role of dietary proteins in the process of growth and development, a sharp restriction (<15% of total daily amount of nutrients) of proteins in adolescents with diabetic nephropathy is not justified.

Other standard modalities for the treatment of progressive renal disease and its complications (e.g., osteodystrophy) must also be used when indicated, such as sodium and phosphate restriction and use of phosphate binders. When the GFR begins to decline substantially, referral to a physician experienced in the care of such patients is indicated. Radiocontrast media are particularly nephrotoxic in patients with diabetic nephropathy, and azotemic patients should be carefully hydrated before receiving any procedures requiring contrast that cannot be avoided. [31]

As for any other patient with ESRD, diabetic patients with ESRD can be offered hemodialysis, peritoneal dialysis, kidney transplantation, or combined kidney-pancreas transplantation.

10. References

[1] National kidney Fondation:Prevention of progression in diabetic nephropathy. Diabetes
    Spectrum. 19: 2006; 18-24.
[2] The Diabetes Control and Complications Trial Research Group, (1993). Effect of
    Intensive Treatment of Diabetes on the Development and Progression of Long-
    Term Complications in Insulin-Dependent Diabetes Mellitus. The New England
    Journal of Medicine 14(329):977-986.
[3] EURODIAB ACE study Group, variationand trends in incidence of childhood diabetes in
    Europe. Lancet 355,873,2000.
[4] Orchard TJ, DormanJS, Maser R, et al.Prevalence of comlicationes in IDDM, by sex and
    duration. Pittsburg Epidemiology of Diabetes Complicationes StadyII. Diabetes 39:
    1116, 1990
[5] Bernardo, J.F., Ellis, D., Orchard, T. (1997). Predictors of microalbuminuria in individuals
    with insulin dependent diabetes mellitus (IDDM). An update, J Am Soc Nephrol
    8:109A.
[6] Andersen, A.R., Christiansen, J.S., Andersen, J.K., Kreiner, S., Deckert, T. (1983) Diabetic
    nephropathy in type I (insulin-dependent) diabetes: an epidemiological study.
    Diabetologia 25:496-501
[7] Rudberg, S., Ullman, E., Dahlquist, G. (1993). Relationship between early metabolic
    control and the development of microalbuminuria – a longitudinal study in
    children with type-1 (insulin-dependent) diabetes mellitus. Diabetologia 36:1309-
    1314.
[8] Shimomura, H., Spiro, R. (1987). Studies on macromolecular components of human
    glomerular basement membrane and alterations in diabetes: decreased levels of
    heparin-sulfate proteoglycane and laminin. Diabetes 36:374-81.

[9] Williamson JR , Kilo C,Basement membrane physiology and patohystology in (eds): International Textbook of Diabetes Mellitus. Edited by Alberty KGMM,Defronzo RA, Keen H and Zimmet P, 1992. John Wiley and Sons LTD, p 1245-65

[10] Chiarelli F, Gaspari S, Marcovecchio ML. Role of growth factors in diabetic kidney disease. Horm Metab Res. May 18 2009

[11] Kostadaras A. Risk Factors for Diabetic Nephropathy. Astoria Hypertension Clinic. Available at Accessed 7/2/09

[12] Zdravkovic S. Dragan: Klinička Pedijatrijska Endokrinologija, 2001, Hronične komplikacije dijabetes melitusa: s.446-459

[13] Markovic-Jovanovic Snezana; Peric Vladan; Jovanovic Aleksandar; Stolic Radojica The Influence of Acid-Base Disturbances on Development of Microalbuminuria in Children With Type 1 Diabetes. Endocrinologist. 18(4):182-186, July/August 2008.

[14] Viberti GC, Wiseman MJ, The kidney in diabetes: significance of the early abnormalities.Clin.Endocrinol.Metab.,151986;p.753-82

[15] Garg JP, Bakris GL: Microalbuminuria: marker of vascular dysfunction, risk factor for cardiovascular disease. Vasc Med 7:35-43, 2002

[16] Klausen K, Borch-Johnsen K, Feldt-Rasmussen B, Jensen G, Clausen P, Scharling H, Appleyard M, Jensen JS: Very low levels of microalbuminuria are associated with increased risk of coronary heart disease and death independently of renal function, hypertension, and diabetes. Circulation 110:32-35, 2004

[17] Parving HH, Smidt UM, Frusberg B et al.: A prospective study of glomerular filtration rate and arterial blood pressure in insulin-dependent diabetics with diabetic nephropathy. Diabetologia, 20, 1981; p.457-61

[18] Viberti GC i sar. 1983). Viberti GC i sar.: Long term correction of hyperglycemia and progression of renal failure in insulin -dipendent diabetes. Br J Med 1983, 2 86: 598-602

[19] The National Kidney Foundation Kidney Disease Outcomes Quality Initiative (KDOQI) National Kidney Foundation. KDOQI clinical practice guidelines and clinical practice recommendations for diabetes and chronic kidney disease. Am J Kidney Dis. 2007;49(suppl 2):s1-s179

[20] DCCT DCCT Research Group. Are continued studies of metabolic controll and microvascular complications in insulin-dependent diabetes mellitus justified? N.Engl.J.Med. 318, 1988, p.246-9

[21] United Kingdom Prospective Diabetes Study (UKPDS), American Diabetes Assotiation, Diabetes Care Implication of the United kingdom Prospective Diabetes Study, January 2002, vol 25

[22] Rohlfing CL, Wiedmeyer HM, Little RR, England JD, Tennill A, Goldstein DE: Defining the relationship between plasma glucose and HbA(1c): analysis of glucose profiles and HbA(1c) in the Diabetes Control and Complications Trial. Diabetes Care 25:275-278, 2002

[23] KDOQI Clinical Practice Guidelines and Clinical Practice Recommendations for Diabetes and Chronic Kidney Disease, 2007 National Kidney Foundation

[24] Standards of Medical Care for Patients with Diabetes, Diabetes Care 27 (Suppl. 1), 2004: S15-S35. 3 American Diabetes Association

[25] Laight DW. Therapeutic inhibition of the renin angiotensin aldosterone system Expert Opin Ther Pat. May 21 2009

[26] Anderson S, Tarnow L, Rossing P, Hansen BV, Parving HH: Renoprotective effects of angiotensin II receptor blockade in type 1 diabetic patients with diabetic nephropathy. Kidney Int 57:601–606, 2000

[27] KDOQI Clinical Practice Guidelines and Clinical Practice Recommendations for Diabetes and Chronic Kidney Disease, Guideline 3: Management of hypertension in diabetes and chronic kidney disease,2007

[28] Lewis EJ, Hunsicker LG, Bain RP, Rohde RD: The effect of angiotensin-converting-enzyme inhibition on diabetic nephropathy. The Collaborative Study Group. N Engl J Med 329:1456-1462, 1993

[29] Wenzel rene et. Al. Avosentan Reduces Albumin Excretion in Diabetes with Macroalbuminuria; jurnal of the American Society of Nephrology, January, 2009, 1-10

[30] Diabetes Guidelines. Royal Free Hampstead NHS Trust. Accessed 7/2/09.

[31] Nephropathy in Diabetes , American Diabetes Association Diabetes Care January 2004 vol. 27 no. suppl 1 s79-s83

Permissions

The contributors of this book come from diverse backgrounds, making this book a truly international effort. This book will bring forth new frontiers with its revolutionizing research information and detailed analysis of the nascent developments around the world.

We would like to thank David Wagner, for lending his expertise to make the book truly unique. He has played a crucial role in the development of this book. Without his invaluable contribution this book wouldn't have been possible. He has made vital efforts to compile up to date information on the varied aspects of this subject to make this book a valuable addition to the collection of many professionals and students.

This book was conceptualized with the vision of imparting up-to-date information and advanced data in this field. To ensure the same, a matchless editorial board was set up. Every individual on the board went through rigorous rounds of assessment to prove their worth. After which they invested a large part of their time researching and compiling the most relevant data for our readers. Conferences and sessions were held from time to time between the editorial board and the contributing authors to present the data in the most comprehensible form. The editorial team has worked tirelessly to provide valuable and valid information to help people across the globe.

Every chapter published in this book has been scrutinized by our experts. Their significance has been extensively debated. The topics covered herein carry significant findings which will fuel the growth of the discipline. They may even be implemented as practical applications or may be referred to as a beginning point for another development. Chapters in this book were first published by InTech; hereby published with permission under the Creative Commons Attribution License or equivalent.

The editorial board has been involved in producing this book since its inception. They have spent rigorous hours researching and exploring the diverse topics which have resulted in the successful publishing of this book. They have passed on their knowledge of decades through this book. To expedite this challenging task, the publisher supported the team at every step. A small team of assistant editors was also appointed to further simplify the editing procedure and attain best results for the readers.

Our editorial team has been hand-picked from every corner of the world. Their multi-ethnicity adds dynamic inputs to the discussions which result in innovative outcomes. These outcomes are then further discussed with the researchers and contributors who give their valuable feedback and opinion regarding the same. The feedback is then collaborated with the researches and they are edited in a comprehensive manner to aid the understanding of the subject.

Apart from the editorial board, the designing team has also invested a significant amount of their time in understanding the subject and creating the most relevant covers. They scrutinized every image to scout for the most suitable representation of the subject and create an appropriate cover for the book.

The publishing team has been involved in this book since its early stages. They were actively engaged in every process, be it collecting the data, connecting with the contributors or procuring relevant information. The team has been an ardent support to the editorial, designing and production team. Their endless efforts to recruit the best for this project, has resulted in the accomplishment of this book. They are a veteran in the field of academics and their pool of knowledge is as vast as their experience in printing. Their expertise and guidance has proved useful at every step. Their uncompromising quality standards have made this book an exceptional effort. Their encouragement from time to time has been an inspiration for everyone.

The publisher and the editorial board hope that this book will prove to be a valuable piece of knowledge for researchers, students, practitioners and scholars across the globe.

List of Contributors

Laura Espino-Paisan, Elena Urcelay, Emilio Gómez de la Concha and Jose Luis Santiago
Clinical Immunology Department, Hospital Clínico San Carlos, Instituto de Investigación Sanitaria San Carlos (IdISSC), Spain

Constantina Heltianu and Simona-Adriana Manea
Institute of Cellular Biology and Pathology "N. Simionescu", Bucharest, Romania

Cristian Guja
Institute of Diabetes, Nutrition and Metabolic Diseases "Prof. NC Paulescu", Bucharest, Romania

Enrica Favaro, Ilaria Miceli, Elisa Camussi and Maria M. Zanone
Department of Internal Medicine, University of Turin, Italy

Adriana Franzese, Enza Mozzillo, Rosa Nugnes, Mariateresa Falco and Valentina Fattorusso
Department of Pediatrics, University Federico II of Naples, Italy

G. Bjelakovic, I. Stojanovic, T. Jevtovic-Stoimenov, D. Pavlovic and G. Kocic
Institute of Biochemistry, Faculty of Medicine, University of Niš, Serbia

Lj. Saranac and B. Bjelakovic
Department of Pediatrics, Clinical Center Nis, Faculty of Medicine, University of Niš, Serbia

B.G. Bjelakovic
Clinic of Internal Medicine, Department of Hepato-Gastroenterology, Faculty of Medicine, University of Niš, Serbia

Miguel Ángel García Cabezas and Bárbara Fernández Valle
Servicio de Pediatría. Hospital General de Ciudad Real, Spain

Petru Liuba and Emma Englund
Division of Paediatric Cardiology, Pediatric Heart Center, Lund University and Skåne University Hospital Lund, Sweden

Yu-Long Li
Department of Emergency Medicine, University of Nebraska Medical Center, United States of America

Francesco Chiarelli and M. Loredana Marcovecchio
Department of Paediatrics, University of Chieti, Italy

Anwar B. Bikhazi, Nadine S. Zwainy, Sawsan M. Al Lafi, Shushan B. Artinian and Suzan S. Boutary
American University of Beirut, Lebanon

Mirella Hansen De Almeida
Federal University of Rio de Janeiro (UFRJ), Brazil

Alessandra Saldanha De Mattos Matheus
State University of Rio de Janeiro (UERJ), Brazil

Giovanna A. Balarini Lima
Fluminense Federal University of Rio de Janeiro (UFF), Brazil

Snezana Markovic-Jovanovic
Pediatric clinic, Medical Faculty Prishtina, Kosovska Mitrovica, Serbia

Aleksandar N. Jovanovic and Radojica V. Stolic
Internal clinic, Medical Faculty Prishtina, Kosovska Mitrovica, Serbia

Printed in the USA
CPSIA information can be obtained
at www.ICGtesting.com
JSHW011456221024
72173JS00005B/1095